A Time to Remember

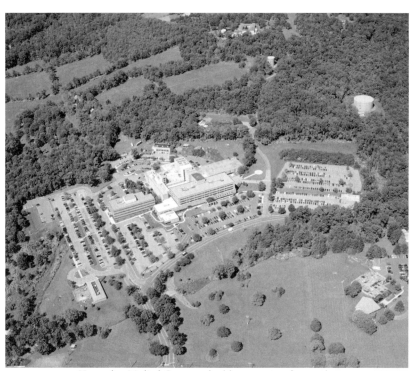

Hunterdon Medical Center, a health care system for people.

A Time to Remember

Hunterdon Medical Center—
A Health Care Ideal for the People

AVRUM L. KATCHER, M.D.

Dear Friend —
Thank you for supporting
the next chapter in the life
of Hunterdon Medical Center

Avrum Katcher

2003
HUNTERDON MEDICAL CENTER FOUNDATION

With love to Estelle, Ruth, Susan, Eva and Daniel

The complexities of life escape and resist one's every attempt to simplify them.
—JACQUELINE DE ROMILY

Contents

Illustrations

Preface

In seven years, from 1946 to 1953, a quiet rural county, working with leading national experts, created the most advanced community health care system in the United States: Hunterdon Medical Center (HMC). Its core was a hospital-based health plan whose objective was the health of an entire community. The mechanism chosen to achieve this goal was to make available for every resident a personal family physician to whom specialists, affiliated with an academic medical center, brought the latest advances and educational programs to stimulate high-quality health care. This work describes how and why, and the people who gave life to the institution. I attempt to show how this project is of broad historical significance for issues in health care policy and practice.

I have been privileged to serve this distinguished community hospital since the spring of 1959. As Director of Pediatrics, I enjoyed working with members of the original Staff and Board and became curious to know how HMC was built. When Frederick Knocke, the first full-time orthopedic surgeon, died in 1995, the year after I retired, I decided to create a record, in the form of an oral history, from surviving key persons. As a pediatrician, I am experienced in comprehensive medical histories designed to obtain information on events of health, disease and behavior. William Fernekes, PH.D., of the Department of History at Hunterdon Central Regional High School and Dr. Howard Greene of the New Jersey Historical Commission introduced me to the theory and practice of oral history.

As interviews accumulated, they revealed patterns of much broader significance than had been anticipated. HMC was an attempt to create a health care system whose mission—nothing less than the health of the community—was to be attained by a unique, comprehensive system based on primary care physicians supported by full-time specialists, regional consulting relationships, and integration of all related services. It became clear that the plan succeeded because the community engaged with determination, expected to help itself, listened to expert opinions, and selected leaders who recognized notions of merit and seized chance opportunities. Therefore, my work plan shifted to add reports of historical events and to try to understand the forces of change in health care structure and delivery. The more I became immersed in HMC's original goals and plan, the more these seemed relevant to contemporary issues.

Recollections of major actors were combined with other sources to explain an early venture of powerful utility for attaining excellence in community and individual health. Ray Trussell, the first Director, whose remarkable achievements will be described below, has told *what* happened with clarity and style.[1] I want to tell *who* did that *what, how* and *why.* The events that led to HMC's creation were arguably the finest hours of Hunterdon County, New Jersey. This rural community, which came together in the years after World War II to make a health care system unlike any other in these United States, has since become typical suburban sprawl. It would be a remarkable event indeed that could rouse this county today as it was roused then.

Key support for material and typing services was obtained from the New Jersey Historical Commission, The New Jersey Council for the Humanities, and the Large Foundation, mediated through the Hunterdon Medical Center Foundation. The Merck Foundation, the Hunterdon Medical Center staff and the Hunterdon County Medical Society all provided generous support. Mr. Terrance Keenan of the Robert Wood Johnson Foundation gave sage advice and insights. Ray E. Trussell, HMC's first Director, and Andrew Hunt, its first pediatrician, gave generously of their time and their wisdom.

No words can express my gratitude to the many who have donated their time, their thoughts, and their hearts by consenting to be interviewed and by offering candid comments and insights. The reader will come to know them by their words and their stories. Of all who were approached, only one declined to participate. Interviewees reviewed transcripts of their comments to make changes as desired. The approved final copy was the source for the record. To all of those no longer available for interview by a living historian, the author dedicates his respect and admiration.

My criterion for selecting those to be interviewed was either that they worked at HMC before I did or were related to someone who had. Interviews with Deborah Wescott Clarke, Bruce Hotchkiss, Edmund D. Pellegrino, M.D., and Ray E. Trussell, M.D., were most invaluable. The interviewees were Albert B. Accettola, M.D., Clara Anthony, R.N., Jeannette Ash, R.N., John B. Bambara, M.D., Bea Barad, Gerald Barad, M.D., Sara Boutelle, Elizabeth Colella, Norman de la Chapelle, Elisabeth Dewing, Louis Doyle, M.D., Jack Elinson, Ph.D, Caldwell B. Esselstyn, Jr., Elise Fidellow, Raymond Fidellow, M.D., Jane Fuhrmann, Pauline Goger, M.D., Edward V. Grant, David Greenbaum, M.D., Lela Greenwood, R.N., Cowles Herr, Esq., Andrew D. Hunt, M.D., Lynn Jenkins-Madina, Ph.D, Mary Lu Katzenbach, C. Buckman Katzenbach, M.D., Lazelle Knocke, R.N., Wesley Lance, Esq., Edwin K. Large, Esq., John Lincoln, M.D., M. W. Looloian, M.D., Trudy Macholdt, Arno Macholdt, M.D., Mary McCarthy, R.N., Mary Mercer, M.D., Kenneth V. Myers, Charlotte Mitchell, Alexander Mitchell, M.D., Christopher Olmstead, Esq., Belle Parmet, Walter Petryshyn, M.D., Nancy Rannels, Aaron R. Rausen, M.D., Peter Rizzolo, M.D., Barbara Roessel, Mary Margaret Rogers, Leonard Rosenfeld, M.D., Catherine Rosswaag, Murray Rubin, David S. Sanders, M.D., Ann Sauerland, Emolyn Sheninger, Don Shuman, Henrietta Siodolowski, R.N., Frank Snope, M.D., Catherine A. Tantum, M.P.H., Frederick W. Woodruff, M.D., and John Zapp, M.D.

Donald Davis, former President of HMC, Anne Somers, Emerita Professor of Health Care at Rutgers, Felix Salerno, M.D., Patricia McKiernan, Susan Morlino, Donna Duncan, George Roksvaag, M.D., President Robert Wise, CEO Larry Grand, Virginia Champion and other HMC employees were all very helpful. Karen Davies, President of Commonwealth Fund, and Dr. Erwin Levold, archivist of the Rockefeller Archives, were generous with access to Commonwealth Fund records. Dr. Karen Reeds was kind enough to review the manuscript and offer suggestions. Kerry O'Rourke, Director of the Robert Wood Johnson Medical School Library, was very helpful in locating information. Karen Sheridan, the librarian of the *Hunterdon County Democrat*, gave generously of her time providing much vital data. Amanda Phillip, reference librarian at the Hunterdon County Library, provided references. Jeanne Dutka of HMC's library not only provided many references but also edited the bibliography. The reference staff at the library of the New York Academy of Medicine were very helpful. Karen Bredenbeck not only gave generously of herself in preparing transcripts of taped interviews, but often clarified what was said when the tape was unclear.

Helaine Randerson, who edited this manuscript, asked questions to make me think and clarify my meaning and verbiage. Her contributions were invaluable. Remaining errors are mine.

Most important of all, Estelle S. Katcher, my wife, provided expert writer's opinion on text, advice on content, and unstinting support and energy to this project. Without her, it would not have happened.

To this work I bring no grand expertise in history or in the larger world of health care delivery. Although I came to Hunterdon by circumstance, my father and grandfather farmed in the early years of this century not over a mile or two from where HMC would be sited. My life experience has been as a practicing pediatrician, with special interest in child development and behavior. After graduation from The Johns Hopkins Medical School in 1948, pediatric training at the Harriet Lane Home of The Johns Hopkins Hospital and Mt. Sinai Hospital of New York City, and private practice in Philadelphia, I succeeded Andrew Hunt as Director of Pediatrics at Hunterdon Medical Center on 1 April 1959. With events subsequent to that date, as with Thucydides, I was an actor, observer, recorder or all. There is no comparable claim for accomplishment. Every effort has been made to tell this story in neutral fashion and to present all sides. Bias may be inevitable. We are all imprisoned by the perspective of our time. Opinion has not been withheld, but has been separated from event and noted as mine. If at any place in the text I did not succeed, it is a mark of my limits, and not of those of my advisers, associates and interviewees.

This volume is lengthy. I have assayed to reach three goals: to explain how and why this health system came into being, to identify those principles of value for health care delivery in our nation, and finally to record the stories of those who made Hunterdon Medical Center. Thus, some may wish to start with Chapter 18, Conclusions, which summarizes what the Hunterdon experience has taught about innovation in health care delivery.

A Time to Remember

Introduction

It is my impression that Hunterdon County is a better community in several respects than any of those in which the Fund put on public health demonstrations. There is more self-reliance, fewer indigent and dependent individuals, and more widespread spirit of cooperation than we have encountered anywhere else. [They] are frankly seeking help to make of it something new, different and more complete than any medical service with which they or we are familiar . . . I feel that it represents an opportunity for the Fund to help to do some of the things that the Board of Directors has expressed as desirable.
    —HARRY HANDLEY, COMMONWEALTH FUND, 1950

All of us who came in the early days were so anxious to have this place function as the community wanted it to . . . I would have done anything under the sun to make a success of this hospital—to make it what the community wanted it to be, and what they had given so much to get . . . This attitude got to . . . all of us . . . It was the spirit of the place.
    —LELA GREENWOOD, R.N., HMC'S FIRST DIRECTOR OF NURSING, 1995

Everything just had to be right. He [Ray Trussell, first Director] just wanted things right. I think . . . the early people felt that it would either live or die—they were responsible in other words for making a go of it. If it didn't go it was their fault . . . I don't care whether they were doctors, administrators or what. Because they had been given the chance to try this and so therefore it was everybody's responsibility . . . They were all in it together.
    —JEANNETTE ASH, R.N., STAFF NURSE, 1996

THESE EPIGRAPHS EXPRESS the three most important features of the Hunterdon Medical Center: first, it was to be a health care system of the highest attainable quality—an exalted standard of excellence; second, in pursuit of that quality, leading national health

care experts and a major foundation were involved; third, it was a
community venture with which an enormous proportion of the
40,000 persons in Hunterdon County were caught up. It was as if
an entire county and the entire staff of a small hospital had all
decided, as Eleanor Roosevelt is said to have believed, that you
never let down doing the best that you were able to do, even though
it might be poor because you might not have much within you to
give, or to help other people with, or to live your life with. That
was what you were put here to do and that was what you were
accomplishing by being here.

Lester Evans, a physician consultant on the staff of the Commonwealth Fund and a key figure in HMC's development, emphasized these notions when he wrote, many years later, "Hunterdon
served as a learning experience for me . . . I had no idea of the
crucial role of community organization and leadership."[1] At
Hunterdon, that organization and leadership, while sensitive to
consulting advice and thoughtful suggestions, nonetheless accepted
responsibility in the face of challenge. As Terrance Keenan of the
Robert Wood Johnson Foundation pointed out recently,[2] "Strate-
gies for change, however well grounded in theory, are likely to
falter when they do not become nested within the experience and
values of the community and elicit a response that carries community ownership."

Two distinguished students of initiatives seeking to generate
improvements in health care systems have reached the same conclusions, separated by 23 years. The HMC project demonstrates the
value of the community perspective for producing change and sur-
mounting challenge. Thus, I will describe Hunterdon County with
emphasis on its people and the actors whose efforts led to HMC's
creation. No one individual was responsible. The contributions of
many were necessary, although no one was sufficient. This volume
examines the process of creation and change in one health care
organization that provides lessons of national significance. It describes how individuals concerned with health care in a rural community responded to circumstance in the post–World War II era
to create an institution that from its start has stood out as a model
for community hospitals. The book illuminates how local events
and national developments in health care become inextricably intertwined, and how groups of diverse background and interests

were able to collaborate successfully. The story includes how a distinguished health care foundation chose to assist a desirable model project by providing expert consulting help rather than by just throwing in money and what useful lessons are applicable to the turmoil of health care today.

Hunterdon Medical Center, the first hospital in Hunterdon County in west central New Jersey, opened on 3 July 1953. At its inception, HMC was the most advanced community hospital of its size in the United States:

- Board, Administration and Staff recognized HMC's mission as nothing less than the health of Hunterdon County residents;

- barriers to health care were overcome by providing a primary care physician with hospital staff privileges accessible to every resident and recognized as gatekeeper before the term was invented;

- every patient was cared for in the same facilities by the same staff with the same amenities, regardless of means or source of payment;

- high quality of care was maintained by full-time specialists in the hospital and tertiary care academic physicians at an affiliated medical school, who supplemented, educated and advised family physicians, thereby bringing health care advances to the community. Staff was prepared to send patients to an academic center when indicated for best quality of care;

- all specialists held a university appointment, attended at the university on a regular basis and led an educational program including residents and medical students;

- the hospital served as central focus for joint planning, pooling of resources and coordination of health and social services—an acute care hospital, an ambulant health center, and a source of specialized programs designed to integrate public and private agencies with an array of health, diagnostic and preventive services. The goal of all this was efficient, economical and effective response to perceived community needs;

- distinguished consultants and an extraordinary staff advised community representatives;

- a survey of chronic illness led to a program of screening and a focus on population health and preventive medicine;

- geriatric and mental health services, organized on a population basis, provided outreach to key individuals and groups in the community;

- a comprehensive approach to child care incorporated behavioral and physical health, including rooming-in for newborn and mother, plus round-the-clock visiting for parents of sick children;

- finally, HMC was fortified by widespread community participation. It was a hospital of, by and for the community. Board, Staff and employees worked with a spirit of idealism and a sense of togetherness.

In sum, as was said by Lester Evans, the intent was to solve the problem of how "to make the hospital a vital factor in the lives of people in the years when they do not have to occupy a bed as a hospital patient." [3] Hunterdon Medical Center was designed as one solution for the problem of bringing the latest medical advances to family physicians and the public. Its goal was to treat the health of a population, not just the sicknesses. It planned preventive care for people who were not sick as well as sickness care for those who were.

Although the Medical Center exemplified "an enlightened and active public spirit which wants the best within reason for its people,"[4] it did not arise as Venus upon a shell of wealth and enthusiasm. The community was economically lean, with strong conservative roots in the harsh disciplines of dairy, poultry and crop farming. Other comparable nearby counties already had well-established hospitals. The citizens of Hunterdon were not the first to adopt new ideas.

None of the vital concepts which imbued the Medical Center with a sense of idealism and a community of spirit were entirely novel. It was the combination of ideas for which the group, not one person, was responsible. The best comparison is tumblers who create a human pyramid. Remove one and the remainder must readjust or the pyramid falls. Those who built HMC may or may not have had a sense of destiny or achievement, but such was the nature of what they did, viewed from the perspective of today.

PART I

The Story of a Health System for People

CHAPTER I

Hunterdon County—The Community and People

THE LAND, THE FARMERS AND THE GENTRY

To understand Hunterdon Medical Center, it is necessary to understand the community from which it sprang. As Meredith Willson, author of the Broadway musical *The Music Man,* wrote: "You gotta know the territory!"

Hunterdon County is old traditional farming. Or, rather, it was. And not gentleman farming. Hardscrabble. Shale, red dirt and stones in a thin layer over rock—which we know today is emitting radon in considerable quantities. My father, who as an adolescent prior to the First World War, helped his father farm here, described what it was like walking behind a one-blade plow pulled by a horse. Regularly, the plow would hit a rock, jolt his arms all the way up to the shoulder. Hold up the horse. Pick up the rock, if he could, and he usually could. Strong for his age and size. Take it over to the side of the field and put it on top of the wall rising there. He had other things to say about farm life, too, but that's another story.

Scattered farmhouses, made of wood. Not many of substantial brick and stone, as found in Bucks County, Pennsylvania, across the river. Farmhouses here are framed of 6 x 6 timber smoothed with an adz, joined with dowels, angle pieces at the corners, boards on the outside, lath and plaster on the inside and dirt, stones, old bottles and anything else that came to hand filling up between. Two stories tall. Peak roof. Dug dirt basement. Stone foundation. Fireplace to heat, cook in, whatever. Shed. Often porch in front. Barn buildings nearby. Not quite connected, as in New England, but near. Cows for milk and some steers for meat. Sheep. Goats. Chickens. Pigs. Hay. Corn. In 1940 more than 18,000 milk cows producing over 12,000,000 gallons of milk. Poultry—over 6,000,000 dozen eggs. Later, peaches and apples. Throughout, resistant to change. Someone who wanted the farmers to try new things called it "The China of New Jersey" way back in the early years of the century.[a]

A significant proportion of the land was marginal; agricultural experts recommended trees rather than crops. Although in 1880 the U.S. Census Bureau labeled New Jersey urban, Hunterdon County remained a farm community. In fact, the number of chickens quadrupled between 1840 to 1880. The first Grange was founded in 1874, the county Board of Agriculture in 1886. In 1893 a Farmers Alliance picnic drew 5,000 people. In 1927, out of a total population of just over 32,000, there were 2,605 farm families. Most of those who were not farmers were employed in agriculture-dependent occupations. This was, then, until mid 20th century, a farm community, rural, conservative, cash-poor, land-rich.

The county population did not pass 40,000 until after World War II. The 1950 Census showed 42,736 inhabitants of whom 28,179 were over 21. There were 14,081 dwellings and 10,555 families. Fewer than two-thirds of the dwellings had central heating; 10 percent did not have a refrigerator. Farms numbered 2,231, manufacturing businesses 73, retail stores 635. Towns were small; businesses local. Telephone calls were difficult. Only 12 exchanges, all manual, served the entire county of 26 municipalities. Almost half the 12,000 telephones were on party lines, with an average of seven telephones per line. One measure of the rural nature of the place is that in 1953, the year the Medical Center opened, Raritan Township, in which the hospital is located, for the first time banned construction of new outhouses.[1] The following week a woman was killed when a cow she was milking knocked her off her feet and trampled her.[2] Richard Thruelsen, a resident writer, describes the community in 1953:

> If there is anything we Hunterdonites cherish it is our illusion of isolation. Though we live within television range of two of the country's largest cities, the average native of these hills is completely unaffected by this propinquity—indeed many of our more relaxed citizens haven't been in "the city" since

[a] Kovi LV. *As ye sow: the story of an American rural community.* Flemington, NJ: Hunterdon County Board of Agriculture, 1961. Of course this rather judgmental comment may say as much about the attitude of the speaker as about Hunterdon.

the horse cars gave way to the electric trolley. This indifference to the questionable delights of the outside world has, fortunately, been repaid in kind . . . When an acquaintance or a persistent relative from the outside does materialize at the front gate, we always wait for the inevitable, "Why I never knew there was a part of New Jersey like this!"

Hunterdon, for a time, seemed destined to become another suburban boarding house . . . Fortunately, nothing like this has happened. About 1910 the county turned its back on the world (or vice versa) and settled down to a strictly rural future. While adjacent areas were adopting all sorts of modern inconveniences . . . Hunterdon sat back and picked its teeth with a straw in a bemused and happy state of retrogression . . . It begins to look now as though we Hunterdon backsliders have reached the end of our halter. With . . . a Medical Center at least twenty years ahead of its times, it appears that we shall have to accept progress and make the best of it.[b]

Stasis vs. Change

Hunterdon County included conservative, resistant-to-change, as well as let's-try-something-new farmers. Students of agriculture described "the inability and unwillingness of farmers to cooperate—even in their own best interest."[3] Farmers resisted introduction of a county agent, joining the Board of Agriculture (fewer than 5 percent were members as late as 1920), and in the 1930s refused to sign up for the New Deal programs for farmers. Some local separatists felt they should live their own lives in their own fashion regardless of anyone else. One such group defied the state police in 1926, leading to a shoot-out, with several casualties.[c]

A change in the community that may have accelerated innovation was the arrival of a new kind of farmer, the wealthy farmer of city background who was interested in quality herds and quality

[b] Thruelsen R. In: *Ladies Auxiliary. 378 recipes from Hunterdon's kitchens.* Quakertown, NJ: Quakertown Fire Co., 1953. In 1999 the dichotomy of life styles persists. The community has become a "suburban boarding house," yet for a high school senior of my acquaintance, taking his first trip to see the Atlantic Ocean, 60 miles away, was an event.

[c] Kovi (p. 31) suggests that, as is so often true, there might have been an alternative to violence. Contemporary accounts indicate that local authorities may have acted precipitously and aggressively against a reclusive family.

crops. "Gentleman farmers" came during the 30s and 40s and after World War II to buy land. Other urban residents arrived to
summer or vacation homes, or year-round living.[d] They changed
things, but not alone. Local men and women, the old crowd, began to make changes on their own. Telephone and automobile
reduced the sense of isolation. New families created a new chemistry. Newcomers and those who lived here for generations, immersed
in the problems of farming, combined to produce boldness and a
spirit of innovation.

The establishment of the Flemington Egg Auction Cooperative
in 1930 is typical of innovation—and resistance to innovation—in
Hunterdon County. Charles Cane and James Weisel, local hatchery and egg production leaders, devised the idea of selling the huge
production of local eggs by auction. Except for the founders, few
local farmers signed on. It looked as if the co-op would fail for
lack of cooperation. But in a few months, when it became known
that selling through the auction yielded higher prices than selling
in nearby cities, there was a dramatic change of attitude; thereafter the Flemington auction became not only the first but also the
largest in the United States. The egg auction may have been a
practical way to help farmers earn more, but it also demonstrated
that the farm community acting through, and supported by, the
county Board of Agriculture, could display bold initiative.

Hunterdon County farmers brought artificial insemination of
cattle for breeding to the United States from Denmark during
World War II. One of them was Lloyd Wescott, who became the
leader of HMC. Other innovations often produced strong feeling
between the advocates of something new, and those who did not
wish to alter their farming methods—farmers who felt that what
worked in the past should not be abandoned, as opposed to those
who wanted to identify and practice the best methods known. Members of both camps went on to take prominent roles in the founding of the Medical Center and to serve on its Board.

Howard Moreau, the publisher of the *Hunterdon County Democrat*,
a weekly newspaper, and the dominant print voice of the community, perceptively commented on the community in 1951:

[d] Andrew Hunt, the first Director of Pediatrics, recounts the view of Lloyd Hamilton, a
leading general practitioner in Lambertville, New Jersey, in 1953: "This area is about as rural as
the Bronx!" Hunt to author 10 March 1997, Hunt file, HMCA. Hunt felt it was the leadership of
the new exurban element that made the Medical Center possible.

A conservative farm group of high caliber, with long-estab-
lished leadership in the hands of landed families, with a recent influx of outsiders, including a number of
foreigners—Czechs, Hungarians, Russians, Poles, etc.—who
. . . in many instances are taking a good share in civic progress.
Snyder, the first president of the Medical Center, comes from
one of the old farm families . . . Three dozen such farm families have continued to hold leadership in the community for
many years . . . The relative newcomers like Wescott have
been well accepted . . . Farm income is relatively stable . . .
[There is] no farm in the county which is not electrified.[4]

Changes were indeed taking place in other ways. In 1948, when
a new county Superintendent of Schools, Eric Groezinger, arrived,
there were 36 one-room schoolhouses. Lacking authority to regulate the 29 autonomous school districts, he had by persuasion, tact,
pressure and reasoning, brought that number down to 18 within
two years.[5] After World War II a network of rescue squads and fire
companies was built.

By the close of the 20th century, Hunterdon County had become affluent—more than affluent: one of the top counties in the
United States, ranked by household income levels. Median income
for a single person in 1996 was $49,000, for a household of four,
$70,000.[6] Taxes are high. Unemployment is in the 2–3 percent
range. This is no longer the community that gave birth to the
Medical Center.

THE HUNTERDON COUNTY BOARD OF AGRICULTURE

The County Board of Agriculture, although for many years composed of a small proportion of the county's farmers, gained sufficient influence between the world wars to become the most important
political entity in the county. Bill McIntyre, former Assistant County
Agent, said: "The County Board of Agriculture was a real eye-
opener to me. I didn't realize how strong an influence a group of
people could have on the welfare of a county. They really had it."[7]
And, through the Board, the County Agent was a very influential
person. Hunterdon County's Board of Agriculture was founded in
1886 by a group of men and women of the five Granges, the Pa-
trons of Husbandry. Granges were community social organizations,
open to farm families. Although Granges offered a social network

to the farmer, the Board was the only countywide organization that represented farm-family interests. Its officers were recognized leaders of the farm community, men who went on to make many contributions in many areas.

According to McIntyre, who later became the County Agent, the Board in the period after World War II encouraged and financed programs of tree planting on marginal lands, unified contentious local fire companies to fight fires instead of each other, brought in as members local bankers, businessmen, representatives from the power company and the state police, and encouraged municipal planning and zoning groups, and eventually a county planning board.

Typical of the stresses on the Board of Agriculture was that produced by Hunterdon County Local No. 3 of the Farmers' Union, an unequivocally aggressive group founded in the Depression when farmers could not market milk. That militant group argued for strikes and "direct methods" of improving prices. They were contemptuous of traditional farm organizations—the Board of Agriculture and the Grange.[8] HMC Board member and attorney Wesley Lance recalled:

> I remember one day I picked up the *Wall Street Journal* and read that the farmers around Freehold, New Jersey, withheld their crops from market that Sunday. I called Herb Voorhees, the President of the Farm Bureau. At that time for a few years I was the attorney for the Farm Bureau. I said, 'Herb, that violates the antitrust laws.' It wasn't if two or three farmers did it, but could be if enough did it.[9]

Minutes of Board meetings range over diverse topics, such as the state constitutional convention, school-bus safety and the state police force and courts. The private, nonprofit Board was the most influential group in the county, not excepting the Chosen Board of Freeholders, the legal governing body. This was informal, unofficial government by the powers of persuasion of the leaders of whom it was composed. Power arose from three characteristics: agriculture as the dominant industry of the county at the time, representation of many other organizations and groups and the quality of the men and women who served on it. Action was by consensus, facilitated by a shared heritage, informed by recognition of common problems and challenges, and achieved by an implicitly understood structure of extensive individual and small group consultation.

The ability to bring about change in the structure of county services became evident in 1946 when a formal proposal for a hospital was brought to the Board of Agriculture. The idea was not new. Prior efforts yielded no results. Now a more solidly founded project appeared, a joint venture of Rose Z. Angell, head of the Hunterdon County Board of Welfare, Louise Bonney Leicester, a New York public relations consultant, county resident and civic improver, and Ann Stevenson, a farmer's wife, who headed the Blue Cross Committee of the Board of Agriculture. The events will be described in more detail.

CHAPTER 2

Starting a Hospital

People and Organization

THE EARLIEST EFFORTS—
THE PHILLIPS MEMORIAL HOSPITAL

Efforts to create a hospital began 30 years before Hunterdon Medical Center was built. In 1918 Edgar T. Phillips, a businessman from the riverfront town of Lambertville, Hunterdon County, New Jersey, bequeathed his estate to construct and endow a hospital in or within a mile of the town for the support of the area's indigent sick. Funds were insufficient to allow any action. In 1926, Edgar W. "Ned" Hunt, an attorney in Lambertville, heard of the Commonwealth Fund initiative, begun that year, to fund exemplary rural hospitals and wrote to ask whether their program "affords an opportunity for rendering useful a bequest made by a client of mine . . . for the establishment of a hospital at Lambertville, N.J., and which must be impossible of fulfillment for a number of years unless the fund can be increased from outside sources."[1]

Henry J. Southmayd, Director of the Rural Hospital Program, responded that the Lambertville situation did not "come within the scope of this program."[2] Later Commonwealth provided crucial help, not so much in money as in advice and consultation for Hunterdon.[a]

Four years later, Carl W. Ackerman, a trustee of the Phillips Memorial, approached an old friend and college classmate, Geddes Smith, an official of the Commonwealth Fund.[3] In the interval a

---

[a] One reason why the Fund initially declined to provide support for the earlier request was lack of community financial backing; with the subsequent development of massive community support in Hunterdon County, not only in dollars, but also in every other conceivable form, the Fund reversed its decision.

house suitable for a small hospital was purchased, additional funds raised, and Phillips, acting under protection of a *cy pres* ruling from the Court of Chancery, now supported an ambulance service, the indigent sick, and public health work in the community. After discussing alumni affairs, Ackerman again brought up the subject of the Phillips estate, by now amounting to $180,000 ($1,895,000 in 2001 dollars). Tactful inquiry about sources of help did not lead to further action by Commonwealth. In 1939, the Memorial was augmented from the estate of John E. Barber.[b]

In 1949, four years before HMC opened, its Board entered into discussions with Phillips, whose trustees offered a large gift, if the Medical Center would obligate itself to take area indigent patients at half cost. The offer was refused, as binding the administration of a hospital not yet in existence, in ways whose future impact could not be foretold. There was no further involvement of the Phillips Memorial Hospital in HMC affairs until more than ten years after opening. Those developments will be described in Chapter 9 on organizing the Family Physician Staff.

THREE WOMEN STIMULATE CREATION OF HUNTERDON MEDICAL CENTER

An unlikely trio of women—a 58-year-old nurse and social worker from the Midwest, a 55-year-old, dynamic, experienced public-relations expert from New York City, and a farmer's wife—these three musketeers at last set in motion the movement to create Hunterdon Medical Center. It will be much easier to understand the course of events by knowing who they were.

ROSE Z. ANGELL

If HMC has a single founder, the person who initiated the movement that created a hospital, it was Mrs. E. D. Angell, known to all as Rose Z. (for Zander) Angell, the Director of the Hunterdon County Welfare Board from 1932 until she retired in 1951 at the

[b] Legend has it that Mr. Barber, about to undergo surgery in a Trenton hospital, called his attorney, the same Ned Hunt, to prepare a will. Hunt drove to Trenton with a secretary and a portable typewriter, the will was dictated, typed and signed. The next day Barber died in surgery.

age of 69. This remarkable lady rose above personal tragedy to invest her life in public service through two world wars. Although she was not from Hunterdon County, her story typifies much of the strength found in the local community.

Rose Angell, born in 1882 and raised in Wisconsin, graduated as R.N. from Trinity Hospital, Milwaukee, in 1903. After two years in charge of the operating room at Madison General Hospital, she began to teach domestic science. In 1916 she was made Director of the Milwaukee Society for the Care of the Sick. She organized and served as President of the Retired Nurses Emergency League to care for civilians during World War I. In 1917, she opened a school for "cadet nurses"—the term for practical nurses at that time—to provide home nursing care for those who could not afford "trained" nurses. Mrs. Angell's husband, Emmett D. Angell, M.D., was, among other things, a physical education instructor, coach, inventor of games, author and a doctor. After service in the U.S. Navy during World War I, he served as ship's doctor for the United States Cruise Lines. Dr. Angell entered private practice in Butler, New Jersey, in the early 1930s, where he remained until his death in 1952.

Robert A. Angell, a grandson, describes how the family came to Hunterdon County:

> In 1920, my grandmother packed her six children (four boys, two girls) into a touring car and left Milwaukee for New Jersey. The motivation to relocate her family was simply that she wanted her family to be nearer to her husband and [their] father when he was not at sea. During this period she worked as a social worker in Garwood, New Jersey. In 1924 Rose purchased a 108-acre farm in the Woodglen area of Lebanon Township.[4]

Three of her four sons died of polycystic disease of the kidneys. Hospitalization of the boys necessitated journeys to New York or Philadelphia.

In 1932, with Mrs. Angell's extensive experience in nursing and welfare, she was asked to inaugurate the Hunterdon County Welfare Department. She had come to the attention of Wesley Lance, a prominent local attorney, judge, political figure and early member of HMC's Board, whose uncle was a leader in Democratic politics in the same part of the county where Mrs. Angell, also a Democrat, came to live. At that time, the Board of Chosen

Freeholders, the county governing body, was also Democratic. Her outstanding ability, combined with being in the right place at the right time, led to her selection. She did an extraordinary job in a demanding position.[c] An annual report that Mrs. Angell prepared for the County Welfare Board reveals her abilities and the conditions in the county at the time. One wonders how many Welfare Directors are prepared to cite Dante: "Of those things only should one be afraid / Which have the power of doing others harm." To this, she appended her own modification of the verse: "Of those things only one should be glad / Which have the power of doing others good."[5]

Angell dealt innovatively with problems of the aged, handicapped, children needing protection, and the chronically ill, for instance, paying some clients to supervise or live with others who could not care for themselves. She negotiated with local physicians and area hospitals to purchase, at the lowest rates the market would bear, needed care for her patients. She also arranged flat rates for daily hospital care and selected surgical procedures—in other words, risk was borne by the hospital, not the county. While conserving funds, she would be sure that all needed care was provided. She stated that "it feels right" for federal and state participation to help with local needs combined with "the ancient concepts inherited from the Elizabethan Era poor laws . . . namely, local responsibility, legal settlement and assistance from legally responsible relatives."[6] She aimed to help individuals to do more for themselves, while at the same time recognizing those she could not help—individuals suffering from alcoholism or unequipped for self-care. A multiplicity of factors made each client unique. In 1942 there were 161 children supervised at home on an average monthly budget of $13.37 per child; 321 applications were received from persons of all ages for help in paying hospital bills; 179 were certified as eligible for free care; and 2,430 patient days were provided.

She developed a central information registry, maintaining close liaison with state and local public health and school nurses. The Welfare Department gave space to the local Cancer Society and Red Cross chapters, Dental Clinic, Blue Cross, an itinerant mental hygiene clinic and maternal and child health nursing services.

[c] Lance W. Interview by author, 30 January 1997. One of the caseworkers on the staff of the division Mrs. Angell headed, Anne Anderson, became Mrs. Lance.

Angell was a charter member of the county Mental Health Association, the Homemakers Society, and the New Jersey Welfare Council. She founded her local PTA and was active in Democratic politics at the county level. On her retirement in 1951 the *Hunterdon County Democrat* wrote:

> To the Hunterdon County work she brought not only an understanding of the obligation to make our sick and infirm aged people who lacked resources feel that somebody with a heart was interested in the[ir] comfort and security, but also an understanding of the limited ability of the people of a rural county like Hunterdon to maintain such a service . . . Mrs. Angell brought to her position a breadth of vision which has comprehended more than a service to the infirm indigent people of our county. In administering the county's appropriation for hospitalization of people who could not pay, she was forced to deal with a problem which nobody had had the courage to challenge—that of providing Hunterdon with a hospital of its own. And she proceeded to look for the answer to this problem.[7]

Rose Angell was a trigger for the Hunterdon Medical Center. She was a necessary, but not sufficient cause. Two other women, Louise Leicester and Ann Stevenson, shared her initiating step; one of them, Leicester, was the key initial actor, without whom the Medical Center would probably not have emerged in the same form. They brought to fruition the work begun 20 years earlier by Ned Hunt on behalf of the Phillips Memorial.

LOUISE BONNEY LEICESTER

Louise Leicester was born in 1891 in Eaton, New York, of French-Canadian stock. Fluent in French, she studied decorative arts in Paris and was "prominent in the fashion world." She wrote radio serial mysteries, including *The Green Hornet*. She was living in Hunterdon County when she worked with Grover Whalen, a politically adept promoter, managing the public image of the 1939 New York World's Fair. She was an excitement maker who arranged a press pass for every agricultural agent within 100 miles of New York City—a gesture that paid off when she needed help from Hunterdon County's agents with problems at the Leicester farm. At the Fair, she met and married a chemist, William "Bill"

Leicester, who had been assigned by the Borden company to demonstrate a glue he invented by constructing a house out of plywood and glue.[8]

Bill had a long-standing interest in farming. The couple purchased a farm to breed Jerseys, near Pittstown, in Kingwood Township. The plywood and glue house was dismantled and re-erected there after the fair was over.[9] This stimulating couple entered a social whirl, hosting sophisticated parties every weekend. Louise would cook her favorite dishes for a wide circle of friends, including many who would be helpful to the Medical Center, such as Bill Lamont, who served as financial expert for the Board, Cynthia McNeille (who helped found the Hunterdon Exchange, a benefit shop that sold what are now called collectibles) and Sara Boutelle, who helped found the Mental Health Association. Louise Leicester attended municipal meetings, Board of Agriculture meetings, businessmen and farmers picnics, and was involved up to her neck in local affairs. In addition to her work for the Hunterdon Medical Center, Louise Leicester was a bold advocate for improved mental health services. A soft-spoken, patient minister, Rev. E. C. Dunbar, who served on the Board of Agriculture and HMC's Board, said: "She would try to argue me down, and many times she was right. But she was always talking about weasel words, and weasel words were anything she disagreed with."[10] One employee described the staff as "her brood" and said she would "mother hen" everyone.[11]

Lester Evans, of the Commonwealth Fund, described her as "a very flamboyant woman in dress, jewelry, style of hat, outspokenness—all in all a most attractive individual . . . She was one of a mere handful of persons who had a comparable effect in molding [Commonwealth's] thinking about health care." She would "pester and pester" him at the office. She might write from the St. Regis Hotel in New York, where she often stayed, or aboard a trans-Atlantic liner. She typed her memos, with errors corrected by hand.[12] Her persistence, intensity, devotion to quality, and sheer stubbornness made all the difference in obtaining consultants, and in the relationship with the Commonwealth Fund, described in Chapter 6.

In 1956 when she resigned, George I. Bushfield, a pioneering HMC Board member wrote, to Board Chairperson Lloyd W. Wescott: "I know that Louise has been a hair shirt to you . . . At the same time, she is a genuine student of medical trends and needs . . . and her knowledge in this field goes beyond that of anyone on the Board, I would say, with the possible exception of yourself."[13] Bushfield went on to urge Wescott to find a structure through which she might continue to be of help. Wescott did not; he and Leicester did not part on good terms. This author believes she was too much of a threat to him. Early on, the question would be, whose HMC was this, his or hers?

At the beginning it was Leicester, with no background in health care, who was indispensable in finding and using distinguished experts, as noted in the section on the Report of the Special Committee and elsewhere. All observers agree she was untiring and liable to fight with anyone for what she thought was best. More will be said on how she and Wescott related to each other in the section on Leicester, Wescott and the Board.

ANN STEVENSON

Ann Stevenson, from an old Hunterdon family, was a teacher and farmer's wife. Her first job was in Mendham, then a considerable distance. She roomed there during the week with an elderly couple. Her daughter, Carol Baker, still has the tender letters exchanged with her husband at a time when mail was always delivered the next day.[14] Stevenson taught 32 years, taking time off only to care for her two children when they were very young; she became a Learning Disability Specialist.

With prodigious effort the Stevensons built their rundown farm, located on very hilly ground, into a showplace with a fine dairy herd, a good poultry flock, and a small orchard. The *Hunterdon County Democrat* reported on 4 July 1946 (the year the movement for the Medical Center began) that the annual picnic of the Board of Agriculture was held there, a sign that the farm was recognized as a model. Richard Stevenson died in 1959 when his tractor overturned; Ann Stevenson then took over, eventually remarried and died in 1992. Her daughter describes her as "a visionary . . . hungry for challenge and adventure. She could envision processes and how things were done. When she felt that something should be accomplished . . . she was aggressive and very determined."

In 1943 Stevenson, now a member of the Associated Women of the Hunterdon County Board of Agriculture, learned from another member, Mrs. Henry Barlow, of the Blue Cross plans established by Farm Bureaus in the Midwest. Stevenson asked the Executive Committee of the Board of Agriculture whether they could form a group to qualify for Blue Cross insurance. "After explaining, I found I had suddenly been appointed chairman of the Blue Cross Committee."[15] Blue Cross agreed, provided 1,000 farmers signed up. The Board opened membership, for purposes of health insurance, to nonfarm families. She met Blue Cross's goals, recruiting enough conservative farmers with little ready cash and local families to form a group. The premium was $9 per month for one person and $24 for a family (in 2001 dollars, $91 and $244 per month, respectively). Comparable premiums in 1994 were actually $229 per month for an individual and $512 for a family. But in 1943, three weeks of hospital care cost $145 ($1,318 in 1994 dollars).[d] The figures show how rapidly health care costs have increased. As mentioned earlier, Hunterdon was a financially lean community. Farmers might be land-rich, but they were cash-poor. These premiums were perceived as steep. Stevenson did a remarkable job in recruiting over 10 percent of the population.

A CAMPAIGN FOR A HOSPITAL

ROSE ANGELL'S EFFORTS

In 1941 Rose Z. Angell began to campaign for a hospital.[16] She wrote on 25 July 1941 to Ellen C. Potter, Director of Medicine for the New Jersey Department of Institutions and Agencies, to thank her for information relative to the need for a hospital, to submit to the Board of Chosen Freeholders. Angell felt local interest was acute at that time; it would be wise to move promptly. The Freeholders apparently did not act. Angell then wrote to Barry C. Smith, the Director of the Commonwealth Fund.[17] The content suggests she was building on earlier discussions. Angell describes in her letter the existing "Hospital Plan," created by the Hunterdon County Welfare Workers Council. Four hospitals in neighboring counties that served Hunterdon County welfare patients had agreed to accept a flat rate per patient day. The burden of risk was borne by

---

[d] As a crude measure for comparison, three weeks of hospital care in 1994 actually cost $26,985, according to W Fry, HMC Comptroller, personal communication, 16 October 1996. Since the concept of a daily rate does not mean now what it did 50 years ago, he divided HMC's total budget by the number of days of patient care rendered to obtain the daily rate of $1,285. This figure includes a wide variety of ambulant care services.

the provider hospital for costs incurred over the usual. A fixed price for maternity and tonsillectomy/adenoidectomy patients and certain others determined by diagnosis was also negotiated in advance. There was an agreed source of payment (the county) and the Director of the Welfare Board verified that the patient was entitled to benefits. Records do not indicate that a medical referral was a prerequisite for hospital care. Hunterdon County had adopted central principles of what is now modern managed care: risk for some elements of health care was borne by the hospital rather than the payer. In Hunterdon County health care events of later years were anticipated, even if their full implication was not understood. Administration was via the Welfare Board, and the Freeholders backed the plan with an appropriation of $9,800 per year, corresponding to $105,500 in 2001 dollars.

After describing the Hunterdon County plan, Angell then appealed to Commonwealth for money to build and establish a hospital in Hunterdon County.[18] Commonwealth indicated in a letter that for a number of reasons they would not be able to help, apparently ending this round of correspondence.

Angell did not give up—a drumbeat of publicity continued. On 29 November 1945, the *Hunterdon Republican*, a weekly newspaper, carried an article headlined "Welfare Director Cites Dire Need for County Hospital." Dr. John Fritz, the President of the Medical Society, is quoted as concurring. On 6 December the newspaper reported "Doctors from every part of Hunterdon, this week raised their voices in agreement . . . that 'the county's need of a hospital was growing daily more desperate.'"

In 1946 Angell's annual welfare report mentioned the problem of finding hospital care nearby. Adjacent hospitals were resisting opening their beds to Hunterdon County welfare patients. The Freeholders filed her report without comment. Had they pushed for a hospital, what might have been? A governmental, rather than a widespread community, effort? Would it have succeeded? If it had, would the hospital have been a model, incorporating so many advances?

In the meantime, Angell wrote to Louise Leicester in her capacity as an experienced publicist. Was Mrs. Leicester aware of the recent publicity? "I would like help in promoting the idea so as really to accomplish the objective. I have thought of you as an advisor. Have you ever given the 'hospital idea' a thought? Would you let me talk with you at your convenience?"[19] Leicester responded affirmatively, and they formed a team. Leicester suggested that a professional survey by a medical authority might be a fair and possibly a decisive factor in persuading the population to support the idea. When it was time to approach the Board of Agriculture, they worked together. Ann Stevenson, who had put across the Blue Cross and Blue Shield plan, joined them at a crucial meeting. Had correspondence with Commonwealth been more fruitful, they might have come with a fait accompli rather than a proposal.

THE BOARD OF AGRICULTURE TAKES A LOOK

On 2 January 1946 Waldo McNutt, who represented the Farmers' Union to the Board of Agriculture, asked the Executive Committee to hold discussions "at one of the meetings on the subject of the County Hospital and that someone with knowledge of the subject be asked in to speak at that meeting. It was decided to discuss this at the next meeting."[20] Accordingly, on 6 February, in the grand jury room in the Hunterdon County Courthouse, the hospital question came up at a meeting that considered, among other topics, strike legislation, fire prevention, the library and consumer education, the Flemington Fair and artificial breeding of cattle.

Present was the Board's Executive Committee, including President Clifford Snyder and Secretary Richard Schomp. Jack Fritz and Barclay Fuhrmann, family physicians in Flemington, spoke of the need, but also of the difficulties, particularly of ongoing finances. Rose Angell and Louise and Bill Leicester supported the idea. Wallace Suydam and Herbert Van Pelt (the most popular local auctioneer) were dubious, and felt it better to support existing neighboring hospitals such as that in Somerville. Mr. Romine, a trustee of Phillips, explained they could not help because of uncertainty about future annual deficits. Discussion was tabled.[21]

At the next meeting on 6 March, Lloyd Wescott (who would become long-time Chairman of the Board and prime mover of the Medical Center), Rose Angell, Louise Leicester and Ann Stevenson sat together. Rose Angell made the presentation, recalling the other pioneering projects of the Board, praising their vision and presenting her data. Would the Board be willing to support a committee to look into the issue, and perhaps conduct a survey? President

Snyder had hoped to close the meeting before midnight. "The seats weren't getting any softer as the evening went on."[22] Kovi describes the scene:[23]

> All they asked for was a hospital. Of the highest quality. McIntyre recounted: "Clifford Snyder was sitting next to Lloyd Wescott and Lloyd said to Mrs. Leicester, 'You know very well that the only people who would support this sort of thing would be people who have more than the average amount of money. And people like that are not going to use a little county hospital that we could afford here. Forget it, this is foolishness. The kind of hospital we might have wouldn't be worth having—anybody who has enough money is going to go to the city hospitals where he can get really good medical care.' Clifford Snyder said to Lloyd, 'I'm going to put you on a committee to study this thing, and I think you better kill it.' . . . [Wescott later remembers] 'I said I really don't think we can make this work.' And Clifford said, 'I know. But it is too important to let it go.'"[24]

One can understand the points of view in the room. On the one hand, by now most of these people had Blue Cross and Blue Shield insurance, and many had the opportunity to use it in a hospital. Their experiences were not all favorable. They had to travel, sometimes considerable distances. It would be a boon to have a first-rate institution near home. But could they do so? It would be an immense effort. Would it be economically feasible, or would it place a heavy future burden of fund-raising to support an institution that could not support itself? It is not hard to understand that an easy answer—"kill it"—might be the first that came to mind; but it is also not hard to understand the temptation to look further—maybe it just might work. Leicester argued against the skepticism of some of the men present, saying that there were "a lot of angles" that should be looked into. Bill McIntyre said that Ann Stevenson, Rose Angell and Louise Leicester were "the strong voices that really convinced the Board to spend some money to research the possibility." Snyder terminated the discussion in his usual fashion by appointing a committee to look into the matter, including Stevenson and Leicester, Wescott as Chairman, Charles Cane, Herbert Van Pelt, Almena Crane, William Lauderdale, Richard S. Schomp and Waldo McNutt, with Snyder *ex officio*.

Who were these people? Some were indeed remarkable, some

the sort of solid local citizen who gets things done, some skeptics, some idealists. The two most involved are described now; brief biographies of the others will appear in Chapter 19.

CLIFFORD E. SNYDER—FARMER AND POLITICIAN

Clifford E. Snyder was President of the Board of Agriculture from 1921 to 1959. With Theodore H. Dilts, Richard S. Schomp, John Hudnett, and John Tine, he represented a group of farm leaders who worked together for many years. Snyder came from a background of independence, as Kovi notes:

> Burris, his father, was a frugal Quaker who believed in simple virtues like pay-as-you-go, and he did not send his son to college. He told Clifford he could borrow an empty field and some of their equipment, for if he wanted to go to college he had better earn himself some money from the field to pay for it.
>
> The adolescent soon became a man, with a well-tilled potato field, who was saving to go to college. He paid back the money his father loaned him, for as one source put it, "if Burris loaned you a dollar, he expected it back, even if you were his son."[25]

Father and son together made the decision for college. Both were certain that farming would be informed by engineering. What was the best engineering school? Massachusetts Institute of Technology. So to MIT he went, followed by Cornell University School of Agriculture. On his return, Hunterdon County farmers regarded him with disfavor: he had been to college! According to McIntyre, many said: "We don't need no bunch of book farmers coming in and telling us how to farm. That's ridiculous."[26]

Snyder accomplished much because he felt that meaningful agricultural research should be local. He pioneered a cooperative feed mill and helped bring about the engagement of a county agent. His influence was crucial in convincing several community farm organizations that they should thrash out their points of view for joint action. His style of leadership was described as determined, demanding, but willing to delegate.[27] When a problem appeared, he appointed a group representing all sides of an issue and insisted they negotiate a single conclusion, which they usually but not always reached. He would follow up with telephone calls if they lagged. This approach exemplified local decision making of the time and contrasts sharply with how issues are settled in Hunterdon County as well as on a national scale today.

Snyder served on HMC's Board until 1953, the year of opening. Lloyd Wescott, who succeeded him as Board President said "it was late in '52 that [Snyder] stopped at the farm on his way from taking the milk to the factory and announced to me that for *very, very* personal reasons—which he explained to me—he was going to leave the Board . . . [I] begged him to stay on the Board, which he apparently did until August."[28] Wescott wrote Snyder about leaving the Board: "I would hate it like poison!!"[29] In 1966 Wescott wrote to Snyder:

> You taught me the techniques of leadership, kindled in me the wish to find a significant place in the community, and it was your belief in me that gave me the opportunity to lead . . . In a very real sense, you were a father to me, and I constantly find myself judging my life by what I feel are your standards and your values. So this is a personal testament of love and devotion. I hope, when I am no longer active, I can look over my life and think "Clifford would have approved."[30]

Clifford Snyder and his wife Melda enjoyed immense respect in the community. They did not have children. On his death, Melda continued to manage their farm near Quakertown; on her death, she bequeathed it to Rutgers University for agricultural research and development.

The Report of the Special Committee

PROCESS OF DELIBERATION

In her typical way Louise Leicester commenced work by pulling the strings of her social network before the committee was appointed. Her personal physician, James Alexander Miller, had just sold, in late 1945, a country home and farm in Hunterdon County.[31] He was well-known in the field of chest diseases, and with Edward Trudeau, a founder of the National Tuberculosis Association. Miller also founded the world-famous Bellevue Hospital Chest Service, and most pertinently, served for 20 years as Secretary to the Committee on Public Health Relations of the New York Academy of Medicine.[32] In the last position, he was working at the side of Edward H. Lewinsky-Corwin, who was to prepare the initial design for Hunterdon Medical Center. Both were involved in many health issues of the day: ambulance service, venereal disease, birth control, medical education, hospital care and industrial medicine. Like Corwin, Miller was involved with leaders in health care and was close to the Commonwealth Fund.[33]

In February 1946 Miller introduced Leicester to Lester Evans at Commonwealth Fund to discuss the necessary steps to establish a hospital, even before there was a consensus to do so. Evans was a pediatrician and public health physician, who had worked for Commonwealth for many years. She met with Evans on 1 March 1946. His notes of the meeting include the following:

> She thinks the project could be engineered [to] proceed with a really good scientific survey of the area by employing a consultant. It was suggested that she get the names of acceptable consultants from the American Hospital Association. She said, however, that she and her friends are now acquainted with people in the hospital field who do such work . . . While this section of New Jersey is not rich, there is plenty of money which Mrs. Leicester thinks can be obtained in the next year or so . . . She seems to think more in terms of regional development . . . Any local facilities should be related to its neighboring and possible consultant centers. There was no indication of any probable request for financial help.[34]

In order to understand the crucial role of Commonwealth in the realization of the ambitious plans for HMC, it is necessary to understand the consultative function of its staff. Commonwealth Fund, founded by Mrs. Stephen V. Harkness in 1918, with money from her husband's involvement with the Standard Oil Company, had a long history of support for seminal programs to foster community psychiatry, public health and construction of rural hospitals.[35] The staff, most importantly Lester Evans and Mildred Scoville (a social worker and experienced mental health administrator), was at times in almost daily communication with the Board of Agriculture's committee assigned to develop the proposed hospital, later with the members of the HMC Board, Director Ray Trussell, and still later with the physician staff. Most particularly, Trussell, along with Andrew Hunt, Morris Parmet and Edmund Pellegrino, the first pediatrician, psychiatrist and internist, respectively, were assisted and advised by Commonwealth staff. They retained a relationship with Evans long after they left Hunterdon, and have spoken of him as a father figure. The Fund was initially reluctant to participate in the Hunterdon project; its financial contribution was relatively small. It was the consulting services and support that were crucial.

Louise Leicester kept the committee at work investigating sources of funds and advice. Even before the final report was prepared a national effort was made to obtain opinions and collect data. McIntyre believes that it was she who brought Wescott around to consider the idea more positively, even though he remained skeptical about the fiscal practicality as well as the degree to which a hospital might be utilized, saying, "Maybe we should look at it, but I think you are going to find it isn't a practical thing."[36] Miller also introduced her to Corwin as a consultant for the future Medical Center and Clarence de la Chapelle of New York University as consultant for an academic affiliation. Miller did not survive to see the results of his advice; he died in 1948.

THE COMMITTEE REPORT

On 3 July 1946, seven years to the day before HMC opened, the Special Committee submitted a report assembled by Louise Leicester and Dr. Emil Frankel of the N.J. Department of Institutions and Management (probably Agencies).[37] The committee performed an enormous amount of fieldwork: surveys of county demographic data, rural and suburban health care systems and health status, nearby institutions, and methods of hospital planning and organization. Reports from the American Medical Association, Commonwealth Fund and many other sources had been consulted, and personnel from the N.J. Department of Health had been enlisted.

The report noted the enormous expansion of health services throughout the nation, which had, to a great extent, bypassed rural areas. Attention was called to disparities in rural health and mortality, as well as in infant and maternal death rates. The report pointed out that not only was Hunterdon the only New Jersey county with no hospital, but that neighboring institutions were already overburdened, with approximately 10 percent of Hunterdon's population expected to use the services of a hospital elsewhere each year.

With these and many other observations, the committee concluded that better facilities for Hunterdon County were needed. This could be done either by helping enlarge and improve neighboring hospitals, or "*by building a hospital of our own.*" In a very characteristic mixture of Hunterdon boldness and caution, the group recommended pushing forward, but also reminded the Board of Agriculture that the project should be fiscally sound. A new hospital was recommended in "an enlightened and active public spirit which wants the best within reason for the people . . . Such a hospital stands a much better chance of operating without a deficit, because public and professional pride stand back of it."[38] These folk did not hesitate to raise the bar as high as they felt they could reach, but at the same time idealism was tempered by a desire to advance the project with local support. To achieve this goal, the committee suggested three steps: appoint a countywide committee representing all interests, retain a consultant to perform a survey in order to reach a final decision, and pay for all of this with private funds.

After discussion, the Board of Agriculture agreed. Wallace Suydam, originally a skeptic, moved "that the report of the committee be accepted and made a part of our record and that a rising vote of thanks be given." In another motion the Board authorized the committee to "proceed further with the problem to the end that a countywide committee will be selected and called together early in the fall,"[39] a complete turnaround for Snyder and Wescott. These men, initially dubious, were now converted; over time, they, together with Leicester, would become principal builders of the project. They then realized how much such a project might cost, and how important it would be to get everyone in the county interested. If this were done, they might be able to swing the project.

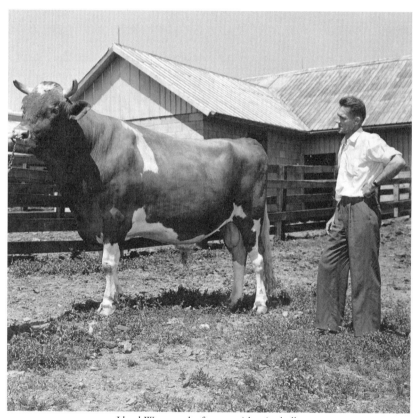

Lloyd Wescott, the farmer, with prize bull.

CHAPTER 3

Lloyd Wescott

Lloyd Wescott was for 20 years not only the leader and one of the engines of HMC, but also for many other local ventures. He stood at the threshold between local and national health care developments, serving as an intermediary in both directions.

Nothing in Lloyd Wescott's background would have predicted that he would have led for 20 years a remarkable community hospital. He grew from an ill-educated farm boy to a consummate man of affairs through his own resources and the help of mentors; to whatever extent the latter were important, it must be said he had the wit to utilize what they offered.[a] He described himself, and is described by others, as a "sponge," absorbing what he saw of value around him. He also felt that his early experiences gave him a flexibility in dealing with people from many different backgrounds and fields of work. Wescott fell by chance into the HMC project when Snyder appointed him Study Committee Chairman. He became the dominant mover on HMC's Board and became Chairman of the Board in 1953, the year the HMC opened, serving until he resigned in 1976.

UPBRINGING AND EARLY LIFE

Lloyd Wescott was born 21 November 1907 in Wisconsin. He grew up on a farm and said he attended one-room schools. He describes his parents as "poor dirt farmers."[1] He was the youngest of two brothers and four sisters; all went on to accomplishment in the

---

[a] Wescott LB. Interview 24–25 January 1982, interviewer unknown; four audiotapes furnished by Wescott estate, HMCA. Where not otherwise noted, quotations in this section are from this interview. Wescott firmly denied having mentors. My own observations were that he used everyone around him as a mentor. During a conference I saw him adopt the ideas and language of almost any profession or science, literally on the spot.

world. The parents worked on "minimal means" for at least three generations on exceedingly poor farmland. Yet he was determined to be a farmer. However, when he graduated from high school, in 1925, he became disillusioned over the adverse economics of farming and expressed a wish to go to college. The farm was sold to fund his education at nearby Ripon College. He worked in a department store in the town for three years to help pay his way, attended college and summer school, but "got the wanderlust" and dropped out to work in New York City from 1928 to 1936,[b] "footloose and fancy free . . . living from one moment to the next." At that point he had no career goal and did not know what he wanted to do with himself.

After clerking in Wanamaker's department store and in an advertising agency, he joined the mail order department at Harper's publishing, where, according to a friend, relatives of favored authors were given jobs. Glenway Wescott, Lloyd's brother (who "loathed" the farm), by then had a reputation as a novelist. One novel, *The Grandmother,* contains much of the Wescott family. Another, *The Pilgrim Hawk,* refers directly, although not by name, to Lloyd's wife Barbara. On his first day on the job, Wescott told a friend he planned to "marry a wealthy woman and do work for the good of the country." His own explanation for a rapid entry into New York society and wealthy, artistic and intellectual homes is illuminating: "I was rather good-looking. I minded my manners. I was respectful of them . . . interested in them as people . . . not that I wanted to emulate or copy them." His brother's position in the world of letters helped open doors.

When Wescott was 28, in 1935, he married Barbara Harrison, a wealthy descendant of well-known southern families and heiress to a sizable piece of the Southern Pacific Railroad. Harrison had lived in Paris for a number of years, where she founded a publishing company. She was acquainted with many prominent figures in the literary and artistic worlds. She came to New York with an introduction from Glenway Wescott to his brother Lloyd. Six days later they were married.[2]

Wescott recalled that Barbara "didn't want to live in New York, and I wanted to farm." After an evening of theater, they picked up

[b] Legislative Manual, New Jersey, 1960: 337. Eventually Ripon awarded him the honorary degree of Doctor of Science on 14 May 1978.

a book from a newsstand on farm animals and pored over it, selecting those animals they would have on their farm. That farm was found in a newspaper advertisement for 600 acres in Union Township, Hunterdon County, located "15 minutes by air from Newark airport." The Wescotts came to Hunterdon in 1936. "When I married a rich woman, the impulse to go away and relax or to play games was very strong. I think it would be hard to underestimate the influence [my mother] had on me to work . . . and I resisted that impulse like grim death." In a 1966 letter to Clifford Snyder he wrote "When I came to Hunterdon, I really had no notion what I wanted to be, what role in life I would find myself. Up to that time, I had been without particular direction or ambition, and the life on which I was embarking was strange and entirely new to me."[3]

Their marriage was one of opposites. Barbara was much more reserved and suffered for years with depression. After they moved to Hunterdon, Glenway and a friend, Monroe Wheeler, who was curator of prints and publications at the Museum of Modern Art, lived on the farm, enabling Barbara to maintain her connection to the world of art. She told Lloyd on their marriage, she did not want to be trammeled by housekeeping; that would all be up to him.

The County Agent described a visit to the Wescott farm:

> There was this young fellow came down [from the silo] covered with stuff all over and he is in there tramping the silage around . . . He didn't want somebody else to do it because they might get hurt . . . He was right in the middle of it. He knew those cows by name, the background, pedigrees and so on. He was a good farmer.[4]

Wescott added that he always felt welcomed to the county,[c] that this area was warm and friendly, and was fond of recounting how he, "a rich man with a beard" had become very close to Clifford Snyder, a farmer from a long lineage of local farmers (but, as already noted, a farmer who attended MIT).

Wescott was instrumental in developing methods for handling

[c] My own family legend is consistent. My father and grandfather walked to Hunterdon from Bayonne, New Jersey, to farm on rented land. As they came up the dirt road to their farm, the farmers in nearby fields all waved them a cheery welcome. A few days later at a cow auction, they were offered an opportunity to sign a note for the animals purchased even though they were strangers.

grass silage, the first wagon drying system for hay in 1950, and an experimental system for loose-housing for dairy cattle. An excellent example of how Wescott was able to seize upon a good idea and run with it was the creation of the first artificial breeding cooperative in the country in 1937, allowing the selection of prize bulls to sire hundreds of descendants. Wescott described his role some thirty years later:

> Mr. E. J. Perry, Agricultural Extension Specialist, found out about [artificial breeding] when on a visit to Denmark—in 1937 . . . He proposed to the Hunterdon County Board of Agriculture and the State Holstein Breeders Association[d] that they sponsor the development here. The County Board put up $500 to bring an authority from Denmark to advise and train the veterinarian. A cooperative was formed and service provided for the first time in America. The bulls used were Holsteins owned by breeders and stabled on the owners' farms. At this point I offered them the use of my Guernsey bulls, which was accepted.
>
> It soon became apparent, however, that to be successful, it would be necessary to stable the bulls at one place. I offered the use of land, and the availability of water, power and of farm help at all times. Fifteen people put up $100 each to build the first bull barn and office for the cooperative. For the next few years, I did devote considerable time and effort to the young organization.[5]

Wescott erected a facade of modesty claiming to be only a dairy farmer and not a hospital expert. He vigorously defended the dairy industry; to the end of his life he was skeptical of evidence suggesting a relationship between cholesterol, lipids and vascular disorders.

MAN OF AFFAIRS

Wescott was involved at many levels, local and state. For 16 years he was the President of the State Board of Control, the umbrella board for human service agencies and prisons in New Jersey. He was President of the New Jersey Agricultural Society, Vice Presi-

---

[d] Actually, Wescott said in an interview on 24 January 1982, that the Breeders Association was not in the least interested, and it was the County Board that sparked the idea.

dent of the State Board of Agriculture, Chairman of the Board of
the New Jersey State Museum and a trustee of both the New Jersey
Ballet and the New Jersey Symphony. He served for 13 years on
the Board of Managers of the Clinton Reformatory for Women.
He was a long-time member of the Board of the Flemington Agricultural Fair. Ken Myers, who served as the group's Treasurer,
noted that Wescott would always have some comment to say about
the Treasurer's report, to improve it, clarify this point, change
that. He listened, and he paid attention, more than anyone else
there.[6] Wescott tells how he came to the State Board of Control:

> It was an odd coincidence. I had Suffolk horses, draft horses
> we had imported. There was an old man . . . named Schley,
> an important figure in banking and social matters in the state,
> and he was the head of the Board of Institutions and Agen-
> cies in the state, had total control of all the programs for
> mental health, mental retardation, welfare and corrections.
>
> His son[e] came back from the War and started a farm about
> 20 miles away and wanted to have draft horses, and his mother
> and his father came over and they bought a couple of horses.
> And he became interested in me—Reeve Schley. About three
> or four miles away there was a reformatory for women, and
> they had a farm operation. Each of those institutions had a
> board of managers. Because they had a farm operation they
> decided they wanted to have a farmer on the board. So he
> asked me if I didn't want to go on the board of the N.J.
> Reformatory for Women.[f] I said I would be glad to.
>
> So that started a whole career in that department. I was on
> that board for 14 years. And then a neighboring senator from
> a community next to mine, that I had known somewhat be-
> came Governor, to everyone's surprise [Robert Meyner]. Mr.
> Schley retired as head of the Board of Institutions and Agen-
> cies. He asked me if I wanted to go on the Board and be the

---

[e] That son, Reeve Schley, Jr., was later appointed to HMC's Board. During a critical fund-
raising period the younger Schley played a key role that enabled the project to go forward, as
recounted in Chapter 6.

[f] A well-regarded model institution in the forefront of criminal treatment, headed by Edna
Mahan, who was widely known for her innovative leadership. She aimed to help inmates turn
their lives around by providing schooling, counseling and other help. Wescott became a part of
this, and for many years his home was managed by a reformatory graduate who had been
convicted of murder.

chairman. I accepted with alacrity and I was chairman of that
for 15 years. There I had a whole career in all of those areas
just because I happened to be breeding Suffolk horses when
his son came home from the Army. I have thought of those
coincidences—it is really quite extraordinary.[g]

Wescott's mind ranged widely. In the 1960s, when Myers was
on the Board of Chosen Freeholders, Wescott said to him, "You
know, we ought to have a park system." Myers pointed out that a
prior referendum on the issue had been voted down. Wescott, seeing the defeated referendum as a challenge, came prepared to accomplish his goal. He said to Myers, "I know but it needs people
that will promote it and you ought to do that. I want you to be
able to say that I gave you 40 acres of land to start the system
off."[7] And that is just what Wescott did. He donated land near his
farm in Rosemont, in southern Hunterdon County, thereby in-
curring the enmity of his neighbors—owners of estates who did
not take kindly to the prospect of public lands close by them and
public visitors coming to the area. But Wescott achieved his goal,
the gift was accepted, and Myers together with another Freeholder,
Vincent Abraitys, a widely known naturalist, put together a County
Park System that has become large, diverse, and popular.

Another example of Wescott's breadth of interests was the development of the Hunterdon County Emergency Call system, 911.
Wescott said to Myers, when Myers was Freeholder:

> You know, 911 is coming up. The County ought to ask for
> some money from the Robert Wood Johnson Foundation be-
> cause they are going to make a grant to four different [areas]
> throughout the country to put together the Emergency Medi-
> cal Services, the police and the fire. Hunterdon County ought
> to apply for that. We could tie it in with the Medical Center
> and maybe we could get that money.

The County applied and was awarded $300,000. It probably did
not hurt that Wescott was on close terms with several members of
the Foundation's Board in its early days, or that Seward Johnson,
Robert Wood Johnson's brother, served on HMC's Board.

In 1968 Wescott heard, via his vast network of friends, that

---

[g] Chance favors the prepared mind. Wescott never failed an opportunity. After he became
Chairman, he also became very active in the New Jersey Association for Retarded Citizens, the
Mental Health Association and the Welfare Association, among others.

federal money was available to build comprehensive community mental health centers. Over $100,000 in construction money and 75 percent of the salaries of new personnel were available. HMC had emphasized mental health since the early planning stages, but the demand had progressively exceeded its ability to provide services, always offered at a financial loss. Ever since 1960 when Morris Parmet, the first psychiatrist, left, to be succeeded by Richard Oliver-Smith, there had been discussions about a community mental health center. I recall being privy to some of them. In 1963 the ideas about how such a unit might function began to coalesce (see Chapter 13). Wescott jumped on the idea of turning talk into action by obtaining federal funds. He went about it in typical fashion by convening a Board meeting on short notice and gained approval to fund a new psychiatrist, Colin Fox, to write an enormously complicated grant due in less than five months. To absent members, he sent a long memo apologizing for acting without them. The Medical Center obtained federal funds for a new wing of the hospital and annual support for a greatly enlarged staff. For the remaining funds needed, probably close to a million dollars, he had at the time not the slightest idea where they would come from.[8] Via the same meeting and memo, he moved along action on two other novel projects, a family practice health center in Lambertville, and an extended care facility. Others had not seen the opportunity. Wescott capitalized on it.

STYLE OF LEADERSHIP

Wescott's skill lay in recognizing good ideas, rather than generating them. He described himself not as a leader but as a person who was able to bring true leaders together. "I didn't have a vision . . . I had a certain amount of know-how." A major strength was his ability to negotiate conflicting aims. He felt that "the times make the man" and that one need not have an overarching goal to take advantage of circumstance. His nephew, Bruce Hotchkiss, who worked with him for many years, said:

> He had within him this capacity for leadership, an astonishing capacity for thought and to think things through and to advise people and to sit there and listen to you and tell you what he thought and to make some sense out of the

nonsense. Money gave him the strength, the power of socia-
bility to get those things done.[9]

Ray E. Trussell, HMC's first Director, said:

> There is no question that he was accepted as a leader. He had
> an enormous amount of energy. He was very supportive of
> almost everything that I wanted to get done . . . The Board
> meetings tended to be Lloyd telling them what was going on
> and getting them to approve. They always went along with
> him, except Mrs. Leicester who was his most active critic.
> The man's willingness to work on behalf of the Medical Cen-
> ter was just unlimited. I think that in the back of the mind
> was the hope that maybe he was going to get so much public
> recognition that he might be considered to run for governor.
> More than once he would say: "If I were the Governor, I
> would do so-and-so."[10]

When asked why he did not run for public office, Wescott said
he would not be comfortable appealing for instant approbation by
the general public. His daughter tells it differently:

> He made Barbara a promise before they married . . . She
> insisted. She said, "I will not marry you unless you promise
> me one thing." He said, "What is that?" She said, "You may
> never break this promise." He said, "What is that?" She said,
> "You may never run for political office." And to his death he
> did not run for political office.[11]

He explained to me on one occasion the dynamics of power in
his position as Chairman of the State Board of Control, mediating
between the governor, at whose pleasure he served, the legislature,
the administrative staff and the public. "The best power," he said,

> is the power that is not yet used. If you must order something
> to be done, you are spending power as if you were spending
> money. But if you suggest, or indicate, why something would
> be desirable, and let it be done on the basis of that sugges-
> tion, you have both accomplished your goal and actually in-
> creased your power.[12]

Wescott was remarkable in his ability to absorb hostility or
anger without necessarily replying in kind. This may have been
because he was such an intense, commanding, indeed overwhelming presence. He would appear to be unstoppable when he decided to push toward a particular goal. It took a brave and determined

person to disagree. I am sure that many who dealt with him were afraid of him, and that he was not unaware of that. He was aware that his appearance could be intimidating. In speaking of himself, he said, "I was presumed to wield far more power than I had."[13] I should add that I never at any time, in an association from 1959 until he resigned, saw him move directly to harm anyone. In contrast he suffered about him some who were frankly incompetent, sometimes for years.

Dr. Edmund Pellegrino, the first Chief of Internal Medicine, said:

> Lloyd was someone I could always go to. He was a business-man. He knew something about the world that I knew nothing about. He had the pulse of the community. I couldn't have thought honestly of a better person to work with. It happens that Lloyd and I were very much agreed on most basic issues. We also shared intellectual interests . . . We agreed on what Hunterdon was, what it should be and where it should go. He was unwilling to settle for the ordinary.[h]

Wesley Lance, who joined the HMC Board after it had been incorporated, said that at one time during the early stages of fund-raising, Wescott became so discouraged that he came into Lance's law office in tears.

> The county was lucky to have a man like him. A lot of people were jealous of him because he did not have to work for a living . . . But instead of devoting his time to horse racing or automobile racing or something else, he devoted it to a worthy cause, and he had the time and the money to do this, which not everybody with equal ability would have had . . . Lloyd Wescott contributed more to the peoples' welfare of Hunterdon County than any single person in the last half century.[14]

A remarkable feature of the early times was how well Wescott and Ray Trussell, the first Director, did work together. Both were dynamos, both charismatic. My own feeling is that each was devoted to the common task and willing to subordinate personal feelings and interests. It was the Board of Trustees that at times was left behind. In 1950, after Trussell was engaged as Medical

---

[h] Pellegrino ED. Interview by author, 27 November 1995. Pellegrino felt that Wescott's qualities stemmed more from his inner nature rather than from his upbringing, granting, however, that both nature and nurture were important.

Director, the pace became overwhelming. Wescott and Trussell ran like railroad engines, with enormous speed and momentum. Some on the Board were acquiescent, others silently rebellious. Louise Leicester was the most vocal and had pertinent things to say. More of this in Chapter 6.

LIFE STYLE

For this man, work was life and life was work—he worked while he played and often played while he worked. He had no hobbies unless one includes the farm as a hobby. Perhaps this may help explain why in 1952, a year before HMC opened, he suffered an acute perforation of a peptic ulcer and had to be rushed to hospital for urgent surgery.[15] He and Barbara had a vast network of friends, socialized frequently, and saw no boundary between their social life and the many programs and activities that interested them. According to Wescott's daughter, their marriage was not close, but there was a strong intellectual bond. It was their daughter who felt neglected, isolated, alone, turned over to the care of servants, given no explanation for her parents' absences. She made plain her vision of him as a man with two personalities: the "Mr. Outside," as described above, and "Mr. Inside," who she saw as a much more unhappy person who not only did not understand her but was also very difficult to live with.[16]

Wescott possessed extraordinary charm, energy, and ability. He never was angry "except on purpose." He won friends everywhere by his warmth, vigorous presence, handsome and muscular appearance, and resonant voice. I remember his late arrival at a charity ball—he was past 70 and widowed. He stood a moment in the doorway. Three charming women jumped up to seek his presence at their tables. Trussell spoke of his energy in the fall of 1950, "I was a little amused at Mr. Wescott yesterday when he told me that now that the [Flemington Agricultural] Fair was out of the way he would have more time to devote to the Medical Center. I assume this means something in excess of his normal 12 hours a day."[17]

For me, their home was a place of wonder. It was my first introduction to such a residence. One came into a living room, perhaps 1,500 square feet. On the wall, to the left, Renoir, Utrillo. Chairs, Mies van der Rohe. A Tang horse. A Greek marble torso by the back wall. On the right, under glass on a countertop, the

"Elles" series by Toulouse-Lautrec. Morandi, Avery, Kandinsky, George Segal. A decade later, color field paintings by Mark Rothko. All of this was the passion of Barbara Wescott, who had an eye, knew everyone in the art world, and was recognized as a connoisseur. Barbara and Lloyd saw themselves not as possessors but as caretakers and sharers. They held one dinner or party after another for the staff, for small groups, for the Board, for someone whose friendship would benefit the Medical Center. When they opened their home, they opened it with generosity and candor. More than once I would watch Barbara or Lloyd for signs of amusement as one guest after another would enter, stop, and with more or less success conceal a stare of astonishment. But if they were amused, it did not show, rather they were genuinely pleased to see the pleasure they gave others. And give they did. Much of their collection was donated to a museum or benefit auction.

LATER CAREER

Wescott was named President of the Medical Center in January 1953, when Clifford Snyder resigned; he retired as President in 1976 after his efforts to institute an HMO failed. Controversy continued over the status of specialists, in particular their freedom to practice independently and have offices where they wished. He remained on the Board until May, 1978, when he resigned, saying in his letter of resignation:

> I am taking this action because I believe most sincerely that if I am not a member of the Board, the Specialist Staff will be more willing to accept decisions that must be made to save those programs which are essential to the survival of the so-called "Hunterdon System." There is little question in my mind that the frustrations they may have felt were attributed, in a measure at least, to what they perceived as my dominance of the Board . . .

> I seem to have become a sort of symbol, not only to our specialists but to other physicians, of what they feel is so threatening—the effective intrusion of government and citizen groups into the provision of medical care service . . . In all the bitter and totally futile confrontations of the past three years, the essential issues have been lost sight of.

> The only people with inalienable rights as far as HMC is

concerned are [the contributors] who will turn to it for care in the future. They did not contribute to build just another doctor's workshop. They built an institution recognized nationally . . . it is to them, AND ONLY TO THEM, that you, the Board members are answerable.[18]

Wescott remained active on behalf of the Medical Center for his entire life. He attempted micromanagement behind the scenes in a barrage of letters to the President (Chief Executive Officer Donald Davis) for years. In later years he was not well; he died 24 December 1990.

CHAPTER 4

Ferment of Ideas

Before describing how the special Committee of the Board of Agriculture approached its task, the result and how ideas were turned into action, it will be worthwhile to consider what was happening on the national scene, and how this set the stage for the creative efforts of the Hunterdon group. This chapter includes selected efforts and important problem-solving approaches to contentious issues of health care delivery in the pre- and post-war era, as well as other notions circulating at the time in the United States.

UNITED STATES HEALTH CARE AT A CROSSROADS

Three great committees, one between the wars, the other two just after World War II, produced reports explicating the best objectives of the time. First was the Committee on the Costs of Medical Care, a voluntary agency financed by eight foundations, one of which was the Commonwealth Fund.[1] A landmark series of reports in 1931 and 1932 lay almost untouched for decades although prescient observers called attention to them.[2] A series of recommendations in the final report of the Committee[3] influenced HMC's planning through E. H. Lewinsky-Corwin, the consultant who in 1948 first outlined an organization plan for the future hospital. The Committee on the Costs of Medical Care called for nonprofit community medical centers characterized by:

- emphasis on preventive medicine, mental health and health education;
- a well-equipped general hospital, outpatient department and pharmacy, including on site the headquarters of voluntary agencies and public health departments;
- a family practitioner of choice for each patient for guidance

in health matters and referral to a specialist only when necessary. The role of family practitioner would be important and respected;

❧ affiliation of rural institutions with a major urban center; and

❧ a professional staff paid by salary responsible for its own conduct.[a]

A second major report originated with the Committee on Medicine and the Changing Order of the New York Academy of Medicine. Several committee members later consulted with the Hunterdon group. Committee reports, which were published by Commonwealth Fund included topics such as medical education, health insurance, preventive medicine and government in public health. One was *The American Hospital,* by Corwin himself, published in 1946, not long before he became consultant at Hunterdon. The final report of the Committee endorsed:

❧ linkage of health centers and hospitals for rural populations, combined with regional systems for all groups;

❧ public health and preventive health services integrated with community hospitals and local physicians;

❧ improved quality of services by isolated local practitioners, including their admission to hospital staffs;

❧ health education programs to empower patients toward thoughtful choices of care;

❧ action on problems encountered by underserved minorities, women and other groups;

❧ voluntary nonprofit and prepayment medical plans associated with group practice, including attention to the medical needs of middle class, medically indigent and indigent families by a combination of plans with governmental subsidies where needed; and

❧ major changes in medical education, including emphasis on

---

[a] Among the Committee's reports was one that focused on the nature of physician practice. See Rorem CR. *Private group clinics.* Publication No. 8. Chicago: University of Chicago Press, 1931, which pointed out that group practice could take many structural forms, was an efficient and economical way to deliver specialist services and that participating physicians could earn incomes comparable to those in private practice. The report also noted that group practices worked best with nonphysician administrators; were in competition with private practitioners and consequently few of them would refer to groups; and, finally, that group physicians were aware of the difficulties of maintaining personal relationships with patients. All of these points were a threat to practitioners and to organized medicine. All were made at a time when group practices were unusual.

careful medical histories and physical examinations before spending scarce funds on testing.[4]

Over 30 years later Bryant et al. found many of these areas remained problematic for a large proportion of u.s. hospitals. Today that is still true. As Bryant et al. wrote: "Few . . . hospitals have been as willing and successful as Hunterdon in accepting an expanded role and responsibility for primary care."[5]

The third major contribution, made by the Commission on Hospital Care and Commonwealth Fund, was a massive five-year study in 1947. Their conclusions, congruent with other committee reports cited, were in the hands of Corwin and the group working on the embryonic hospital. All of the recommendations from this report were incorporated into the plan of the Hunterdon Medical Center—perhaps the only institution in the United States at that time that combined so many features of importance. The Commission recommended that:

- general hospitals (now known as community hospitals) should serve as the focal point through which the community's health services are integrated and should participate in community-wide educational programs to assist the public to fully understand the importance and methods of maintaining a high level of health. Such health education programs should include rehabilitation;

- hospitals and health departments should coordinate efforts, jointly use facilities and integrate functions. Public health officers should have hospital staff appointments;

- community hospitals should affiliate with a medical college to make consulting faculty available to the hospital staff for "informal discussion of professional affairs" as well as for educational and consulting services. General and specialized hospitals should establish integrated programs to optimize personnel and equipment usage;

- hospitals should establish diagnostic clinics and make office space available for physicians and combine their efforts with the medical profession for the extension of group medical practice. Scientific research involving all staff should be conducted on an ongoing basis;

- continuous self-improvement should ensure "the most effective and comprehensive service possible [for] all patients";

- patients with communicable diseases, tuberculosis, nervous and mental disorders, and chronic and convalescent disorders should be cared for in general hospitals (read community hospitals) rather than specialized institutions wherever possible. Treatment of mental conditions should be integrated with community hospital services, and closer relations developed with professional personnel of psychiatric hospitals;

- the formal medical staff organization should also include a dental staff and service headed by an oral surgeon;

- short-term convalescent patients should be cared for in the general hospital;

- medical social service should be a separate department financed through regular budget sources. "The primary function of the medical social service department should be to provide the physician and others responsible for the patient's care with adequate information concerning the patient's socio-economic status and environment, and to interpret to the patient . . . physician's advice."[6]

As if all this was not enough, the Commission also called for racial integration of every aspect of health service, federal financing of care for the indigent, nonprofit prepayment health care programs, and use of criteria of need for enlarging health care services!

It is not surprising that in 1950, when it appeared that Hunterdon was to be the one community hospital in the United States adhering most closely to the spirit of all these recommendations, Commonwealth Fund decided to support the venture. It is surprising that it required several years, and multiple written, telephone and personal encounters before the Fund reached a decision.

For comparison with Hunterdon, six other innovative programs for improved health care are reviewed—Kaiser, Roosevelt Hospital, Rip Van Winkle, Bingham, Rochester and Mary Imogene Bassett. Each program differs from Hunterdon, but offers useful insights.

KAISER FOUNDATION

Kaiser-Permanente was a prepayment plan that grew out of a scheme devised by Dr. Sidney Garfield in 1933 for workers on the Los Angeles Aqueduct, adapted in 1938 for those on the Grand Coulee

Dam, and then by him and Henry and Edgar Kaiser for their wartime shipbuilding program.[7] The premium, in the 1930s, was 5 cents a day, later raised to 7 cents, 25 percent more for children. Garfield created the notion of groups of physicians who contracted to deliver comprehensive care for a single premium. Hospital and sickness care would also be covered. Garfield recognized that health education and prevention would reduce expenses. He wrote about the "worried well" who needed understanding of the source of their concerns rather than expensive diagnostic study and useless treatment. The plan has since grown into a vast network, but Kaiser confines care to subscribers. It does not offer care for an entire community, nor is it integrated into either public or community agencies.

FRANKLIN D. ROOSEVELT HOSPITAL

World War II also stimulated another, innovative but short-lived institution, the Franklin D. Roosevelt Hospital in Bremerton, Washington. This small city increased in population by over 98 percent from 1940 to 1943 as a result of the wartime ship-building boom. Prior hospital services were scant. The county government and public health department combined to construct and operate a 140 bed municipal hospital. It was combined with the health department; both under one head emphasized individual health education to prevent disease and ameliorate existing disorders. The local medical society and the public health department joined in planning and operation. The description of the program[8] appears to be more reactive than proactive. After the war, when the local population fell as dramatically as it had risen, the local hospitals, by then three in number, merged; this institution, and the concepts it espoused, did not survive.

RIP VAN WINKLE CLINIC

In 1946, not long before serious planning of HMC began, another innovative health care system was established in Columbia County in southern New York state.[9] Inspired by the determination and thinking of its founder, Caldwell B. Esselstyn, M.D., specialists were brought into a poor rural community to establish a group practice funded in great part by Esselstyn's own funds and by some large donors. A central ambulant care facility in the town of Hudson was surrounded by seven satellites. In each a pediatrician, an internist and a dentist practiced.[10] Esselstyn estimated this group could care for 80 percent of the medical needs of the community. Consulting specialists were stationed at the central unit; they appeared on rotation at each of the satellites. It was estimated that no citizen of the county was more than five miles from an office. A bitter storm of opposition blew up from the existing local physicians; letters were written to prestigious journals, such as the *New England Journal of Medicine*, about the evils of this group practice. Esselstyn aimed to demonstrate that specialists would settle in rural areas. To prove that research could be done he commenced a longitudinal study (said still to be in operation) of young children with aggressive behavior. Unfortunately, several satellites closed because of poor acceptance by the community; dissension with other physicians over remuneration appeared, and the founder, who could not handle this, retired. The group practice closed its doors in 1963.

BINGHAM ASSOCIATES

In 1932 the wealthy, reclusive William Bingham donated money for a regional plan tying New England Medical Center (NEMC) in Boston with hospitals and physicians in the state of Maine. Features included postgraduate training for primary care physicians in isolated rural areas of Maine, supportive consultations by specialists, and a network of primary, secondary and tertiary hospitals. By 1960 two regional centers in Maine and 60 primary care hospitals were affiliated with NEMC.

The Bingham Associates program emphasized a two-way relationship: institutions at all levels benefited by educational programs and patient flow. Explicitly recognized were the needs of primary care physicians and the detriment to quality of care when physicians practiced in isolation. Bingham provided little by way of subsidy or construction money at the local level. Instead he gave generous funding for construction at the NEMC. There was little participation by community groups except for approvals by hospital boards and physician organizations. This was not a grass roots venture; it was seeded from above. Bingham's private physician and key personnel at the NEMC generated the underlying concepts.[11]

For decades a substantial percentage of physicians practicing in Maine were trained at the NEMC.[12] In 1944 U.S. Surgeon General Thomas Parran recommended to Congress a nationwide plan of regional medical programs based on the Bingham model. More than 20 years elapsed before Congress took action by establishing in 1967 the Regional Medical Program. The Bingham Fund was liquidated in 1974, perhaps as a result, and its assets transferred to NEMC Hospital.

Bingham provided a "trickle-down" form of medical advances for local physicians, rather than structural linkages of physicians and a community-wide horizon for health initiatives. Hospital and physician treated disease, rather than promote health. In contrast, Hunterdon explicitly recognized the health of the entire community as an objective and constructed an administrative framework of staff and regional relationships to attain its goals. Bingham relied on links of a less direct, more didactic nature. It would have been fascinating to compare outcomes of patient care.

ROCHESTER REGIONAL PLAN

The notion of regional hospital organizations can be traced as far back as 1920 to the Lord Dawson report in England.[13] In the United States the Commonwealth Fund proposed in 1943 to finance such a program. After a competition, Rochester was selected. Whereas no one hospital in this regional collaboration is directly comparable to Hunterdon, the overall program has many similar features. The Rochester plan included all hospitals in an 11-county area of upstate New York.[b] It grew from awareness on the part of local hospital leaders of the need to improve the professional quality and functional administration of rural hospitals.

The Rochester group set up in 1945 the Council of Rochester Regional Hospitals, a voluntary association of hospitals and their medical staffs. The large city hospitals, the medical school, and 24 rural hospitals were members. Surveys were conducted to determine what services might most usefully be offered, looking at hospital operations department by department, as well as indices of

[b] Kaiser AD. "An experiment in improving medical care in rural areas on a regional basis." *Pediatrics* 1948; 1: 829–35. This article was not about pediatrics per se, but about regional care, with introduction by the revered Edwards A. Park, who edited the section on the Pediatrician and the Public, because of the importance he attached to ending the isolation of many practitioners and enable them to take advantage of health care advances.

medical care. For example, it was found that deaths from appendicitis varied by 200 percent in the 11 counties, neonatal deaths by 100 percent.

The association offered a menu of services from which hospitals could select. They included purchasing programs, training for administrators, and educational efforts for all departments. For physicians, there were a variety of ingenious arrangements to promote quality of care, including evaluation of outcomes. The regional program became well established, and the process associated with it firmly constructed. Improvements in several hospital areas were demonstrated, but not in postgraduate education of physicians. The intimate consulting and educational efforts of Hunterdon's program were not offered in Rochester. On the other hand, education for, and improvement of, hospital departments was not in the Hunterdon plan. At Hunterdon there have been no formal, comparative studies of health care outcomes conducted by groups outside the institution, although there have been studies of resource utilization in the form of hospital admissions. Until recently, Hunterdon has had no significant involvement in research.

About 20 years ago HMC began to measure community satisfaction in ongoing fashion. An outside research firm has conducted telephone surveys by selecting names at random from the telephone book. A consortium including HMC and public and private community agencies, the Hunterdon Partnership for Health, has surveyed community risk factors, such as risky adolescent behaviors, for four years. Morbidity and mortality data have been subjected to internal study for a number of years, in order to obtain information about outcomes.

MARY IMOGENE BASSETT HOSPITAL

Among efforts to create an ideal community hospital, the Mary Imogene Bassett Hospital in Cooperstown, New York, which evolved into a complex combination of hospital, physician and health services, stands out.[14]

BACKGROUND

Cooperstown, New York, the home of the Baseball Hall of Fame, in Otsego County, west of Albany, lies in a relatively low income rural area; average household income in 1995 was $25,000. Cooperstown itself is small (3,500 population) but affluent. One or more centers of the Bassett Healthcare system are located in nine contiguous counties with a population of approximately 750,000. Jane Schlesser, Director of Public Relations for Bassett, estimates that 25 percent use the Bassett system.

From 1868 Cooperstown was only intermittently served by a hospital. In 1927 the Clark family[c] reopened the hospital, with a group of physicians from Columbia Presbyterian Hospital in New York City. The leader of the group, George Mackenzie, was a dominant personality, director of the hospital, physician-in-chief, and director of the laboratory. He had his own ideas on how medicine should be structured. Hawn said, "Mackenzie ran it all. The Clarks met the deficit. [Staff] never knew the real costs. Information was withheld. It was just the way it worked."

FEATURES OF BASSETT

All members of the medical staff were on salary, at levels slightly under prevailing salaries by specialty, supplemented by bonuses such as rental of homes at low cost. A surgeon established a radium treatment center for cancer patients. The surgeon-in-chief served on the hospital's Board. George Mackenzie described the relationship of the hospital staff to the community physicians: "When the doctor of choice deems it advisable he refers the patient, *with the patient's consent*, to the physician better able to care for him."[15] Four physicians from the area joined the salaried staff. Mackenzie described the goals of the hospital:

> An institution devoted to giving patients the best possible medical and surgical treatment by a staff familiar with the rapidly developing and rapidly changing science of medicine; to function as a focus in a rural district for dissemination of information . . . to contribute even in a small way to the progress of medicine and surgery . . . to offer to the physicians of the region facilities for the study and care of their patients . . . [At Bassett] free choice [of physician] has been greatly restricted, and fee-for-service, as far as the physicians are concerned, completely done away with.[16]

---

[c] The Clark family wealth arose from the Singer Sewing Machine Company. Other donations of importance include the Clark Art Museum at Williams College.

In the same article he boldly attacked the concepts of freedom of choice of physician and of fee for service, a venturesome position to hold in 1942—and now. It was a venturesome position to place before a suburban county medical society, but this utopian approach was well received. The editors of the *Bulletin* pronounced it a "most reasonable and persuasive statement" (p. 7) and added that it would be regrettable if discussion terminated with the publication of the address.

Mackenzie called for all physicians of the area to have hospital staff positions: "Any physician who is incompetent to hold a position on the hospital staff is also incompetent to practice medicine independently." He proposed salaries for all physicians, at levels corresponding to commissioned personnel of the armed services. The staff would offer "general medical care or specialist services" for patients at home, ambulatory, in hospital or in "outposts" to which members of the staff would be assigned for periods of duty upon which they would return to the hospital health center. Emphasis would be laid upon a scholarly approach, continual internal mutual self-review of work, preventive medicine and health conservation, extensive health education for the public, and combined efforts with the local health department, housed in the hospital. The local health officer would be a member of the staff and also the school physician. Finally the hospital staff would "lecture" the community on general aspects of science and "particularly the social relations of science . . . It would be the community center for healing, for health, for science and the scientific attitude."[17]

From the start the hospital has taken residents and medical students in Medicine and Surgery from the Columbia University College of Physicians and Surgeons. An Advisory Board was formed of professors of medicine, surgery and deans, from Columbia, Johns Hopkins and Albany Medical College. A research division was established due to the efforts of Mackenzie, with the support of the Clarks. Staff pioneered in use of marrow transplantation for treating patients with leukemia. One staff member won a Nobel Prize for this work. The staff of the hospital has always been closed (a closed staff is one to which physicians are only admitted on approval of staff and Board of Trustees, regardless of qualifications). The salaried physicians, whose average income in 1946 was $15,000, have functioned as a group practice. In 1951 there were 18 attending physicians and 13 residents, representing the usual specialties;

no family physicians were on the staff. There was one family physician in Cooperstown.[d]

Mackenzie saw the financial basis of such a structure in a prepayment health care program and "taxation as a source of funds for medical care for all the people."[18] The controlling agency would include representatives of the lay public, the medical profession, government and universities. In 1931 the hospital established a prepaid health insurance plan. The physicians on staff agreed to provide care for $100 per year per family.[19] This apparently was abandoned at the behest of New York state officials who were anxious to avoid competition with the Blue Cross plans they were attempting to encourage.

From the beginning Bassett has been a child of the Clark family. Not only did the family foundations construct the buildings, but also met the operating deficit each year, including that incurred by the medical staff. Even during the Depression of the 1930s, the staff was encouraged to continue activities in providing health care and medical education, and members were offered leaves of absence to increase their knowledge of the latest developments. In 1946 the Clark family endowed Bassett Hospital with a permanent fund, which has provided up to $7,000,000 per year in support.

SUBSEQUENT DEVELOPMENTS

The hospital has been generally well accepted. In 1986 Bassett began to establish a series of community health centers in the region, and at the same time affiliated with a prepayment health care plan by the Community Health Plan (CHP). By 1995 there were 30,000 persons enrolled in the Bassett portion of CHP. In 1993, with changes in accounting, it became possible for the first time to view physician finances separately from those of the hospital. Up until that time there was no distinction. Physicians remained on salary; the staff remained closed; but it was now possible for administrators to consider separately income and expenditures for these two segments of the complex. The organizational structure remains highly integrated: management and physicians did not distinguish between the hospital or physician group. Adminis-

---

[d] In his telephone interview Clinton Hawn, who came to Bassett as Pathologist-in-Chief in 1947, indicated that 20 miles away, in Oneonta, was a small hospital with a traditional staff organization of specialists and general practitioners.

trative functions for the group and hospital were consolidated into corporate services. The CEO is always a physician, as specified in corporate bylaws. At present, a large and representative menu of local health services is available, with major programs in the fields of cancer, cardiovascular and pulmonary disorders, and additional programs in many other areas, most in collaboration with public and private community agencies. Family physicians have been brought on the staff; internists, pediatricians and other specialists provide primary care.

Summing up the similarities and differences between Hunterdon and Bassett: Bassett was grafted upon a much older institution; Hunterdon began *de novo*. Bassett was supported by a wealthy family; Hunterdon by many small community donations. The objective at Bassett was the best result for an individual patient; at Hunterdon it was that plus the best state of health for the entire population. Bassett concentrated on inpatients, each to be taken care of by a salaried, geographic (i.e., maintaining an office only on the hospital campus), full-time specialist. Family physicians did not at first have privileges. Hunterdon concentrated upon the health of each community resident, working to provide a primary care physician in the form of a family practitioner for each. The salaried, geographic, full-time specialty staff functioned in a consultative, supportive and educational role. Hunterdon emphasized mental health; Bassett maintained a program but not with the same central role. Bassett staff engaged in major research projects; the physicians at Hunterdon, except for one initial survey, did not. Both had university affiliations; Bassett still does. At Bassett the specialists dominate the Board. At Hunterdon only recently did staff physicians serve on the Board. Most important, the tightly integrated administrative structure of Bassett seems to have been maintained despite serious efforts to adapt to changes in health care. At Hunterdon, which began with such a structure, a grueling and disruptive transition took place in the 1970s, as will be described later. At that time most specialists left the salaried staff; several left the institution campus. Only in the last five years has the number of salaried physicians increased.

CHAPTER 5

The Countywide Committee Swings into Action

GETTING GOING

To get going, Clifford Snyder organized a series of dinner meetings with representative citizens throughout the county, the first in November, 1946, the last, in April, 1947. At the behest of the Board of Agriculture, a larger countywide committee was formed. On 6 November that committee reported that federal funds were now available through the postwar Hill–Burton legislation, which financed construction of hospitals throughout the country.[1] In February 1947, the N.J. Department of Institutions and Agencies, whose Board Chairman, by a remarkable coincidence, happened to be Lloyd Wescott, gave Hunterdon top priority for federal aid for construction.

On 19 March 1947, one year after her first visit, the indefatigable Louise Leicester was back at Commonwealth Fund, this time to see Henry J. Southmayd, another senior staff member involved with hospital programs. In the interim she had laid down a steady barrage of telephone calls to the Fund about Hunterdon's progress. Now she presented a copy of the report of the Board of Agriculture's Special Committee and indicated they hoped soon to be eligible for Hill–Burton funds. According to Southmayd's notes that day, the Hunterdon group was engaged in retaining a consultant (E. H. Lewinsky-Corwin) to conduct a survey. Leicester was particularly interested in a survey of epidemiology—a study of the frequency of various diseases.[2] She asked for a grant of $1,000 but was put off by a referral back to Lester Evans.

The Board of Agriculture wrote to 250 leaders in the community. Almost all asked to be included on the founding committee. On 2 April 1947, Wescott reported on the final dinner meeting, and on engaging a consultant on health and hospital organizations, stating that opinion was changing from the idea of a small local hospital to the idea of having a branch hospital which would be tied in with a large teaching hospital in the City and that this idea appeared to have several distinct advantages. Corwin was settled on as consultant; the following March, 1948, the Board of Agriculture's Executive Committee voted $1,580 for him to perform a survey.

Lester Evans met with Leicester on 5 October 1947—she wanted help in meeting Corwin's consulting fee. Evans noted: "It is not clear just what sort of a consultant job Dr. Corwin is doing." Leicester was at that time interested in a morbidity study, with particular reference to chronic illness, and hoped to mold the services developed "to fit the needs of the community." She also discussed the needs of young practitioners for group association. Evans again turned down the requested funds although he was impressed by what she told him. His memo concludes: "I wish we had a Mrs. Leicester in each of our areas."[3]

On 9 October 1947, Evans and Southmayd exchanged handwritten notes. Evans: "Are you interested? You can see I'm not." Southmayd: "Agree. If they are going to raise over a million why can't they raise Corwin's proposed salary on prospects. Agree too that it is a worthwhile project in good hands."[4] Two weeks later a formal letter turning down the application was sent, with the tiniest crack in the wall—"we look forward to hearing of further plans."

Leicester was back in Lester Evans' office on 10 March, "to continue to talk to us . . . in such a way that the Fund might at some time and for some reason be inclined to help."[5] Corwin had completed his survey, but not his report. She was already thinking of incorporating the Health Department into the Medical Center, providing better ambulant care, and "[giving] emphasis to mental hygiene and chronic illness in some way." She described community enthusiasm. Evans notes, "The job has been carried along by Mrs. Leicester and a man whose name I do not recall" [this could only have been Snyder]. Evans emphasized the importance of assuring that the affiliation with New York University not result in dulling local initiative, an issue of which Leicester was quite aware. Of the visit, Evans' note says: "I still think there is some very good local thinking going on here." An unidentified colleague added:

"You may find part of Corwin's survey interesting. However there is really nothing new in it."[6] That was true. There was nothing new—merely a synthesis of leading ideas in health care that had been floating around for the last quarter century but had seen little implementation.

In time, Commonwealth Fund through their staff consulting work was a support, a guide, a touchstone of accuracy for those who developed the Medical Center. Initially however, fund representatives could not see how the plans at Hunterdon were of significance to them. Despite the ways in which the Hunterdon structure, as envisioned, created a unified approach to the health care issues of the day, showing on a small stage what might be done in the country at large, the staff at Commonwealth saw the plans as conventional. After lengthy lobbying by the Hunterdon group, Commonwealth staff attitudes changed, and when they changed, it was in a dramatic fashion.

CORWIN AND THE CORWIN REPORT

EDWARD HENRY LEWINSKY-CORWIN, PH.D

E. H. Lewinsky-Corwin, who designed a structure for the Hunterdon Medical Center, was born in Poland in 1886 and came to the United States as an adult, obtaining his PH.D. in 1910 at Columbia University in economic, social and biological sciences. This remarkable individual's enormously influential career in the field of public health terminated only with his death 8 May 1953, just before HMC's opening.

Commencing in 1911, Corwin was for 41 years Executive Secretary of the Committee on Public Health Relations of the New York Academy of Medicine. He exposed shocking conditions in contagious disease hospitals, organized an association of outpatient clinics, and the first set of medical standards for dispensaries. In 1924 he conducted a survey of hospital facilities in the region, a standard reference in the field, leading to organization of an information bureau, which he directed for 12 years. He initiated a similar agency concerned with convalescent care. In 1928 he and S. S. Goldwater organized the first International Hospital Association. Corwin also pioneered a systematic medical nomenclature, studied

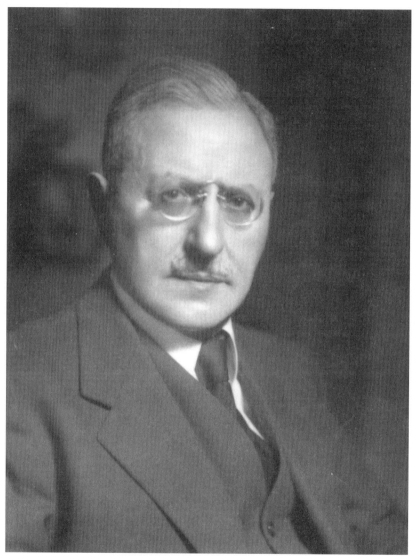

Edward Henry Lewinsky-Corwin PH. D.

public health implications of marijuana, improved standards for blood transfusion, surveyed infant and maternal care, and measured hospital productivity. By 1927 Corwin proposed a study (not carried out as far as I can determine) of family budgets for health care and insurance, which included looking at the adequacy of care compared with social status, at costs by specified illness, and at costs per capita. He recognized that health care costs are disproportionately borne by few families. He felt that insurance had to be carried by all responsible and should provide for periodic examinations for all subscribers.[7]

In 1946 Corwin completed a survey of American hospitals.[8] He compared length of stay and total hospital days with community affluence, described successful regional hospital programs, prepayment plans, the importance of hospital affiliation for physicians, and integration of outpatient departments with hospitals and teaching programs. Individual and family were "the center for the practice of preventive medicine" (in today's terminology "health care"). He advocated that all community health agencies, public and private, should associate with local hospitals until "so interwoven with each other and with the woof and warp of the social fabric as to become indistinguishable as separate entities." Evaluation of the results of medical care was called for.

Early in 1947, just a few months after the report from the Special Committee had been accepted, Hunterdon engaged Corwin as consultant with financial support from the Board of Agriculture. In a letter to Louise Leicester dated 2 December 1948, Corwin said that he had prepared six reports of his work at Hunterdon.[9] (Two of them, the basis of talks he gave on 8 May 1947 and on 28 October 1947, have not been located.) On the earlier occasion, at a meeting at the Clinton House restaurant, he was authorized to proceed with a survey. On the latter occasion, he met with the Hunterdon County Medical Society through the efforts of Ray Germain, a family physician, to discuss a preliminary report of a survey.

THE HEALTH AND HOSPITAL SURVEY

Next, on 15 January 1948, Corwin reported to a group of leaders at the Grange in Clinton on the final report of the "Survey of Health and Hospital Needs in Hunterdon County." The survey had two objectives: (1) to ascertain the available health resources and how they could be improved and (2) to determine whether or not there was a need for a hospital, and if so, with what characteristics. Funds were not available to do a survey of a sample population. Instead, he would rely on demographic and vital statistics.

Corwin established that of three counties examined—Hunterdon, Somerset and Sussex—Hunterdon was the most rural, had the more elderly population, and the lowest per capita income. It is unclear why he did not include even more rural Warren County. Although the population of Hunterdon used hospital services to a greater extent than the other two counties, the death rate was higher; automobile and self-inflicted injury were leading causes of death (still true), and the infant mortality rate was higher. Health services in Hunterdon's schools and public health services were sketchy, or nonexistent, and services totally uncoordinated.

At the time, there were 32 family physicians in Hunterdon County. Eight had graduated from medical school nearly four decades previously; 5 over three decades previously. Although only 5 of the 32 had hospital appointments in the neighboring institutions, 8 percent of the people of the county were inpatients in those institutions every year. Those hospitals had waiting lists and gave preference to residents of their own communities.

Corwin called for a combined health center and hospital, coordinating all the health services of the county and providing an array of specialized public health and clinical services. He suggested that the proposed health officer could double as hospital administrator, recommended that mental health services be incorporated into general medical services and advocated affiliation with New York University (NYU) Medical College.

He summed up by saying:

> if Hunterdon County were to build just another hospital, I would be lukewarm to the proposition, but if this hospital is projected in terms of a progressive institution with a university affiliation, a model of its kind, aimed to bring what is best in medicine to the residents of a rural area, and has associated with it an active full-fledged health center and a good follow-through social service, I would be strongly for it.[10]

The insistence on quality thus recurred. Corwin sums up the trend of the times.[11] Records of the time, and Corwin's report, do not make clear whether Corwin chose this language because it echoed the call to the Board of Agriculture by Angell, Leicester, and Stevenson, as well as the report of the Special Committee, or was a product of Corwin's own vision.

Corwin estimated the operating costs for a hospital of 125 beds, the projected size, would be upwards of $400,000 per year (in 2001 dollars, $2,913,000). Actual expenditures for hospital care in neighboring hospitals by residents were probably close to this figure. Finally, it was noted that the Medical Society, at the prior October meeting showed "no general enthusiasm." Physicians were concerned about the financial burden on the community, interference with the practice of medicine, losing their privileges elsewhere, the burden of medical staff duties and, finally, the impact of bringing in specialists from outside the community. Nevertheless, the Medical Society believed that these difficulties could be overcome. It voted to cooperate in every way should the community resolve to proceed, "particularly if it is to be a hospital run on a high plane of medical competency in association with a large medical center." One wonders if today's physicians would have such courage to back such a potentially transforming venture.

THE CORWIN REPORT

Three versions of the Corwin report exist—a draft copy of 29 June 1948, a "final report" of 27 July 1948, and a "final version" of 3 August 1948, amended by action of the Board of Trustees on 19 November and 5 December 1950.[12] The changes in the document suggest a series of busy negotiations. The conclusion of the amended final version emphasized five principal advantages to the proposal: (1) direct linkage with a university medical school; (2) strengthening local physicians and providing them with additional support services; (3) building a center that would attract patients and new physicians to enable the hospital to become self-supporting; (4) being a potent force for raising health standards throughout the county; (5) attracting physicians and nurses to train at a model for hospitals throughout the country—in other words, creating a center for excellence as a means for serving the community.

The alterations in wording from draft to draft reflect changes wrought by the give and take of negotiation. Corwin's concern for quality led him to write at first "gauging the work done in hospitals." He changed this to "safeguarding," a stronger term. In the draft report, he referred to the importance of a full-time Medical Director, and of regionalization of hospitals in order to raise standards.

> Nowhere to our knowledge has an experiment been worked out whereby a rural hospital is under the direct control of a medical school, where the responsibility for the staff is left entirely to the teaching faculty, and where a systematic effort is made to raise the level of practice in the surrounding community by bringing the local medical practitioners into active association with those who are at the wellsprings of medical science and advancement.

This language was diplomatically toned down in the final report to: "whereby an isolated rural hospital is directly under the wing of a medical school, with all that it implies in the way of opportunities to the local profession and to the community." Corwin may not have considered the somewhat looser organization of Rochester regional program comparable, because of its voluntary aspects in contrast to the "built-in" structural features, which he proposed at Hunterdon.[13]

The hospital would be neither a "medical hotel or nursing home" on the one hand, nor a "Mayo Clinic"[a] on the other, but a "true community hospital which will provide *adequate* hospital care to the inhabitants of the county, a *health protection service* and a *diagnostic service for the convenience of local physicians*" (italics added). Because the care of the sick in rural areas fell upon the general practitioner, the Medical Center should provide for them "utmost opportunities for professional development now and in the future." His language might be compared with the more restrained and subtle words of Reginald Fitz.[14] Corwin described negotia-

---

[a] At a later time this issue arose more than once in considering the development of specialty services. Should they be constructed solely on the basis of the projected need of Hunterdon County or with the intent to draw patients from outside of the county? The then-Medical Director, Robert Henderson, and the Board, led by Wescott, were fearful of raising funds within the county to support services that would be perceived as in good part for out-of-county patients. They did not take the point that regional development of services would improve quality and diversity, thereby benefiting local residents. This was a problem in the development of the Pediatric Service, which will be discussed at greater length in Chapter 16. Today HMC has expanded to provide several special services intended to draw from as wide an area as feasible.

tions with NYU-Bellevue Medical Center for an alliance, quoting Clarence de la Chapelle, leader of NYU's regional medical program, about how important this proposal was for them: "The more intimate the relationship of the two institutions . . . the greater the advantage which will accrue to each unit." The main thrusts of Corwin's proposal and their modification through various versions, are summarized below:

1. "Members of the local medical profession, in good standing, licensed in New Jersey, who express a willingness to serve on the visiting staff of the hospital, will be appointed to positions of different grades on the attending staff depending on their qualifications, experience and readiness to give their time . . . Their work will be guided and supervised by the heads of the various departments." In the final version, the wording became "all members of the local medical profession," and it was specified that that appointments would be made by the Board of Trustees, and that the Medical Board would determine qualifications.

2. "Attending staff [would be] appointed by the Hunterdon Medical Center Board of Trustees on nomination of the NYU-Bellevue Medical Center. The heads of . . . medicine, surgery, pathology and radiology would hold academic rank . . . [and] a straight salary arrangement without privilege of a private consulting practice . . . The departments of obstetrics and gynecology, pediatrics, anesthesiology, psychiatry and such other specialties as it may be thought desirable to maintain . . . will be on a rotating basis in charge of senior residents . . . supervised by the corresponding department chairmen of the University faculty. Their salaries will likewise be paid by the Hunterdon Medical Center." The staff would be responsible for performance in the hospital and supervise the Health Center (see item 6).

3. House staff in all departments would rotate out from the university liaison and educational programs. Medical students would work in the hospital, the Health Center for outpatients and with local practitioners. A nurse's training school affiliated with Bellevue would be established.

4. A Medical Board would be composed of specialists and local physicians (initially with a majority of specialists, in the final version with equal numbers) to formulate and recommend to the Trustees medical policies and rules and oversee professional efficiency.

In the final version, a representative from NYU was added to the Medical Board.[b]

5. Admission policies were to be outlined by the Trustees jointly with the Medical Board, with all patients referred for admission by their respective physicians. All patients would have the benefit of consulting service by the heads of departments, "not only with regard to ward patients but . . . private and semi-private patients as well." Patients requiring care beyond the scope of the hospital would be transferred to NYU Hospital.

6. A Health Center would be established as a part of the hospital, adjoining both the outpatient department and the laboratories and radiology services. Clinics would be under supervision of chiefs of service. The Health Center would also house visiting nurses, and health and welfare agencies of the county. "Prevention of disease, early diagnosis, and adequate medical and social treatment of it are the foundations of a successful health program."

7. "Stress will be laid on the prevention and treatment of ailments associated with middle life and the aging process . . . Care of the chronically ill, as differentiated from the care of invalids, is inseparable from general medical service . . . Psychosomatic medicine will be stressed, for . . . as much illness is due to social, emotional and occupational stresses as to organic causes."

8. An administrator with "good judgment, tact, experience . . . good public relations and a diplomat" would be a nonvoting member of the Medical Board.

9. Specifications for a working library and medical records department were briefly outlined.

10. A clinical laboratory and radiology department would each be headed by a well-trained, full-time chief, with the privilege of "a limited amount of private work" (later deleted).[c] Both services would be allowed to serve private physicians or hospitals without full-time chiefs, if this could be done without detriment. In the

---

[b] That representative turned out to be Clarence de la Chapelle, who headed the NYU regional plan, and who served faithfully, wisely and with the respect and affection of the Hunterdon staff for many years until his retirement. Along with Lester Evans, he is regarded as one of the two professional father figures of the specialist staff.

[c] These were the only members of the specialty staff with this privilege. No reason was specified, but presumably it related to the attitude of specialty societies at the time to salaried employment in these fields, as well as to the difficulty of recruitment. Frederick Woodruff, who came to the Medical Center as the junior radiologist not long after it opened, commented that his initial salary was competitive, and he was aware of no problem with the concept of a salary.

final report a morgue was included to enable the pathologist to perform autopsies and county medical-legal duties.

11. A study of charging: "The generally accepted method of charging for hospital care puts a penalty, as it were, on thorough medical work-up. To offset this many hospitals have adopted various types of inclusive or fixed-rate payment for specialist and auxiliary services, some in connection with pre-paid insurance plans. The Board is at present conducting a study of this problem as it will apply to the Hunterdon Medical Center and the people of the county."[d]

12. The distribution of beds was suggested: 25 private, 60-65 semi-private (two or three patients) and 35 to 40 in four to six-bed rooms.[e]

The innovation of Corwin's design is better understood by comparison to the perceived wisdom of the time about hospitals. A good example is the monograph by James Howard Means, long-time chief of the Medical Service at the Massachusetts General Hospital. Writing in 1953,[15] the year Hunterdon opened, he made plain that the hospital was a place where complex medical care "can be given under the most efficient circumstances." Means makes no reference to an institution accepting overall responsibility for the health of all members of the community, an institution that set its goals, planned for action, and made decisions informed by the larger vision of function of a health care organization.

Further changes were recommended by the Medical Center Board of Trustees.[16] The Trustees wrote to be responsive to concerns voiced by the County Medical Society (the general practitioners), who, although they voted to cooperate, were reluctant to endorse the hospital project. An acceptable redraft of Corwin's proposal specified that practitioners would not be required to attend clinics, dissatisfaction with actions of the Medical Board would be submitted to arbitration and patients could be referred to a specific individual rather than to the institution. All references to the radiologist or pathologist engaging in private practice were deleted. Later, in November of 1950, after the arrival of Ray Trussell, and probably acting at his recommendation, HMC's Board of Trust-

---

[d] See below for the fate of the prepayment program.
[e] Later this was changed to all doubles, with a few single beds for sicker patients.

ees reiterated licensure in New Jersey. At that time an important paragraph was adopted:

> As a basic policy, all specialist and surgical services (except minor surgery) will be given by fully qualified specialists on a full-time basis in the Center. As a guarantee to the community of high standards of service, such specialists must qualify for academic positions on the faculty of a center of medical education, designated through affiliation by the Board of Trustees.
>
> Exceptions to the above policies will be made only in exceptional cases. The basic nature of such exceptions will be determined by the Board of Trustees after study and recommendations by the Medical Board and the Director of the Medical Center.

These changes, some of them clearly substantive, came about after considerable negotiations among the interested groups. All parties gave a bit to obtain the final result. Already the Medical Center project had gained such popularity that it could not be blocked. The result was to strengthen the role of the Medical Board, while disentangling its powers and function from those of the administrator. A significant change in the role of the university altered responsibility for appointments to the specialty staff from initiation and control to review and approval. Each adjustment influenced subsequent developments after HMC opened.

There is a striking contrast between the tone of negotiations that resolved these issues and later negotiations over fundamental changes in staff structure in 1977, as well as constructing a physicians' office building in 1985. On later occasions discussion revealed a spirit of intransigence and acrimony matched only by the political rhetoric of the U.S. Congress of the 1990s. One reason may have been that the participants initially viewed HMC's structure as a constitution, inviolate for the ages. Neither the Corwin reports nor the opinions of those present at the creation of HMC seem to have recognized the need for mechanisms for amendment to adapt to changing times, or distinguished between fundamental principles and structures that may change.

With a covering letter to Lester Evans in January, 1949, Corwin enclosed a prospectus, listing the features of the proposed institution. Shortly thereafter Leicester, Corwin and Snyder met with Evans to romance the Fund. In his usual tactful way Lester Evans complimented the visitors, indicated how impressed he was with

Snyder, "a most intelligent lay leader,"[17] and then noted that they had not inquired about Commonwealth support. But this time he did not say there was no interest.

Local reaction was mixed. Ken Myers, a later member of HMC's Board, widely known in the community and active in fund-raising, said, "Corwin's report was impressive. I read it and I understood it to some extent, I think. But I'm not sure it got general circulation except that it was talked about. The fact that there was a relationship with a New York [hospital] convinced some people that this was a reliable institution." He also said, relative to bringing all county family physicians on staff, "There were two sides to that question. Some . . . said, 'I'm not sure that when I get sick, I want two doctors. I'd like to have the specialist.' . . . It was not clearly understood by everybody up and down the street as to how this thing was going to work."[18]

Trussell, an astute student of public health advances, told me he was not impressed with Corwin's work. A more advanced structure could have been devised. What seemed remarkable to the Board did not seem so to Trussell. President Truman's proposal for national health insurance in 1946 had been shot down by the Congress. Trussell felt it was a difficult time to innovate: He commented, relative to Corwin and his reports:

> He was a very gracious man. He was a respected figure in the field of medical care but you have to remember that the climate in those days was pretty much anti-thinking about anything other than the existing fee for service, open-ended free enterprise and unrestricted building of hospitals. If you could get the money, you could build a hospital. A health officer that interested himself in the National Health Insurance [in England] was liable to get fired.[19]

A special open meeting was held on 7 December 1948. Sponsors included, in addition to the Board of Agriculture, almost every other health and social group in the county. The N.J. Commissioner of Health, Daniel Bergsma (who later on was to be of immense help for the project), Harry S. Mustard, who was both the Commissioner of Health of New York City and the Director of the School of Public Health at Columbia University,[f] Clarence de la Chapelle and Corwin all attended. Not everyone was convinced, however. "One knowledgeable person who looked the

[f] Trussell later succeeded him in this position.

audience over said he 'couldn't see $30,000 in the whole crowd.'"[20] When the report was mailed out to 3,000 influential citizens, only 15 percent expressed active interest. In time many volunteered.

Presenting the Corwin report was a vital step in the creation process for Hunterdon Medical Center. Although Myers described an uninspired response, the community was extensively involved from the start. When only 15 percent of those circularized expressed active interest, a vigorous educational program was mounted around the fund drive. A core group of enthusiastic supporters bound to themselves ever-greater numbers from the wider community. In 1952, as part of a Chronic Illness Survey, half the community completed questionnaires about what they wanted in their new Medical Center. This group identified and overcame many challenges to community-wide health care access—challenges that continue to concern professionals in the field.[g] Ultimately, the Corwin report was sufficiently malleable to flesh out the program that eventually became Hunterdon Medical Center. That flesh was provided by the influence of the Commonwealth Fund, Ray Trussell, the Director it helped to bring on board, and later the specialist staff.

Corwin did not live to see the hospital he proposed open. He died in 1953, approximately two months before HMC opened its doors. Long before then, events began to move much more rapidly, in part because of the influence of the consultants sent by the Commonwealth Fund.

---

[g] Hutchins VL, editor. "Pediatricians' involvement in promoting Community Access To Child Health (CATCH)." *Pediatrics* 1999 Jun; 103(6 Pt 3): 1369–1432. See, in addition to many thoughtful discussions, a table of challenges and responses, p. 1386. Although these articles addressed a pediatric context, the authors make clear their generalizability to other areas of health care.

CHAPTER 6

Carrying Out the Plan

FIRST STEPS

This chapter describes the first steps to create a new hospital, working from Corwin's recommendations. On 25 March 1948, incorporation papers were signed by Clifford Snyder, President, George Hanks, Vice President, James Weisel, Treasurer, Lloyd Wescott, Secretary, and Samuel L. Bodine, Louise Leicester, Raymond Germain, M.D., and Waldo McNutt. In 1949, Father Edward J. Dalton, Rev. Edward C. Dunbar, J. Seward Johnson, Joseph E. Moskowitz, Wesley L. Lance, George I. Bushfield, Herbert D. Stem and Mrs. Charles E. Wagg were added. More will be said about them in Chapter 19. Dr. Germain soon went off the Board; in the future physicians would not be allowed to serve because of a perceived conflict of interest.[a] In 1951, George Hanks went off, and Alfred E. Barlow, Frank Dalrymple, Cyrus R. Fox, William S. Lamont and Reeve Schley, Jr. came on. In January 1953, Clifford Snyder went off; Lloyd Wescott was elected President, Samuel Bodine and Seward Johnson, Vice Presidents, Joseph Moskowitz, Secretary, and William Lamont and Reeve Schley Jr., Treasurers. Dwight M. Babbitt and W. Luther Stothoff came on the Board. Typical of Hunterdon County we find among these personages a politician, a physician, a union organizer, two clergymen, a man of wealth, a businessman, a lawyer, an advertising agency executive, a realtor, a dentist's wife, head of a small steel company, a butcher, a lumber dealer, two financiers, a farmer, the agricultural agent and a well driller.

It is not easy to state exactly how the Board of Trustees functioned with such strong personalities as Lloyd Wescott, Louise

---

[a] This provision remained in force until the 1970s when a consent decree resulted in a reorganization of relations between Board and Staff.

Leicester, or Ray Trussell as the Director. Much of the Board's work was handled by the Executive Committee. Much of its work was done by Wescott and Trussell, with Leicester snapping at their heels. The Committee and the Board appeared to rubber-stamp much of the work. Nevertheless, much was accomplished by the Board. I often saw Wescott call on them for expert knowledge or advice, seasoned judgment, or their network of friends or business associates. Often their contribution was critical, often amusing.

In one instance, in the 1970s, HMC was negotiating an affiliation with Rutgers (now Robert Wood Johnson) Medical School. Wescott was conducting a clause-by-clause review with members of the Executive Committee of an imposing contract prepared by the attorneys. One particularly sticky paragraph gave him real hesitation. He turned to Cowles Herr, an attorney then on the Board, for an opinion. Would the Medical School group accept removal of the errant wording? Could they be talked round? Herr had no idea how important this was to them, but he told Wescott, "Just take a pair of scissors and cut it out. It is down at the bottom of the page. They'll never notice." This was one of the few occasions when Wescott was nonplussed. "Do you really mean it?" "Sure," said Herr, "they never look at that sort of thing." And the deed was done.

These men and women who served on the Study Committee and the Board shared in common qualities that characterize those in every community who serve, move, and work to better the quality of life. First, they were all hard workers, with a record of accomplishment. Second, they all had their own lives and professional skills. Third, many, but not all, were kind people, sweet in social discourse, easy to get along with. Fourth, they were reliable; they kept a bargain. Hunterdon County has many like them today, but no one comparable goal to unite them.

The first draft of the proposed Constitution and By-Laws gave as the purpose of the Corporation to:

- "furnish within the boundaries of Hunterdon County, New Jersey, hospital and outpatient services to the sick and disabled;

- maintain the highest standards of professional medical, surgical, obstetrical and pediatric care;

- offer facilities for the advancement of the science of medicine and the training . . . [of health professionals];
- provide in association with university hospitals and the local medical profession, complete diagnostic and consulting facilities, a disease prevention service . . . [and rehabilitation and psychiatric guidance]."[1]

In April, 1948, the Board met with Edwin A. Salmon, Director of NYU-Bellevue Medical Center, who excited them further by terming the plans "revolutionary."[2] Later the same year the Board accepted affiliation with NYU-Bellevue. In April Barclay S. Fuhrmann, a well-known family physician, agreed to obtain personal endorsements from all physicians in Hunterdon County. The Board approved a Medical Advisory Committee, consisting of Fuhrmann, Lloyd A. Hamilton from Lambertville, Arthur M. Jenkins from Frenchtown and P. W. Baker from High Bridge. After extended discussions about Medical Staff eligibility, the Board decided that physicians in good standing "all or part of whose practice lies within the County of Hunterdon"[3] could be admitted, signaling how strongly the Board felt that this was an institution for the county. The Board was not interested in becoming a regional resource; they worried about floating a hospital for Hunterdon County.

A memo by Evans about a meeting with Leicester on 11 January 1949 concludes:

> Mrs. Leicester no longer asked for Fund help in this project. She has been told on many occasions in the past that we were not assisting in local hospital developments. However, the thought very definitely crossed my mind, particularly as I listened to her on this occasion . . . that here may be a local unit so conceived that it would justify help such as the Fund might give to further the experimental aspects . . . I have nothing specific to propose and I made no indication of such to Mrs. Leicester, but I do think . . . we might give further thought to this particular situation.[4]

One day later the Board at NYU voted to affiliate with Hunterdon. An exchange of memos continued to reveal mixed opinions on the part of the group at Commonwealth. Geddes Smith, another senior staff member, noted: "LJE's memo indicates that local thinking has gone well beyond Corwin's rather conventional suggestions. That would justify keeping in touch with this as it develops."[5]

Harry Handley, on the other side, wrote, "Except that it is nearby, I can see no reason why the Fund should be interested in this."[b] These comments illustrate how dramatically, in a short while, their opinions changed. There is no evidence that any major features of the Hunterdon plans changed, but the perception of the advanced nature of the project by the officials at Commonwealth underwent dramatic reversal. The start of such reorganization of thinking was with the memorandum, just quoted, authored by Lester Evans. More will be said about how Commonwealth changed its thinking, and what came of that later in this chapter.

Other telephone and personal exchanges were of a more positive nature. On 13 January 1949, Corwin wrote to Evans, enclosing a draft of one of his reports, summarizing the situation, and revealing uncertainty about fund-raising and how workable some of the ideas would prove to be.[6] He visualized a five-year "trial and error" period to test out some of the concepts. Leicester, Corwin and Clifford Snyder met with Evans in New York on 1 February 1949, for discussion of plans. Evans notes that Commonwealth might be ready to consider outside help after the fund drive.[7]

Meanwhile, on 19 January 1949, an office was established at 57-½ Main Street, Flemington, on the second floor, over what had been a livery stable, in a building since replaced by a shopping and office complex. Marguerite Moore was hired as executive secretary. Moore had been a helping teacher in Hunterdon County, but retired to avoid a conflict of interest when her husband Harry was appointed County Superintendent of Schools. Her job as executive secretary led to a 21-year career with the Medical Center. Moore had worked for the United Nations, was a member of the Board of the N.J. Federation of Women's Clubs, and had just been hired by the Hunterdon County Public Health Association. She was initially hesitant to take the HMC offer. Mrs. Moore described the situation in her own notes. At the time, she was busy and tired. She was finishing up a UN special assignment, had responsibilities as member of NJFWC Board, and had just accepted a position with the Hunterdon County Public Health Association. She felt uncomfortable walking out on a new job and also doubted her ability as a fund raiser. Her predicament was solved when the Presi-

[b] Harry E. Handley, M.D., was a pediatrician and public health worker who had been on the faculty at Vanderbilt and in the Tennessee Department of Health prior to coming to Commonwealth.

dent of the HCPHA "lent" her to the HMC Board.[8] That same month Rosalie Hodge was employed as a secretary-typist. Hodge had worked in Lloyd Wescott's office and was asked to transfer to the new position. In May, Beatrice Walter was hired as bookkeeper. Walter applied for the job as bookkeeper and also remained with HMC for 21 years. It was said of her by Moore that "she gave two days of work in every 24 hours."

As described in detail by Trussell in his book,[9] the Board now devoted seven months to a series of meetings with an outstanding group of consultants for the purpose of defining the best possible kind of program for the new medical center. On 14 March 1949 Leicester was back again in New York to see Evans, as he put it, "for one of her more or less usual visits."[c] She tried to convince Evans to fund Corwin as an ongoing consultant; he turned her down. On 3 May 1949 Leicester and Wescott discussed with Edwin A. Salmon, Winthrop Rockefeller and Donal Sheehan[d] of NYU the possibility of underwriting specialist staff expenses for five years.[10] Four chiefs of service would be backed by six residents and four interns. The Hunterdon group requested $150,000 to be potentially available on a declining scale over a five-year period. This request was also turned down. Fund-raising began that month and continued all that year.

LEICESTER, WESCOTT AND THE BOARD

Struggles between Louise Leicester and Lloyd Wescott were overt. Both were involved from the start, Leicester more prominently. Both felt ownership. She as much as anyone set the venture on its path by the quality of her vision, the expert consultants she was able to acquire and eventually by convincing Commonwealth Fund of the value of this enterprise. Given the absolutely crucial role Leicester played in moving the project along at the start, in obtaining

[c] Evans LJ. Memorandum of meeting, 14 March 1949. RAC, CF. Commonwealth 1949 file, HMCA. Commonwealth records indicate she was in and out of Fund offices up to twice a month in 1948–1950.

[d] Salmon was the administrator, and Rockefeller the Chairman, of NYU Medical Center. Sheehan, a basic scientist without a medical degree, had been the Third General Director of Commonwealth in 1947–48 before he returned to academic medicine at NYU as Dean and Professor of Anatomy. He strongly believed in the notion of "comprehensive medicine." By this, Sheehan meant that patients could not be understood without evaluating their physical and emotional constitution, their own past and present environments, as well as a knowledge of the cultural patterns of their society. He pushed the idea of educating physicians with such skills as the direction Commonwealth should promote.

the distinguished consultants, and above all, in establishing the Commonwealth Fund connection, given all of this, the proprietary character of her interest and the structural basis for conflict with Wescott are understandable. She was there first. Wescott, initially skeptical, was won over later. It was destined that they compete; she lost the competition.

Mention has been made how Wescott ran the Board. Leicester fought back. The fight was over whose Medical Center this was going to be. Leicester and Wescott both possessed great personal charm, enormous energy, enthusiasm and scintillating communication skills. Differences between them determined the outcome. Leicester was dramatic, intense; Wescott distinguished, suave. Wescott had far greater reserves of money from his wife Barbara. Leicester was more than comfortable (on her visits to New York she stayed at the St. Regis) but not in that financial league. Initially, she had the health care contacts—James Miller, Lester Evans, Corwin and finally Commonwealth Fund. Over the long haul, Leicester's contacts, enthusiasm and forceful manner were bested by Wescott's political savvy, his ability to seize the moment, and his enormous statewide network. In personality, he came across as the leader; she as the critic who asked key questions but was not as able to identify key answers. He made friends everywhere. She came across so strongly she turned people off. As mentioned earlier, Wescott was untiring; both had enormous energy but he did not stop. Work was play and play was work. One other difference was crucial. Wescott was a man; Leicester was a woman. In those times, that counted more. How it would play out today might be harder to say. Ultimately, Wescott felt sufficiently secure to describe her as "my hair shirt."[c] When Leicester retired George Bushfield, prominent and active Board member, put the "hair shirt" in context:

> I know that Louise has been a hair shirt to you and others at times, for her raising of questions, her tendency toward detailed discussion, her reluctance to take decisive action or to make definite decisions. At the same time, she is a genuine student of medical trends and needs in relation to communities, and her knowledge in this field goes beyond that of anyone on the Board, I would say, with the possible exception of yourself. Her devotion to the community's interest in this respect, comes first always.[11]

[c] He made this observation in my presence on more than one occasion.

She dispatched long boldly worded memoranda on little or no provocation. Her concerns were with content—what services the hospital might offer or how they would be financed—and with process—how the Board should be functioning in relation to leaders such as Wescott and Trussell. By improving process she hoped to involve others in a way that would result in improved function. As one example, she wrote a memorandum,[12] in which she summarized administrative powers and Board responsibilities as she viewed them: the administrator must act within policies established by the Board. At Hunterdon Medical Center, establishing many new patterns in health care, the Board had the responsibility to make those patterns "sound and workable, and relating them to the community, without relying upon normal checks and balances of experience." The making of policy and programs are so intertwined to require the closest possible collaboration between Board and Director, so that the Board has a vital role in making policy and does not simply approve that which has been already made. Leicester made a series of recommendations:

- One or more members of the Board should be attached to each important project. "Projects now reach the Board as finished products, planned by the Director, often with the collaboration of outside agencies, and submitted to the Board for approval . . . so chock full of policy, but so complicated, that it is almost impossible for a Board member to isolate and evaluate these considerations at a single presentation . . . Active participation of the Board . . . *would expedite rather than retard the routing of Projects* through the Board."

- Important programs or policies should be submitted well in advance of presentation, and final drafts should always be formally approved.

- There should be appraisal of the community's ability to pay for a program if and when outside support is withdrawn.

- Conferences between the Board and outside agencies would help "get the feel of the community"—the community could make a contribution to lay or professional planning.

- An Advisory Committee of the Board should oversee each project.

Another example of Leicester's energy occurred when Trussell, soon after his arrival in 1950, asked the Board members what they expected HMC to be and do. Leicester's laundry list was seven pages (described by her as a "quickie" in her cover note)[13] and included, among others, rooming-in on maternity, a focus on chronic illness and a countywide survey of morbidity, every service being self-funded, attention to mental illness and degenerative disorders, school health and home care. No one else on the Board prepared anything comparable.

In those times a feeling of urgency propelled all. Large sums had been provided from widespread community participation. The executive office (Trussell, the Director, and Wescott functioning as co-chiefs) saw opportunity and felt the need to move. The Board strongly aware of its fiduciary responsibility and concerned whether the future institution would be too much for the community to bear, vacillated between acquiescence and objections, boldness and fear. However, the Board rarely scrutinized issues with the same passion and determination as Leicester or Wescott. This remained a characteristic for many years. Pat Klopfer, a Board member from 1957 to 1960, repeatedly raised the identical issues as Leicester, but in far more sophisticated and tactful language, directly with Wescott as well as with others on the Board. She was no more successful, receiving answers of apology and soothing language. It was a long time before the Board was capable of standing up to its President.

Commonwealth Fund archives for 1950 show a revealing change. For the first half of the year, most memoranda by Fund staff describe visits to or from, or communication with, Leicester and Wescott. When Trussell arrived, he became the principal intermediary. But also, when an HMC Board member is mentioned, it becomes predominantly Wescott; Leicester's name comes up rarely.[14]

After Trussell left in 1955, Wescott became the Board: the sparkplug, the engine and the accelerator. All that he did, he did with dedication, with first thought to the good of the community and the stability and progress of the institution. But what he did, *he* did, and the Board, usually, approved. At times in his dealings with the Board of Trustees, it was easy to say that the others sat back and let him manage things. One former trustee wrote a blistering letter on this point.

It is also important to recognize the interplay of personalities. If Wescott more than once described Leicester as "my hair shirt," it must also be kept in mind that she was engaging, charming, but also a very persistent and determined person. Seward Johnson commented, on learning she was to be introduced at a meeting: "We'll never get out of here now." In the early 1950s she became marginalized. Her memoranda became more strident. In June, 1956,[15] she resigned, leaving another long note containing much wisdom about how Medical Center affairs should be conducted. Board members George Bushfield and Bill Lamont both issued communications emphasizing how her ideas were worth careful consideration. Wescott again recognized the worth of other's ideas, and looked carefully to see what should be adopted.

RAISING MONEY

The process of raising funds offers insight about how the county at large, and some of the major players, worked together.[16] Initially the Board of Agriculture contributed $5,000 for Corwin's work and report. "The 'country club' group and the 'city people'" strongly opposed the project,[f] fearing burdensome operational costs. Thus, influential groups and individuals had to be recruited. A flying squad of cheerleaders led by Wescott, Leicester and McIntyre talked to any group that might be a source of funds. Solid investigation and planning brought about an incredible breadth of community participation and determination, at times in the face of adversity. Granges, unions, schools and many other groups organized every conceivable kind of event. On one occasion, a volunteer committee held a "gourmet dinner" at the Stanton Grange. Three hundred attended, and HMC garnered $1,701.40 from the occasion. The "gourmet" menu, which illustrates the nature of the county, included Swedish meatballs, scalloped potatoes, chocolate dipped grapes and French vanilla ice cream.[17]

Campaign chairmen from local municipalities included farmers, doctors, real estate brokers, political activists such as a freeholder and municipal officials, a grocer, a well driller, an undertaker, fire and rescue squad leaders, teachers, druggists, and a road equipment salesman. Educational handbooks and a film strip were provided, and methods to deal with responses from potential donors

---

[f] Nicolai CS to LB Wescott, n.d. Wescott file, HMCA. Nicolai, in advertising in New York, was engaged by HMC's Board to advise on fund raising; he created the filmstrip mentioned below.

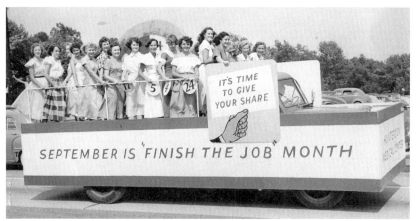

A group of young women creating interest and excitement to raise money for HMC.

outlined. Key points from the Corwin report reiterated the central role of the family physician. The County Medical Society issued a press release encouraging community support for the project.

As one example of crisis and response, the Board had applied for Hill–Burton assistance in raising funds. When Hill–Burton representatives examined records, they found half the pledges not legally binding, and therefore unacceptable to the representatives. Volunteer solicitors returned to donors to re-sign a legally binding pledge. Donors representing 5 percent of the total refused, amounting to about $58,000. Trussell recalled his solution to the shortfall:

> In those days, $58,000 looked like a lot of money. Seward Johnson, who was the Vice President of the Board, never in public put forth any gesture of generosity. I learned that the way to deal with Mr. Johnson was to send him a memorandum at his home. So, I sent him a little memorandum about this particular problem, and I was invited to his home and met his wife. Rather a very gracious lady. He was sitting in his study looking at this piece of paper and said, "Well, if I back it, it's only a loan." And he, very quietly, signed the necessary papers to cover the $58,000.[18]

No actual loan took place. Johnson was never asked to put up the cash.

In these early years, there were, of course, skeptics. Reading Gebhardt, a leading local attorney, wrote to Henry Southmayd of Commonwealth in February, 1948, to inquire whether or not a supervisory relationship with an institution such as NYU-Bellevue had ever been done before. His letter suggests other doubts: "I am a resident of . . . a rural county. There is movement on foot here to try to establish a rural hospital . . . This is a county of approximately 38,000 people with very few industries, indeed."[19] Another attorney, Italo Tarantola of Flemington, remained strongly opposed for years. He barraged the Board, Wescott and many others with letters finding fault with the whole idea.[20] Another skeptic was Herman Lazarus, Jr., owner of the *Bayonne News*, who wrote to Board President Snyder during the fund drive. Lazarus took a different tack. He quoted extensively from Corwin's documents to support his belief that "a hospital for Hunterdon County is an adventure in finance which we cannot afford or maintain." Lazarus feared a farm community of limited resources could not handle the fiscal drain. Finally he made plain he did not wish an argument; rather he aimed to rest his mind by presenting a different point of view. "Experience will indicate whether I was right or wrong . . . I shall hope with you that I am wrong."[21] Records do not indicate whether Lazarus changed his mind. However, the institution's opening convinced many skeptics and garnered the "blessings" of many prominent local citizens, including Lloyd Fisher, a Flemington attorney who had been prosecutor in the trial of Bruno Hauptmann for the kidnapping of the Lindbergh baby. Fisher was treated at the Medical Center shortly after it opened and wrote a very warm letter to Wescott to express his admiration of HMC's efficiency, effectiveness and the courtesy extended to him.[22]

In all, the first fund drive raised almost $1.5 million over several years—in 2001 dollars $10,917,000 or $909 per family. Of the first $905,000, 20 percent was in sums of $1 to $99. Only 63 gifts exceeded $1,000.[23] The Riegel Paper Company of Milford, New Jersey, on the Delaware River, pledged the first major gift: $50,000 to be paid in thirds over three years. With that in hand, Wescott went to Seward Johnson and said:

> "You're the richest man I know." He said, "OK, I'll give you $1,000 a year for 2 years." I said, "That's the second biggest gift so far, but it's not what I want. I want $25,000 in cash now." He went to his brother, Robert Wood Johnson, who was dubious but said, "OK."[24]

By April 1953, almost 10,000 families of an estimated 12,000 in the county had contributed! The breadth of this support was a major reason why Commonwealth decided to help, and much of HMC's success is attributable to the strong level of community support. The community manifested a proprietary interest in the hospital. A major reason why my wife and I elected to relocate to Hunterdon County in 1959 was our perception of the bond between community and Medical Center.

Another crisis occurred in 1951. Architectural plans had been drawn up and put out to bid. In August, when bids were opened, they exceeded cost estimates by more than a million dollars. The Korean War and other building programs had driven up costs far more rapidly than had been anticipated. When Commonwealth's Lester Evans heard of the problem, he, along with Mildred Scoville, stepped in. He immediately wrote a supportive, emotional memorandum[25] to Malcolm Aldrich, Commonwealth's President, pointing out that the bids were actually in line with costs of neighboring institutions and that the local group seemed motivated to proceed. He reminded Aldrich that "we have in Hunterdon County a field laboratory for progressive health developments thus far unexcelled in our long experience in dealing with communities." He wrote an assessment of what might happen, and outlined ways in which the Fund might be of assistance. An unknown hand (Aldrich?) annotated the memorandum with skeptical comments.

Evans' memorandum reveals as much as any document extant the temper of Hunterdon at that time. He reports the dismay of the Board over the situation. Almost $900,000, in addition to $1,800,000 on hand or committed, would be needed. Despite this, the prevailing attitude was not "let's quit" or "scale down plans," but rather "we have got to do something about raising more money." Evans called for immediate discussion to determine if Commonwealth could consider bricks and mortar money. This would have an immense salutary effect on the HMC Board. On the side, he told Aldrich, he had indicated to Wescott and Trussell (Leicester is by now out of the center of action) that Commonwealth would not be surprised should their Board ask the Fund for a grant—but of course he could express no judgment on the likelihood of any added assistance. The key to Evans' response is his belief that the community would never shirk its responsibility. The belief in Hunterdon County, that it was *our* hospital, *our* responsibility, was evident, and the march of events confirmed that this belief was real, and was widely held.

Visits by Commonwealth staff followed to vet the Board's finances, review the plans and bids, and to take the temperature of the community. The interview of Ellsworth Higgins is worth quoting. Described as a wiry, weather-beaten farmer, interviewed as he was running a corn-stripper on a large mechanized farm, the laconic Higgins said it was not possible to quit and give the money back: "Can't curtail without losing what they've got from outside. Nothing to do but go ahead. The world wasn't built by going backward." He was not afraid of the hospital going into debt:

> Hell, no. I never knew an outfit out of debt that didn't go backward. I never got ahead till I got a little capital, found out what I wanted to do, borrowed what I needed and went ahead. What if it does take twenty years? We got to have something to keep the young folks interested.[26]

Higgins' wife Sarah served on the Board of the Hunterdon County Heart Association with me in 1959 or 1960. Ellsworth Higgins, still wiry, still weather-beaten, smoking like a chimney, would drive his wife to meetings. With a chronic lung problem, her speech was interrupted by the need to take a breath. At one meeting, someone asked her, "Sarah, why do you work so hard, come out to all these meetings?" She replied, "I'd rather wear out than rust out"—the same sentiment voiced in Tennyson's *Ulysses*, his variation on the touching story in Dante's *Inferno*: "How dull it is to pause, to make an end / To rust unburnished, not to shine in use!" Or as Shakespeare has Ulysses say in *Troilus and Cressida*: "To have done is to hang / quite out of fashion, like a rusty mail / in monumental mock'ry." These were the good folks of Hunterdon who backed up the swells and made the hospital happen.

Meanwhile the Board considered the options: abandoning the project, building a smaller, conventional hospital, shrinking the plan's community health portion, or proceeding as planned, with an eye to every possible saving that would not sacrifice programming. To their credit, the vote was unanimous for the last alternative. At a meeting of community councils, 118 of 120 in attendance voted the same way. Money was borrowed by means designed to lead to further contributions from the community. Under the leadership of Reeve Schley, Jr. of the Somerset Trust Company and of

Malcolm Aldrich, President of Commonwealth, a consortium of ten local banks was put together.[g] These banks agreed to a bridge loan of $300,000, with Somerset Trust to take the lead at $84,000. The other nine banks, all in Hunterdon County, contributed the remaining in proportion to their resources.[27]

Seward Johnson, possibly with help from others, including Wescott, put up collateral for an additional $350,000 borrowed from Chase National Bank. As Wesley Lance noted on the occasion of an earlier fiscal crisis, Johnson "could have bought us all out."[28] But that was not how Johnson operated. Wescott in later years commented that Johnson helped the most not by giving money but by providing the notion that it was available.[h]

Wescott now formally asked Aldrich at Commonwealth for bricks-and-mortar money.[29] By this time, late in 1951, Commonwealth was committed to the Hunterdon project, as described in the next section. Within days the Fund gave $250,000. One can only surmise the activity in person or by telephone that underlay these fast-moving events. The community power structure flexed its muscles and called in its markers. One letter says all. Reeve Schley to Malcolm Aldrich, to thank him for the grant, "Reeve" to "Mac."[30] The loans, and the grant from Commonwealth, made it much easier to go to the community for the final $350,000. Ground was broken that fall.

Years later, looking back, Wescott said: "After the War there was a feeling on the part of many people that now we have saved the world and now we ought to do something about ourselves. This is for Hunterdon."[31] Exactly. It was a single focus of achievement for all. No single cause has involved such a large proportion of the community since, although many work for Hunterdon today, but for many different causes. No single cause has captured the imagination or created such excitement. And no single cause has stirred such pride of ownership and involvement. I do not

[g] Schley, a gentleman farmer, owned a large farm on the border of Somerset County. His business interests were in banking and Monmouth Park Racetrack, of which he was President. He joined HMC's Board through his friendship with Wescott. In public he said little, but looked the part of a business leader. By chance at one of Wescott's parties I learned that during World War II Schley was in the OSS, spoke fluent French, and parachuted into Occupied France on several occasions.

[h] Mark Twain's story, "The £1,000,000 Bank-Note" about a young man with a note so large that no one could cash it but who lived well on the strength of it, is an apt comparison. Mark Twain: *The complete stories*, ed. C Neider. New York: Doubleday, 1957.

believe this project could be done today. Proposals of far smaller impact routinely elicit bitter polemic at meetings and in the letters column of the newspaper.

FURTHER PROGRESS

ELABORATING THE DESIGN

The events of 1949–1950 show how the Hunterdon group, concerned with creating a hospital of high quality to improve the level of health of all residents, proceeded locally while maintaining awareness of national thinking on health care delivery. This section describes: the interaction of the Hunterdon group with a variety of distinguished consultants; how the local group, informed by these experts, further defined the basic elements of the program; and how and why the hard work of the local group resulted in a commitment from Commonwealth Fund, and the recruitment of a distinguished Director, Ray Trussell.

During much of 1949 the Board, under Clifford Snyder's leadership, conferred with Corwin and a long list of eminent consultants about programs and design. Among them were Stanhope Bayne-Jones, Daniel Bergsma, Clarence de la Chapelle, Lester Evans, George Baehr,[i] Harry Handley, Edwin Salmon and Donal Sheehan. Trussell describes how the elements of the program emerged out of these conferences.[32] Corwin prepared a preliminary statement of choices, floating proposals for rooming-in on maternity, a mental health program integrated with the hospital, nurses' training and the problems of chronic disease. Wescott and Leicester wrote to Sheehan on other topics they saw as calling for a new approach:

- ➤ a hospital of the highest quality, with the specialist staff supplementing the primary care physician, and serving everyone in the community, not just the well-to-do;
- ➤ integration of the hospital with public health and disease prevention programs;

---

[i] Baehr, Co-Chief of Internal Medicine at Mount Sinai Hospital in New York, was involved in almost every significant health care development in the mid 20th century. He was a founder of HIP, a pioneering health insurance plan in New York. He published widely on the benefits of group practice (e.g., Economic Aspects of Group Practice. The Kingsley Roberts Memorial lectures, 1948. New York: Medical Administration Service, 1949). He was also involved with the Committee on Medicine and the Changing Order of the New York Academy of Medicine.

- architecture that would not be a small-scale replica of large city hospitals, but would lower both building and operating costs, improve patient well-being by a psychological approach, and emulate the modern chain store and factory to solve problems in parking, traffic flow[j] and efficiency; and

- consideration of costs to the patient, which indicated a combination of voluntary insurance and a set scale of fees to cover adequate salaries.

What was happening was a merging of ideas. They came from the fertile mind of Louise Leicester and her army, from Snyder, Wescott and others on the Board, from the deliberations with the team of consultants, from Corwin. It is now not possible to tease the strands apart, to say from whence each concept came. What can be said is that the canny leaders, Snyder, Leicester, Wescott and a few others, were able to fit together a collage of novel notions to create an extraordinary innovative community health care institution.

Enough progress had been made for two other major steps. The Board created a committee on architecture to invite candidates to submit qualifications, and Lester Evans suggested a search for a hospital administrator. Seward Johnson agreed to underwrite the salary for a year. Corwin and Evans addressed an open meeting for the community held by the Board on 1 December 1949. Corwin emphasized the ability of the proposed institution to provide leadership on all health matters, space for any health service needed, outpatient services and to relate to family physicians. Evans praised community involvement, adding, "the big problem is to make the hospital a *vital factor in the lives of people in the years when they do not have to occupy a bed as a hospital patient*" (emphasis in original).[33] He added that the architect should translate ideas into buildings, not the other way around.[k]

Louise Leicester wrote Evans at the end of the month to arrange a meeting of HMC representatives with the Commonwealth group. She thanked him from "all of us." She concluded dramatically: "I feel as if Dr. [James Alexander] Miller[l] were looking over my shoulder as I write this." Of Evans' talk in December, 1949, she wrote:

[j] Parking and traffic flow have become recalcitrant problems far beyond what any founder might have envisioned.

[k] Board minutes of 6 January 1950 show the representatives of the U.S. Public Health Service present to discuss Hill–Burton monies for construction, pushing for early engagement of the architect, precisely the reverse idea.

[l] Miller had died in 1948.

> You should have a Large Gold Medal for that simple but
> masterly presentation you made during the last 10 minutes—
> of our problems and . . . needs . . . If the project is thought
> through along the lines which you laid out—we shall have an
> institution of major significance. We have done our best . . .
> Now we need help and authoritative confirmation of progres-
> sive policies and programs.[34]

Plans were made for a team visit from Commonwealth.

COMMONWEALTH IS COMMITTED

In January 1950, a rapid series of events indicated that the Commonwealth Fund team was becoming active. Harry E. Handley,
who earlier felt that there was nothing at Hunterdon of interest
except geographic propinquity, summarized the situation at
Hunterdon. He raised tough questions that needed to be answered.
He and others from Commonwealth met with N.J. Commissioner
of Health Bergsma on improving local public health services. Bergsma
reported that legislation to allow local municipalities to combine
to engage full-time professional staff had failed. They discussed
health insurance. Evans again advised Leicester and Wescott to
give priority to choice of an administrator, not an architect.

In February Handley and Evans made a site visit to sniff out
the terrain and the people. Handley covered the ground from Hampton and Califon in north Hunterdon to Lambertville in the south.
He spoke with representatives of agencies, government, schools,
and almost the entire power structure of the county, political, financial
and agricultural. It was an impressive survey, reported in candid
fashion. Snyder, Wescott and Leicester rounded up not only project
supporters, but also those who expressed opposition, including
Howard Moreau, publisher of the *Democrat*, the county's leading
newspaper, who had been initially opposed, but was now one of
the strongest supporters. Lou Young, an officer of the New Jersey
National Bank in Lambertville, and a trustee of the Phillips Memorial Hospital Fund, was described by Handley as "the most
Dickensian character I saw." Young was bitterly opposed to the
entire project.[m] Edward Hunt, also a trustee of the Phillips–Barber Fund, which now amounted to a third of a million dollars,

---

[m] DJ Zahler, personal communication, 13 February 1997. He described Young as a quiet
man, a nice man, but fiscally conservative. "If you had $400,000 he might lend you $1,000."

and who had originally written to Commonwealth 24 years previously, was also opposed. Phillips–Barber had offered $50,000 to the Medical Center in exchange for beds dedicated to residents of Lambertville, but was turned down. Nevertheless, Handley, in a resounding editorial statement, said:

> It is my impression that Hunterdon County is a better community in several respects than any of those in which the Fund put on public health demonstrations. *There is more self-reliance, fewer indigent and dependent individuals, and more widespread spirit of cooperation than we have encountered anywhere else. [They] are frankly seeking help to make of it something new, different and more complete than any medical service with which they or we are familiar* [emphasis added] . . . I feel that it represents an opportunity for the Fund to help to do some of the things that the Board of Directors has expressed as desirable and that in this group of people we may invest money with complete confidence that it will be used to the best advantage.[35]

The money Handley referred to proved to be partly for bricks and mortar and partly for the expenses of Commonwealth staff, such as Evans, Handley, Scoville and any number of consultants. Commonwealth did not build a hospital. It helped by bringing the latest in health care developments, by providing personal backup, encouragement and support to the Board and Staff, and by fostering an aura of distinction instrumental for recruiting such distinguished men as Trussell, Edmund Pellegrino (first Chief of Internal Medicine) and Andrew Hunt (first Chief of Pediatrics). The joint visit of Handley and Evans 8–11 February 1950, documented in their memoranda, marked the turning point—the fulcrum against which the lever moved. Information gathered on these visits convinced Commonwealth that this was the place to invest Fund efforts.

Evans was also impressed by the Board's willingness to face those who opposed the project in order to debate pros and cons. Nowhere else had Fund representatives been exposed to such varying points of view: concerns over the community's ability to provide financial support, and even whether a hospital was needed at all. At the same time, Fund representatives' suggestions were incorporated into the thinking of Board members. Evans wrote: "Any feeling I had of the rich potentialities in this situation was accentuated by this visit . . . This is the best community situation with respect to health, hospital, and medical development we have ever been exposed to." What was needed was visible evidence of action—selecting an architect, digging a hole in the ground, and moving along. Evans outlined a process to reach a decision about a grant for the Hunterdon group to obtain "outside counsel and advice they can use." He hoped they would formulate a proposal of such quality that Commonwealth might be justified in providing risk money to underwrite selected portions, mentioning specifically, "health insurance plan, social service, home care, a broad service for ambulant patients including private doctor's facilities at the hospital." He visualized $75,000 to $100,000 per year for five years.[36]

After years of dancing, first with Louise Leicester and then with Snyder and Wescott, the Fund realized that this was their dream hospital. It was not so much that Hunterdon was trailblazing new concepts, but rather that, in one place, just about every feature considered characteristic of advanced health care was being put together in one institution. It was the combination, the totality of the vision, together with the clear evidence of deep roots throughout a community that ultimately brought in Commonwealth. Thus the intertwining of local and national events: after some years in which the Hunterdon group learned from national experts, now national figures were to learn from Hunterdon what could, and was, being done. The relationship that followed lasted for two decades.

At a meeting with the Board on 10 February 1950, Evans and Handley strongly hinted at their very favorable impression, but said that this was "confidential" and "off the record." This was the "best rural county in which we have had experience." The Board, they said, should concentrate on functions, the financial picture and building plans in that order. This contrasts with the reaction later that year when Trussell (by then the Director), the Board and Commonwealth personnel visited a group practice in Hudson, New York, the Rip Van Winkle Clinic (see Chapter 4). The structure of that center was greatly admired. Of this visit Evans wrote:

> [The] group is professionally run and stimulated. No public
> involvement. [Therefore] much less easy to find a way in which
> an organization such as Commonwealth Fund can help . . .

> When the impetus for better organization, integrated service,
> comes from the lay public, as in Hunterdon, we can readily
> find ways and means of assisting.[37]

Now the Board proceeded to engage a top-flight individual to
serve in a dual role: first, as executive secretary to the Board, perhaps for nine months, and later as administrator and consultant.
Commonwealth could not provide consulting services to the degree needed. It was important that the local group work things
out for themselves, rather than be told by experts. A locally based
consultant could assure that the planning process was responsive
to local needs and wishes. Evans, Handley and the Board began to
accumulate candidates for the consultant/administrator. Meanwhile,
they developed a short list of five architects with whom they had
met; at least one or two seemed promising. On 1 March Handley
told Wescott and Leicester the most important step was to select
the best person available for administrator. The Board, Handley
recorded, wanted an administrator who could coordinate what was
new with tried and true practices—a sign of their ambivalence.
He also emphasized that formulating the master functional plan
must precede planning the building. Form follows function. Again
a prepayment health plan was mentioned.[38]

Later that year Carolina Randolph of the Fund performed another survey of the county's public health services and health characteristics, including many revealing interviews with nurses and
other helping personnel. Although available services were scant,
incomplete data on morbidity and mortality suggested only two
major problems. There were no maternal deaths, perinatal death
rates were below other New Jersey counties, deaths from tuberculosis less than two-thirds the national rate, but deaths from cancer
and trauma were significantly higher. She slogged through thick
emotions in an all-day meeting in Flemington to get a better understanding of exactly what services were available from school
nurses. Her memo makes plain the fears and resentments of some
professionals already working in the community about this "experimental and demonstration" Medical Center.[39]

By 8 March 1950 Clifford Snyder formally requested financial
assistance from Commonwealth, with a preliminary budget. He
emphasized integration of services, many of the concepts previously described, including "nation-wide significance in reestablishing
the importance of the general practitioner," and, for the first time,

mentioned departments of rehabilitation and geriatrics[n] as well as mental health. Snyder included in a list of questions to be answered, essentially points raised by Leicester.[40] On 13 April Commonwealth voted "$25,000 or as much as may be needed," for consulting services and planning. By 20 April HMC's Board was in touch with Ray Trussell, as well as several other candidates.[41] On 22 May, at a public meeting, attended by New Jersey's Governor Alfred E. Driscoll, the grant was announced. At that meeting Evans spoke of new ways to provide for community health, built upon the observation that "medicine, including health services . . . in its simplest terms is fundamentally a relationship between two people, the patient and the doctor, the former seeking help from the latter for the solution of some physical or emotional problem."[42] This crucial observation was built upon the words of Sir James Calvert Spence, Nuffield Professor of Child Health at Newcastle, England, who said:

> The real work of a doctor is only faintly realized by many lay people. It is not an affair of health centres, or public clinics, or operating theatres, or laboratories, or hospital beds. These techniques have their place in medicine, but they are not medicine. *The essential unit of medical practice is the occasion when, in the intimacy of the consulting room or sick room, a person who is ill, or believes himself to be ill, seeks the advice of a doctor whom he trusts. This is a consultation and all else in the practice of medicine derives from it. The purpose of a consultation is that the doctor, having gathered his evidence, shall give evaluation and advice...not the diagnosis or the technical treatment* [emphasis added].[43]

Spence and Evans stood with one foot on either side of the threshold that separates disease-focused from health-focused care. Evans understood and believed in the importance of anticipatory health care founded on patient education by a physician with limited powers, where patient life style, attitude and habits are crucial. Both also show in their writings ties to the traditional model of physician–patient interaction: the physician prescribes; the patient complies. One cannot know whether or not they could have

---

[n] Until a few years ago, geriatrics as a medical specialty was not represented on the staff nor were there geriatric-focused programs. Recently, a graduate of the family practice residency obtained special training, became certified in the sub-Board, and joined the health center in Lambertville. In 1999 a full-time geriatric physician, double-Boarded in geriatrics and internal medicine, came on salary at HMC.

conceived of a collaborative relationship wherein the physician provides opinions and suggestions for the patient to consider. However, I believe these two thoughtful men, if presented with such a model, would have endorsed it.

Buoyed up by the excitement of this fresh backing, the Board shifted to looking for a Director (someone who could manage the complex and novel combination of programs) rather than an Administrator (someone to run a hospital). The Board selected Ray Trussell. In a memorandum to Malcolm Aldrich, Evans indicated how pleased he was with Trussell's selection and recommended reallocation of the Commonwealth grant to facilitate that appointment.[44] Evans did not say so explicitly, but the appearance of Trussell was extraordinarily fortunate for Hunterdon. This might be an appropriate place to say more about first Evans and then Trussell.

LESTER EVANS,
PRINCIPAL COMMONWEALTH CONSULTANT

Lester Evans was born in Kansas, graduated from the University of Arkansas and Washington University School of Medicine in St. Louis in 1921. He took his pediatric residency at St. Louis Children's Hospital from 1921 to 1923. For the next five years he worked in Fargo, North Dakota, as Medical Director of the Commonwealth-created Child Health Demonstration Project, and staff member of its Child Health Committee. The aim was to bring together current beliefs about child health into one program. At that time (and later) the training and practice of pediatricians emphasized the care of the sick child. Although a few distinguished pediatricians wrote about, and worked in, the area of health care and prevention of illness, for most practitioners the treatment of disorders was their principal activity.°

Evans joined the Commonwealth Fund staff in 1928 and spent his entire career there, retiring in 1959. He became Executive Associate for Medical Affairs, the senior and most influential of the Fund's staff. Harvey and Abrams write that Evans had a real missionary spirit, energy, diligence and patience and that his "phi-

---

° My experience was typical. After training and military service, I opened an office for general pediatrics. Very quickly it was apparent that while I might be a capable sick children's doctor, I knew very little about the world of healthy children. As a result, I learned on the job from my patients, their parents and my wife.

losophy of medical education and health permeated the thinking of the Fund's staff and of the larger world of American medicine. If one of his ideas did not at first appeal to Aldrich [Malcolm Aldrich, the Fund's President] Evans would not be discouraged but would put it on a back burner until he could recast it to give Aldrich another view. Evans was masterful at asking questions and stimulating conversation without manipulating events directly." Nor was Evans ever burdened with precommitments about outcomes. "His helpful appearance created an ambiance that led people to talk freely with him, confident that he would not use any information he gained to their disadvantage." He would elicit an institution's capabilities to develop innovative programs.[45]

Evans' idealistic approach is well-defined in the summary of a talk he gave in 1938 on what he hoped for in a rural community hospital. It is worth quoting, not merely for its content, but also because it shows why he ultimately found in Hunterdon his ideal:

> This hospital [is] one from which the public expects good work; one where the board and the interested public are cognizant of their obligation to provide adequate facilities for the care of patients; one where the doctor must show his qualifications before receiving the privilege of working there;[P] one where the staff maps out plans of procedure for the complete study and treatment of all patients; one where the physicians as individuals and as a group give critical study to their experience and one which assures itself of continuous help and advice from outside medical and educational centers . . . The educational value of this experience is what the doctor makes it.[46]

Evans also answered Leicester's questions, mentioned earlier, about comprehensive care. He said:

> There is nothing new or complicated in the concept . . . [It is] compassionate, personalized, birth to death attention—preventive, advisory, rehabilitative, as well as diagnostic and

---

[P] This point should be kept in mind in light of several intense discussions, described later, about whether all family physicians in the community should be admitted to HMC's staff. Although Pellegrino, who was appointed Director of Internal Medicine in 1952 and who later succeeded Trussell, yielded to no one in his admiration for Evans, he felt strongly about inclusiveness, because he believed a physician *on the staff* was more likely to improve than if *isolated* in the community. Also remember comments of George Mackenzie, the chief at Bassett, who said if a physician was unqualified to be on the staff of a hospital, he should not be allowed to practice.

therapeutic—that the ideal family physician [gives] within the limits of his knowledge . . . What is new and complicated is adapting the concept to the uses of urban society and specialized skills; so that medical care does not become increasingly an episodic, impersonal and even haphazard matter of a patient's shopping in bewilderment from specialist to specialist, none of whom may know the emotional and environmental problems interacting with his organic complaint. The aim should be to combine the concentrated knowledge and skills of the specialists with the broad understanding, vision and continuing care of the generalist.

Pellegrino summed up the crucial role Lester Evans played. He was a

father figure who would visit from time to time . . . If there was some problem here or there, Lester always had an upbeat view about its solution and the future. He believed in the Hunterdon Medical Center and communicated his confidence in the idea to all of us "young Turks." I was the youngest chief there. But we chiefs were not that far apart in age. We all needed a professional father figure and Lester provided it, in some ways more substantially than Clarence [de la Chapelle] who came out intermittently. Lester was the visionary; Clarence the down-to-earth counsellor . . . He was a very nonaggressive man, and very gentle in his approach, but clear on what he was about . . . [Evans] saw in Hunterdon the fulfillment of his hope for a community hospital as a community health center, combining preventive and curative medicine, community health, and bringing together community health organizations under one roof.[47]

Typical of Evans' supportive approach is a 6 June 1952 visit with HMC's Board. Wescott recorded several assertions Evans made: the county could support a health department, the specialist staff would become self-supporting, the occupancy rate would grow rapidly, the integration of hospital, medical and health services was a logical step that would result in savings, and finally that more young doctors were tending toward general practice and that this program would be attractive to them.[48] Six months later Wescott wrote to Evans to ask for a performance appraisal of the Medical Center. It is typical of the relationship that Wescott felt comfortable in doing so; it is typical of Wescott that he utilized this occasion to reconfirm his perception of what was of most interest to the Fund.

These perceptive remarks bear closer examination. The Board needed this encouragement. Members alternated between entrepreneurial excitement and fear of their ability to support the vision. They must have felt like the cartoon character who races along to the edge of a cliff, runs out on air, suddenly looks down, and falls on realization there is no support. At that time, it was received wisdom that even small governmental units should open health departments. The burden of multiple services was far less. Today the minimum population size recommended for a department is much greater. Then, Evans spoke for stepping out as few similar institutions and population groups had done. Integration of services was then and now rational, subject to legal, political and attitudinal constraints. His comments on a self-supporting specialist staff and expansion of the "generalist" staff (primary care physicians) were farseeing. The specialist group was quickly self-supporting as a result of shared earnings between surgical and medical specialties. Within ten years this led to internal friction; soon after the twentieth anniversary high-earning specialists became independent practitioners. All specialists worked in open but not destructive competition with the generalist staff, now known as the family practice staff. Again, at the time, generalists were seen as dying breed. The future world belonged to specialists. Instead the primary care physician staff has expanded progressively and a vibrant and highly successful family practice residency program has provided many new family physicians for the community. All of Evans' predictions proved justified.

Another measure of Evans the man is found in a letter he sent in 1976 to Lloyd Wescott upon his retirement from the Board and Fred Knocke's resignation as Medical Director. Wescott had, correctly, identified these changes as the end of an era, and the commencement of new leadership and directions. Evans wrote:

> A lot happened in those early days and of course it is flattering
> to think that I may have been of some help—what you don't
> know is how Hunterdon served as a learning experience for
> me. While I had some idea of where the program might go, I
> had no idea of the crucial role of community organization

and leadership, and that was what I learned. It took your leadership along with others to set the medical program in the right direction, it would never have happened under professional sponsorship—I think this is what the country either has not learned or will not accept. Our National health program should have progressed as smoothly as yours—instead it gets chopped into pieces with the ever stronger pressure groups seeing that they get their share of the cake first—with the person as patient being lost further and further between the stools.q

q Evans LJ handwritten letter to L Wescott, 30 August 1976. Wescott file, HMCA. On 23 May 1950, Evans had prepared a memorandum for Aldrich of the text of his talk, already mentioned, to a large public meeting in Hunterdon County. His comments then show how long before this letter he had used experience to drive his beliefs: "We know from our experience with field workers that those who are learning on the job turn in the best records." Indeed, Dr. Evans, indeed.

CHAPTER 7

Ray E. Trussell

The First Director

Ray E. Trussell, M.D., M.P.H., the first Director of Hunterdon
Medical Center, inherited the rich treasure of concepts and
principles of HMC's founders. But Trussell was much more
than an actor filling a role scripted by others. He immediately
made major contributions to the guiding notions, organization and
the very structure of the institution—even more than Wescott,
the driving force from 1953 on. Trussell arrived at Hunterdon prepared by temperament, ability and experience for a task unlike
any other in the history of hospitals and medicine in this country.
His performance of that task yielded great dividends on the investment in existing plans that he found on arrival, to which he
added so very much of his own devising. It is true that no one
person alone created the Medical Center, but it is also true that
Trussell is one of those few whose contributions were necessary.

UPBRINGING AND EDUCATION

Ray Trussell was born in 1914 and raised on a farm in Iowa. Both
parents died when he was a child, and he was raised by a grandmother. He graduated Phi Beta Kappa from the University of Iowa
in 1935 with a B.A. in Chemistry. Trussell knew in college that he
wanted to go to medical school, although he no longer remembers
why. Perhaps it was his talent as a Boy Scout treating minor injuries.

Soon after entering University of Iowa Medical School Trussell
became a half-time lab instructor in the Bacteriology Department.
He says, "The University was so broke that they employed upper
level students to become lab assistants. Then the professor of

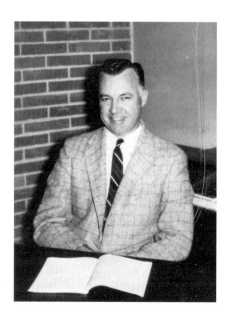

Ray E. Trussell, MD, MPH, first
Director and administrator of
Hunterdon Medical Center.

obstetrics . . . wanted to [know] . . . whether *Trichomonas* was a
harmless commensal or was it truly the cause of vaginitis. He took
me on as a half-time assistant."[1] Trussell was a half-time medical
student, half-time instructor in bacteriology, and half-time researcher
in obstetrics and gynecology for six years. By graduation he had
published a substantial number of papers and written a book on
infectious diseases.[a] He also managed to participate in investigations of scarlet fever and Rocky Mountain spotted fever epidemics
at the behest of the Iowa State Health Department Laboratory.
He received his M.D. in 1941 and was elected to Alpha Omega
Alpha, the medical honorary society. He interned at University
Hospital in Iowa City for nine months and then took a position as
Instructor in Preventive Medicine.

MILITARY SERVICE AND EARLY CAREER

Trussell served in the Army from 1943 till 1946, assigned as epidemiologist to study epidemics in New Guinea and on Leyte in the
Philippines. He was awarded the Bronze Star for this work. He
subsequently assisted with a two-month survey of research in the

---

[a] In a letter to Lloyd Wescott dated 1 May 1950, he enclosed an informal résumé that
mentions "25 articles in scientific journals." HMCA. One day later he hand wrote a note to
Lester Evans regarding that résumé. "The attached 'pedigree' has about as little relation to the
future as possible since it looks like strange and interesting seas to me." RAC, CF.

medical schools in Japan.[2] He returned to Iowa as Associate in the Department of Preventive Medicine. With a Rockefeller Foundation Fellowship in Epidemiology at Johns Hopkins, he received the degree of Master of Public Health in 1947. Then, as epidemiologist for the New York State Department of Health, he developed a statewide program to improve standards of newborn care. In 1948 he became the first full-time Professor of Preventive Medicine at Albany Medical College, where he introduced a social component to physician training by having students work with public health nurses and social agencies. Trussell, who became active in the Conference of Professors of Preventive Medicine, was elected the group's Secretary and there met Harry Handley of the Commonwealth Fund.

First Contacts with HMC

Handley suggested Trussell as administrator to HMC's Board. The Board meanwhile was vigorously pursuing the selection of an architect, feeling less urgency and more uncertainty about the choice of an administrator. Thus, the Board revealed a lack of sophistication by pursuing a structure before defining what functions it would serve. According to Commonwealth's Geddes Smith, the Board's "final decision was to look for a fairly young man who would serve as executive secretary of their governing group . . . In addition there should be a top-flight coordinator supplemented by several consultants."[3] Lloyd Wescott now wrote to Trussell to ask whether he would be interested in the position of Director of the future Medical Center, a letter worth quoting as an example of the Board's thinking.

> We have committed ourselves to produce a unique institution, one that will set an entirely new pattern in rural medicine. The challenge is enormous, but the task is staggeringly large.
>
> The task immediately ahead of us is drawing up a detailed program, closely relating our project to community needs and resources, and translating this program into architecture. We are planning to hire an architect immediately, and also an administrator or director . . . Dr. Handley of the Commonwealth Fund has suggested that as one of the outstanding men in the field, you might be interested . . . We are indebted to Dr. Handley for the suggestion. It is probably through

> this kind of personal understanding of our needs that we shall
> find just the right man . . .
>
> If you are not interested in the long-term connection, do
> you want to be considered as a consultant?[4]

At that time Trussell had no experience in hospital administration. He would learn on the job, often under the tutelage of Miss
Lela Greenwood, the first Director of Nursing.

Board records first mention Trussell's name in mid-April, 1950.
Trussell thought he might have gone "down to talk to these people
out of curiosity more than anything else." At an evening meeting
with the Board committee, Trussell sensed that even though Clifford
Snyder was Board President, "it was clear that Lloyd Wescott [Board
Secretary] was the dominant figure in the meeting." Trussell felt

> very much at home with many of the people in the room
> because we had similar backgrounds and similar roots. Wescott
> . . . was originally the son of a Wisconsin farmer. The group
> had a certain human quality and enthusiasm that was very
> infectious. So it ended with my being offered the job. I re-
> quested a proposed salary level a little higher than they had in
> mind. On the other hand, Wescott knew he needed some-
> body very badly.[5]

At the Board's request, Trussell met with Lester Evans, who
told Malcolm Aldrich: "We have had our eye on him as a person
in public health and medical education who is able to visualize the
kind of thing that we are interested in in our experimental health
services." Trussell then wrote Wescott to determine the strength
of the Board's interest:

> Through [Evans] I have been able to see even broader hori-
> zons in your projected adventure. We concluded that I should
> explore the matter further with you provided that is also your
> wish. I would not want to put either of us to the time and
> expense involved unless you feel that it is clearly indicated . . .
> I am deeply interested but must study the situation thoroughly
> before I can reach any decision one way or the other.[6]

Trussell held discussions with project consultant and N.J. Commissioner of Health Daniel Bergsma, representatives from NYU
School of Medicine and several key people in his own field. He
planned a second trip to Hunterdon County, commenting (in a
letter to Lester Evans): "One of the critical issues will be the reaction of the medical profession." Trussell made clear he would come

only on a full-time basis and that he wanted to be involved in teaching. Unless general practitioners were brought more fully into the planning process there might be some isolation, he emphasized in the letter to Evans.[b] After a climactic meeting, the Board agreed to hire Trussell on a full-time basis with the title of Director and a salary of $15,000 per year (approximately $109,200 in 2001 dollars).[c] Leicester described the meeting as "a little difficult" and "something of an ordeal for Trussell," according to Smith's notes. This was all about the disparate expectations of the Board and Trussell. The Board had in mind a limited consultancy, perhaps part time, to set up the hospital, followed by the hiring of an experienced hospital administrator to manage the organization. Trussell, fully aware of the importance of this venture for the future of health care in the United States and to Commonwealth and potentially to his career, prepared himself well and went in expecting a salary commensurate with the job he planned to do— nothing less than the job of a lifetime. The Board may not have realized what a locomotive they were dealing with. Trussell, in turn, may have elicited some of the Board's latent ambivalence, of which Commonwealth was made quite aware from their key visits of February 1950, but which Trussell did not as yet fully understand. The encounter might have foundered that night. It is a tribute to all involved that they persevered, managed to reconcile expectations, and focus on the job to be accomplished.

REASONS FOR ACCEPTING HMC OFFER

Some of Trussell's reasons for accepting Hunterdon's offer have been already mentioned—the feeling of community he felt with the farmers, both the older county group exemplified by Clifford Snyder, and the immigrants of wealth, represented by Wescott. All projected an infectious enthusiasm that kindled interest and was hard to resist. It looked like a fun place to work.[d] Another

[b] Trussell RE to L Evans, 2 May 1950. RAC, CF. Characteristic of the writer is that in the same letter he also extensively discussed the process of establishing a School of Public Health in Albany.

[c] Smith G. Memorandum of telephone conversation with L Leicester, 27 June 1950. RAC, CF. Commonwealth 1950 file, HMCA. Today, a physician/CEO of a comparable institution might expect a salary of $250,000–300,000 plus a bonus of $50,000.

[d] By the time of my arrival in 1959 some of the early staff and Board had departed, but my wife and I recognized this infectious enthusiasm. It was as if we were being invited to join a wonderful club. We have never regretted the decision.

important influence was Commonwealth, in particular Lester Evans. Like the broom handlers in a curling contest on ice, Evans and others smoothed the way, creating a network of associations and facilitating progress—something for which no amount of grant money could substitute. Trussell told me, with reference to this point:

> Hunterdon was one of these places where you go in to fill in a vacuum and you have a Foundation that is there to help you fill it in. The degree to which they [Commonwealth] financed that operation is greatly overstated. They really provided strategic grants and there was never any general support of the Medical Center . . . They helped by making it possible to bring in some staff earlier than usual, and then, of course, the Chronic Illness Survey was a separate item that enriched the place. There were some people who felt that Hunterdon was an aberration because they had all this Commonwealth Fund support. Well, there was no general support at all. It wasn't like what Kaiser got started during the war: he had the United States Government behind him to keep his workers working. We had nothing like that in Hunterdon.[7]

In addition to Wescott, Trussell mentioned Clifford Snyder, Mrs. Donald Klopfer,[e] Louise Leicester and others on the Board as personalities of warmth and helpfulness who influenced his decision. Trussell was also very impressed by the amount of money that had been raised for the proposed hospital, the extent of community participation, the standards the Board had set, the quality of its consultants, and, of course, the relationship with Commonwealth.

Co-workers at Albany discouraged him from considering Hunterdon, a place they regarded as a backwater. Trussell could not articulate specific reasons underlying his final decision to come. He knew that at Albany he was on a fast track in the academic and public health world. He had never had to worry about a job. He had no particular career path in mind. Although he was pleased because he had added a social component to preventive medicine, he also felt that he had been credited with abilities and accomplishments that he did not deserve. He says of his decision: "I

[e] Donald Klopfer co-founded, with Bennett Cerf, Random House Publishing. During my recruiting interviews, my wife, our three-month-old daughter and I were invited to the Klopfer home for a dinner gathering of the Board and the Selection Committee, an evening that still glows in my mind four decades later.

sensed that I needed to do something more, get a little broader exposure." He found it hard to give specifics, and apologized for not explaining himself more precisely. This was one of the few occasions during our interviews where Trussell was vague.[8]

LEADERSHIP STYLE

Trussell had an enormous job. As the Medical Center was planned, and for the first few years of its existence, almost all responsibility flowed through the Director's office. During his first two years, he was the sole professional on the staff. He generated dozens of position papers, outlines, reports and other documents and consulted regularly with Commonwealth's staff, particularly Lester Evans, but also others. In addition, the nature of the Director–Board relationship required working intimately with Lloyd Wescott. Wescott brought many supportive qualities to his position; other aspects were not so positive, as noted elsewhere. Trussell said, "I did not concern myself with the structure or function of the Board nor was it my job."[9] At the time Trussell told me this, he appeared quite definite. By the time I had interviewed others, and annotated many documents, I came to believe that his memory had coated reality. He could not have accomplished his tasks without taking into close account, and manipulating as best he could, Wescott, Leicester and other key Board members. Nonetheless, Trussell and the Board were not infrequently at odds. With Bill Lamont, the Treasurer, there was a continual butting of heads, according to Murray Rubin, who came in 1954 as chief financial officer.[10] Trussell and Wescott, two powerful engines, inevitably clashed from time to time, for they did not always agree. It was the genius of both men to be able to focus on the task at hand and figure out how to work with one another to accomplish it.

Board minutes and Trussell's own comments, do not suggest eagerness to provide great monetary rewards, although in December, 1953, Wescott arranged for a Christmas bonus for Trussell, using leftover Commonwealth money.[11] The market for top administrators then was very different from today, when salaries well into the mid six figures are not at all unusual. One wonders whether the parsimony of Wescott and the Board may have influenced their relationship. After Trussell left, there was a distinct coolness between Wescott and Trussell, which contrasts with the frequent, warm communications between Wescott and Pellegrino, Trussell's successor.

Two men served as administrators while Trussell was there, but as Ed Grant, who came as administrator when Pellegrino succeeded Trussell, said:

> Ray was not in any sense a Medical Director.[f] Ray was Director, so he was also Administrator. That's just a change of title . . . Ray was Director . . . [Running everything was] his way, but he accomplished getting the Medical Center open. They needed a bull in a china shop if you will, and that's not meant unkindly. He was a strong personality.[12]

The demands of the job were huge; the resources that Trussell brought to the challenge were commensurate. Trussell wanted very much to be in charge, as well as to start with a clean canvas. It is doubtful that he could have carried out the requirements of his position otherwise.

Trussell described those years:

> I was very busy equipping the Center, getting staff, getting it functioning, getting the Chronic Illness Survey on the way, responding to national and local demands to appear at meetings and talk about the place. Before the place opened, I spent an endless amount of time going to local meetings to explain to people what it was going to be like and how it was going to work . . . But here I am all by myself and I'd never built a hospital. I had never made an equipment list. I had never made a hospital budget and on top of which we were doing something that in itself was a full-time job . . . I would meet with Lela Greenwood [Director of Nursing] every morning for coffee at 8 o'clock and she would go over the preceding 24 hours of problems at all levels and then make suggestions on what might be done about them. I was getting a postgraduate course in hospital administration.[13]

Absorbing comments about Trussell, reading the books he wrote, and observing the man himself 45 years later, one sees a bear for work and a mind of far-ranging erudition and remarkable judg-

---

[f] Pellegrino preferred the title of Medical Director as more descriptive of his areas of interest. He requested, and the Board agreed, that if he were to succeed Trussell, it would be with the understanding that a trained hospital administrator (Grant) would be engaged.

ment. On each of his interviews with me he packed enormous amounts of information into the time allotted. He was precise, clear, and efficiently communicative. In addition to everything else, that man was methodical, careful and complete. For example, on one occasion, six months before opening, he sent to the Board's Executive Committee a list of items "which must be worked through before we open," including everything but the kitchen sink: equipment, budget, opening ceremonies and relationships with agencies.[14]

David Sanders, a resident in pediatrics at Hunterdon in 1953, and later a psychiatrist and colleague of Trussell's at Columbia, was impressed by the intensity of his focus which, added to his seemingly effortless precision of communication, led to extraordinarily effective management. "He had a wonderful way of cutting through bureaucratic nonsense. He would answer memos by just writing on the memo 'yes' or 'no' or 'I don't think so' or 'talk to me about this.'" Trussell was so articulate that he could dictate a letter or speak spontaneously so that the only editing required was for punctuation. Sanders added: "If he liked you, you were terrific, and I was on that 'like list.' If you were on the 'not liked' list you could have a lot of trouble . . . When he got angry he got very angry." Sanders believes that what made Hunterdon happen, in the last analysis, was "the force of Ray's personality."[15]

Aaron R. Rausen, the first medical student to be a clinical clerk at Hunterdon, said: "[Trussell] was a very imperious Medical Director. I remember him as being . . . very . . . patriarchal . . . He exuded leadership," a view counterbalanced by nurse Jeannette Ash: "If you went to a meeting where he [Trussell] was, you were very proud that you were connected with the Medical Center because he was there."[16]

Edmund Pellegrino described Trussell as similar to Lester Evans— "another visionary but a hard-headed one," and as a man with bold ideas, courage and the capacity to get things done.

> His personality wasn't always pleasant, but he engendered
> respect. I personally always felt he was a good person to work
> with. His view of life was different from mine. I was a clini-
> cian. He was a public health person. We met in the middle
> because Hunterdon combined both of these things. We comple-
> mented each other rather than having an antagonistic

relationship. Ray held the place together in crucial times in that first year when everything was so much up in the air. There were so many unanswered questions. Would we get any patients? What would happen to the first patient? He had the courage to persist, and also the very good sense to leave us alone. He didn't micromanage as far as I could see.[17]

The essence of Hunterdon for Trussell was the vision of the health of the community, centered on an institution prepared for involvement in every aspect of community health and welfare. To this challenge he brought unusual abilities: brilliance of mind, clarity of communication, decisiveness, extremely broad interests, vigor and ability to influence others. He was also single-minded, sometimes brusque, and although he was always respected, he could be irritating. Finally, he looked at the community as a whole. His perspective was not that of the clinician, whose objective is the best interest of a given patient at this moment, regardless of resources required. Trussell saw resources as allocated for the health of all the patients, the entire population of the community. This unavoidable conflict is at the heart of the great debates of today about the u.s. health care system. How do we apportion our resources for health care? Who gets what?

LATER CAREER

Early in 1955 Trussell resigned to become Dean of the School of Public Health at Columbia University. Recipient of several excellent unsolicited offers and feeling that HMC was well established, Trussell was relieved of administrative duty as of 1 April 1955, in order to write two books, one on the Chronic Illness Survey and the other about the Medical Center. Somewhere along the way, he and Wescott grew more distant. In many contexts Wescott makes clear he never had doubted Trussell's ability or accomplishments. But a decade later, in a letter to the then Medical Director of Hunterdon, Wescott wrote: "He has been difficult to stop on practically anything he attacked . . . I rather doubt that he ever really understood Hunterdon County and its people."[18] These two incredibly strong-willed and energetic men shared the highest mutual respect, yet at other times their relationship was one of highest dudgeon.

Trussell remained as Dean at Columbia for 13 years, directing large-scale studies of medical care and health insurance and also establishing innovative programs. During this period he headed the Department of Hospitals of the City of New York for four years when Robert Wagner was mayor. Repeatedly the center of controversy, Trussell displayed the ability to stick to his principles under criticism. In 1965 he was one of nine physicians in an advisory group to President Lyndon B. Johnson to help shape policies for Medicare. Finally he served as General Director of Beth Israel Medical Center in New York City until his retirement. David Sanders said, "He left Hunterdon to take on the world."[19] Trussell died in 1999.

CHAPTER 8

Building a Medical Center

FUNCTION PRECEDES FORM: A HOSPITAL AND HEALTH CENTER FOR PATIENTS

This chapter describes frenetic activities of the Board, representatives of Commonwealth and consultants, as a more detailed and specific programmatic description was created, financing secured and design of the physical plant worked out. The Board, joined in mid-1950 by Ray Trussell, moved from ideas to reality. Although most of the key elements of the plan were retained, along the way the prepayment insurance program, the integral health department, evaluation, research and packaging on campus of community agencies and non-profit activities all fell by the wayside. Previous chapters have presented the Corwin reports of 1948 which provided the first outlines of a program, the fund-raising of 1949, which showed the extraordinary extent of community involvement, and the results of the extensive Board meetings with numerous consultants in late 1949 and early 1950, which offered a detailed plan.

Alternative agendas competed at the end of 1949 and early 1950. Should the Board hire an architect and fit the plans into the subsequent building design? Should the Board hire an administrator or planner first and design the building around the final mix of functions? In some ways they attempted to do both.[a] Initially, on 1 December 1949, Clifford Snyder, as chairman of the Committee on Architecture, wrote to the architectural firms interested in the project. He outlined main features, including sections for diagnosis and temporary treatment of "chronic and mental cases," inte-

[a] Community pressure to start construction was very evident. Community representatives made this point clear to Handley and Evans during their joint site visits 8–11 February 1950, recorded in simultaneous but not joint memoranda, dated 8–11 February 1950. RAC, CF. Commonwealth 1950 file, HMCA.

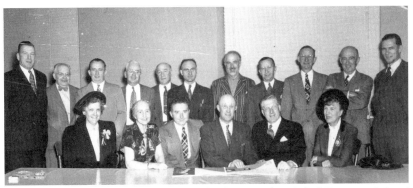

Board members, dedicated friends and workers for the Hunterdon Medical Center watch Board president Clifford Snyder in 1950 sign the contract for architect Vincent Kling (not present) to begin designing the building. Seated, left to right, Marguerite Moore, Margaret Wagg, Waldo McNutt, Clifford E. Snyder, Samuel Bodine, Louise Leicester. Standing, George Bushfield, Rev. E. C. Dunbar, Frank Dalrymple, Herbert Stem, Joseph Moskowitz, Wesley Lance, David Jensen, architect with United States Public Health Department, E. Chapman Romine of Lambertville's Phillips Memorial Fund, James Weisel, George Hanks, Lloyd Wescott.

grated services of a hospital, health center and public health and welfare activities of the county, flexibility[b] of the physical plant to allow easy expansion or alteration to meet rapidly changing social and economic conditions, medical advances and basic conceptions of hospital organization, planning, administration and construction. Snyder also mentioned provision of professional and physical services adequate to support the mentioned principal departments, consideration of new relationships such as between inpatient and ambulatory care and hospital organization and finally he named some of the consultants with whom the Board had been working and expected the architect chosen to continue such collaboration. He also added: "We do not want to seem pretentious, but we are convinced that our project will have national significance."[1]

On 6 January 1950, New Jersey and federal representatives from the Hill–Burton program met with the Board to urge them to proceed forthwith on a search for an administrator.[2] Commonwealth ever so gently worked to brake the headlong plunge into building. Robert Jordan of Commonwealth Fund, who was knowledgeable about hospital construction, met in New York with Leicester and Wescott. He also advised them to obtain their

[b] Regrettably, flexibility for future alterations and additions was one feature lacking in the final building plans.

administrator first.[3] The same advice was offered to the same persons by Handley and Carolina Randolph, another Commonwealth staff member.[4]

Simultaneously the Board corresponded with several administrative candidates. As mentioned earlier, Trussell's name first appeared in the minutes in April 1950. On 7 April 1950, Board minutes show the architectural firm of Vincent Kling and associates was chosen; that firm also designed Lankenau Hospital in the western Philadelphia suburbs.[c] Trussell was less than enchanted with Kling. He made plain in our interviews that he felt the real work on this project was done by a member of the firm named Eschbach.[5] On the other hand, Lester Evans commented: "We are more than pleased with the architect . . . He said he had built hospitals for medical people but never before had he been asked to build a hospital and health center for patients."[6]

The basic design elements were threefold and related to the proposed Medical Center programs. The dominant feature, a hospital wing, included conventional beds as well as a dozen or so beds for convalescent patients who did not need full hospital facilities.[d] A small ambulant care wing called the Diagnostic Center included scanty offices for specialists and family physicians to see patients, for mental health, social service and other services. A connecting wing included supporting services—library, auditorium, and laboratory and radiology services. The design appeared logical and straightforward, but obviously emphasized inpatient care. After all the to-do, HMC harked back to the original call of Angell, Leicester and Stevenson—a hospital building to house the sick! As far as I can determine from the documents of the era, this ambivalence over what the Hunterdon Medical Center was really all about arose as much as anything else from Board anxiety over money and community reaction to the idealized new programs contemplated. There is no doubt about what Trussell had in mind. On the Board, not even Wescott quite understood the structural implications of programmatic concepts.

Competition for a site was between a location on State Route 12, between Flemington and Frenchtown, and one about four miles north of Flemington, towards Clinton, on State Route 69 (now

---

[c] The physical appearance of Lankenau is a large version of Hunterdon.

[d] Many years later a Continuing Care floor built with a major contribution from the Large Foundation replaced these.

N.J. 31).[e] Kling's firm found many advantages to the first in terms of economy of construction and exposure to breezes in a building lacking air conditioning. The principal advantage to the northern location was that it was closer to the mass of the population.[7] An advisory committee of realtors split on the sites, but the Board by eight to four voted for the location which would be convenient for most citizens.[8] At the same time Trussell, as indicated in his Director's report for November, was struggling to refine the construction budget to lower costs, and crowed over an estimated saving of $175,000. The Route 31 site, a farm owned by the Butler family, was purchased for $25,000.[f]

Problems emerged later. The original building was planned economically as an entity in and of itself, with little thought for later needs. When it became necessary to expand radiology and laboratory in the center wing in the middle of the building, these areas could not be expanded readily—a problem to this day. Additions for more physician offices and other ambulant care services required an ingenious design to piggyback a new building atop the old one.

PLANNING A PROGRAM

One of Trussell's first acts was to request Board members to write him individually expectations for the hospital and for his performance in his job. By the 7 July 1950 Board meeting he had ready a list of considerations he felt should receive attention. This was a characteristic Ray Trussell list, methodically identifying every problem he felt might need attention. A look at this list indicates that on his arrival at Hunterdon he was ready "to take on the world." The 27-item list included: general physicians; dentists; bedside nurses; public health, state and local nurses; school nurses and teachers; voluntary health organizations; local welfare; all community

[e] So many youngsters ripped down the signs to use as trophies in their rooms that the N. J. Department of Transportation changed the number for cost conservation.

[f] Although not everyone agrees, most informants say the Butlers gave the Medical Center a good buy. My father remembered them because they were kind to him and his family when they farmed nearby. One holiday season, before World War I, my grandfather managed to accumulate enough money (not a frequent occurrence) to purchase a goose from the Butlers. The next morning, when my father went out to get the animal for slaughter, it was nowhere to be found. The family was devastated, for they had no more money for another. My father was dispatched to the Butlers to see if another goose could be obtained on credit. Mrs. Butler greeted him with roars of laughter and pointed to their goose, which had gone home for the holidays. The old Butler farmhouse is still on the grounds. For many years it was painted pink and called "the pink house" and used for the Family Nurse Service.

organizations with any kind of health program; nursing homes; tuberculosis sanitarium; mental hospitals; state health department; Hill–Burton funds; local boards of health and health officers; Commonwealth Fund; community; auxiliary personnel—social workers to occupational therapists; Medical Center Board and Director; Veterans' Administration; insurance program; industrial medical programs; every known professional society—local state and national; pharmacists, optometrists, and osteopaths; and national voluntary health organizations.[9]

The Board responded with a six-point directive:

1. patient-centered planning to promote health in the broadest possible sense;

2. provide facilities, services, leadership and organizational connection to enable the general physician to render comprehensive and continuing service and to foster full use of the Center to achieve goals;

3. assure needed specialist services;

4. move to comprehensive, integrated countywide community health services;

5. emphasize planning, continuity of medical care, coordinated services, training, research and health education; and

6. be financially self-supporting when special funds are no longer at hand.

On 13 July 1950 Vincent Kling, the architect, Trussell, and Harry Handley, Robert Jordan, Carolina Randolph, Mildred Scoville, and Geddes Smith of Commonwealth met.[10] Trussell strongly believed that program plans should precede any serious consideration of structure. Trussell and Scoville raised the issue of full-time chiefs of pediatrics and psychiatry. There was uncertainty whether a full-time radiologist and pathologist were needed. Perhaps part-time consultants would suffice. It was suggested that Jack Fritz, a respected family physician in Flemington, might obtain training in obstetrics to serve as consultant. In some fields, such as brain and chest surgery, it was quickly agreed that all work should be referred elsewhere. They also discussed practical issues of which other agencies could be incorporated into the campus, and how.

Less than a month after that meeting, Trussell submitted his first extensive Director's report to the Board and to Commonwealth. Trussell respected the Board but regarded them as amateurs who had picked up smatterings of advanced health care ideas but without the perspective to put them into place. His words were cautionary:

> [Much of this] is material stemming from exploratory conversations with advanced thinkers in the field of health and medical care. Careful professional study and planning and community education are necessary before many of the social advances suggested can or should be translated into reality. It must be kept in mind always that Hunterdon Medical Center is now nationally known and the subject of much interest and discussion. Several aspects of the proposed program are considered to have real social significance.[11]

Trussell laid out a schedule built around the need to complete a definitive program statement by mid-August to allow Kling time to make preliminary drawings for an October application for Hill–Burton money, which would allow groundbreaking by the summer, 1951. He underscored the Board's responsibility to obtain support by interpreting the program to the community, an activity that "will in large part determine the outcome of this venture."[12]

The files contain a document entitled, "Considerations Governing the Hunterdon Medical Center Staff Appointments and Organization," dated 1950, marked "Rough Draft, Latest Copy" and "Superceded [sic]" with Trussell's signature. I believe he wrote it and that it was an early version of the Summary Statement of Objectives of 1952, described below. The text establishes how early his concepts were formulated. This document emphasizes continuity of care by the "family physician," community-wide education and education of all patients, and the participation by each in care to make possible "joint interaction" and "individual responsibility and opportunity for health maintenance." In addition, he recommends integrated planning, resource pooling and coordinating the efforts of all organizations with related activities. Trussell saw hospital care not as an isolated event but one in which the social and emotional aspects of the individual should receive care and attention. Unit health records of individuals linked to families should further this.[g]

---

[g] In Chapter 6 I wondered whether Evans would have accepted a doctor–patient relationship in which the physician's role was to advise the patient about alternatives and educate them on the advantages and risks of each. I rather thought he would. Here Trussell demonstrates how well he understood this issue, as well as the importance he attached to understanding the social context in which a patient is nested, and, at least intellectually, the relationship between the clinical aspects of health care and the public health aspects of community health.

By late summer, Trussell had:

- lined up support for materiel, salaries and consulting to create a single medical record incorporating both *health and medical care* activities from the N.J. Department of Health, with the expectation that a County Health Department would be created;

- discussed with both Commonwealth and the Department of Health a combined approach to financing a mental health program;

- initiated plans to promote mental health, medical care and education, and preventive services via ambulatory care delivered at HMC by both family physicians and consultants;

- signified that he and Commonwealth strongly believed a prepayment insurance program should be started, which would be "the answer to many of our problems."[13] Wescott was enlisted to delay the Board of Agriculture's proposed Blue Shield program until this was settled.

- arranged for tentative provision by Commonwealth of risk money to underwrite new experimental programs, perform a countywide survey, and delegate staff freely for consulting services;

- moved with consultants Salmon and de la Chapelle for NYU to provide consulting help in hospital planning, design, an educational program, and to complete negotiations with architect Kling;

- activated a Public Health Advisory Committee chaired by Howard Moreau, publisher of the *Democrat*, the county's leading newspaper, communicated individually with family physicians and the County Medical Society and obtained a resolution of support and cooperation;

- planned a survey of health needs, funds spent and services given, to be followed by a survey on health of the community at large;

- opened negotiations with Dr. Morton Levin of the National Commission on Chronic Illness about a survey in Hunterdon County;

- scheduled meetings, which were enthusiastically received, with the county dentists to plan an extended dental program to supplement the existing dental services clinic;

- performed a study of the Public Health Department of Hagerstown, Maryland, to learn about the integration of hospital, voluntary agencies, public health services and nursing, and school health services;

- reviewed the functioning of Johns Hopkins Hospital's Medical Care Clinic in Baltimore. The clinic provided support functions in the form of reports and recommendations to general practitioners, but did not offer treatment.

- emphasized Hunterdon's need for a "stable and adequately financed position"[14] because the venturesome quality of the program would inevitably increase costs.

In September Wescott sent a planning progress report to Commonwealth. Evans supplemented it with one of his laudatory memoranda, to Malcolm Aldrich, Commonwealth's President:

> [The] community holds potentialities beyond those previously experienced by the Fund . . . [It] coincides . . . with a major area of interest to us—the general area of the needs of the ambulant patient both in the clinic and in his home. It is through and around the ambulant patient that integration of the hospital OPD [outpatient department] clinic and diagnostic facilities and public health services can be brought about . . . Hospital facilities and personnel can be extended community-wide into the home . . . When there is complete integration and continuity of medical care for the individual person in the home, the clinic and the hospital . . . creation of an all inclusive voluntary insurance plan . . . [which] may need underwriting . . . may even run to $100,000 a year for a few years.[15]

By the end of the month Commonwealth's Board was so pleased with the venture that Aldrich wrote:

> We see in it potentialities for experimentation in the integration of all phases of medical and health work as they affect the individual citizen in his medical and health needs . . . We are prepared to give very earnest consideration . . . to the ways and means by which the Fund can give further financial assistance to the Center for the more highly experimental and demonstration aspects of the services which do not logically rest with the local community at the start.[16]

This accolade, to which is attached the key to the treasury, may well have been unprecedented in Fund ventures. It is even more remarkable that the Hunterdon group made sparing use of this offer, relying primarily on the expertise of the Commonwealth consultants who shuttled out ceaselessly from New York.

In the autumn of 1950 and through all of 1951, the Board, Trussell and the Commonwealth staff worked long, busy hours on many topics such as staff organization and interrelations, financial support and integration of community social and health activities. They called once more on connections. The aid of Winthrop Rockefeller, Chairman of NYU-Bellevue Medical Center and also highly influential at the Kress Foundation, was utilized to open negotiations with the latter. The goal was to provide $150,000 backup support for the salaries of the future specialist staff. This was accomplished in time; the support was never needed; eventually Kress turned over the money to the specialist staff treasury, as noted later.

Trussell laid out a series of principles, including emphasis on social and emotional features of illness and the responsibility of the individual to work towards his or her own health by adjustments of life style and active participation with the personal physician.[17] "Hospitalization and other services provided in a Medical Center are not isolated incidents but are part of the entire life experience of an individual."[18]

The same document, referring to actions by the HMC Board on 19 November and 5 December 1950, defined the professional staff. It would consist in part of specialists serving as heads of departments who would hold academic rank on the faculty of an affiliated medical school, with teaching obligations primarily, although not exclusively, at HMC. They would be salaried by HMC and would charge for services to patients. Income so derived would be accounted for separately from hospital operations and used for specialist salaries, auxiliary personnel who aided them, overhead, travel and salaries of residents. The goal was that neither account would subsidize the other. (More will be said about this later.) They would have supervision, with responsibility for quality, over work in the hospital and also in the health center. The other part of the professional staff would be local general practitioners (the terms family physician or primary care physician had not yet come into use) who served residents of the county and who were licensed to practice in New Jersey. If willing, these physicians would be appointed to different positions of different grades on the staff depending upon their qualifications as determined by the Medical Board,[h] experience and readiness to give time to the institution.

The general practitioners would have admitting privileges and would carry responsibility for care of their patients in hospital, supervised by the specialists, to whom consultations would be directed, and by whom care would be rendered when appropriate, such as patients requiring surgery or with serious illness. Specialists would perform all surgery.

In support of these principles, Wescott met with Lester Evans and Geddes Smith at HMC offices.[19] His intent was first to obtain support for the professional staff policies as described above. He emphasized that "The ruling consideration is that the whole service—whether given by general or special men—is to be keyed to patient need."[i] Smith described Wescott as very concerned with balancing protection for the prestige and income of the generalist against possible competition from the specialist, on the one hand, while *at the same time* protecting the patient against incompetence in medical care. A prepayment plan was discussed; he was not ready to support one. Smith described Wescott's view that day as differing from the statement of principles noted above: Wescott did not see a reason to segregate specialist's income and expenses from general hospital funds; he favored the Bassett model described in Chapter 4, where until recent years there was no distinction between the accounts. Both points of view changed subsequently. Wescott's second goal was to obtain additional funds. Costs of building had risen sharply, the Board needed additional funds to be able to proceed. Both of Wescott's concerns met with support from Commonwealth.

Trussell prepared an extensive report for Evans describing progress through the end of November, saying, "the basic problem here is to provide health promotion, health protection and comprehensive medical care for a rural population of 42,000."[20] By then he had, in addition to the above, secured agreement from Eric Groezinger, superintendent of schools, to include school health

[h] The Medical Board, defined elsewhere, would be composed of equal numbers of primary care physicians and specialists, and was charged with responsibility for quality of care, and for recommending staff appointments to the HMC Board.

[i] In the 1950s they all thought of males. Rarely did the notion of professional women come to the fore. This explains a portion of internist Pauline Goger's strong feeling about sexism, as noted in the chapter on the specialist staff.

services in HMC's community health program; obtained strong expressions of interest in working out of the Medical Center from the public health nurses, and from three voluntary agencies (Cancer, Red Cross and Public Health); outlined the financial needs to carry through the proposed programs; indicated that an "all-inclusive" prepayment insurance program would be studied in 1951; called for ongoing professional education; discussed progress towards a County Health Department; planned ongoing evaluation of the results of all these programs; and presented detailed plans for the Chronic Illness Survey.

The Board, working overtime, formed an Executive Committee to carry out business between regular Board meetings and to smooth the decision process. By the end of 1950, the shape of the program was becoming much more defined. A report for Commonwealth's Directors presented 11 January 1951, outlined the program, emphasized the gatekeeper role of the family physician, staff relationships, preventive health services, evaluation of needs and outcomes, integration of community services, and the enormous extent of community participation and support.[j] Commonwealth's Directors voted grants of $50,000 for planning, consultation and preparatory expenses, and $60,000 for the Chronic Illness Survey.

By the end of January Trussell wrote Evans of his progress on staff organization and on getting on the good side of the family physicians.[21] He had met with a senior physician in the New Jersey Medical Society who was quite comfortable with the notion of a closed specialist staff and was continuing to confer with a roster of distinguished consultants. He was about to ask Ethyl Ginsburg, a well-known authority on mental hygiene, to develop ideas for a program.

With Commonwealth's about-face, Louise Leicester could not resist rubbing it in. She wrote to Evans, from the posh St. Regis Hotel:

> A month or so [for a belated Christmas thank-you] isn't very long compared with four or five years. And I seem to have felt confident, that you know how much Commonwealth's action has meant to me personally. Do you? Remember the

[j] Except for the Chronic Illness Survey, the proposed evaluation of community health needs and of outcomes in terms of public and individual health did not take place. Hunterdon County Medical Center, Report of the President and Staff to the Directors of the Commonwealth Fund, 11 January 1951. Commonwealth 1951 file, HMCA.

times when you had to say, "I'm sorry, Mrs. Leicester, but—"
I'm to be in town next week—here, right around the corner
from you. Perhaps you'd like to see a member of the "community" . . . Then I'd like to call on all my friends at Commonwealth, too . . . to say "Happy New Year" for all of us, or
something like that.[22]

SHAPING PLANS INTO A PROGRAM

Much of 1951 was occupied by planning. In addition to everything
else, Trussell was deeply immersed in preparing for the Chronic
Illness Survey, of which more will be said in a later chapter. Planning began for the Mental Health program (a key element in the
combined hospital and health center which he visualized), to continue to improve relations with the family physicians and now
with the New Jersey Medical Society and to oversee the architects
who rapidly produced drawings. It was time for the formal proposal to the Kress Foundation for backup funds for the specialist
staff. In the midst of all this, an unexpected fight developed.

In late 1950 and the spring of 1951 a surgeon with good training
moved into a community in Hunterdon County, applied for staff
privileges in surgery and was refused. The occasion was the first
test for the Board policy of a closed specialist staff. A furor ensued
as local citizens, feeling that the doctor had been frozen out, came
to a meeting with Trussell. He quieted them by pointing out Board
policy—all specialists had to be approved by NYU, work there one
day a week and be engaged in teaching and consultation—and by
showing that the doctor had been invited to join the staff as a
generalist. The affair ended well, but consumed enormous amounts
of time.[23]

In the same letter Trussell also reviewed the hectic pace of hospital planning, commenting that this was the least interesting part
of the program to him because the hospital itself was just a conventional hospital approach. However, he noted that when the
preliminary drawings were released they produced much favorable
community response. This response was badly needed comfort for
the Board, because many tart comments about the lack of tangible
results had been coming in from donors to the fund drive. Community donors often did not understand that form follows function; program design should control building design. The Board

hoped the construction contract could be put out to bid by early summer.

By now the Hunterdon plans had produced national attention; Trussell was repeatedly interrupted by visits from the great and the near great. Planning began on a school health program. A network of Community Councils was created, not merely to help with fund-raising, but also to have a way for the community to voice concerns and thoughts to the Board, and for the Board to show the community what was going on. And, as if he had nothing else to do, Trussell obtained a grant for and began to plan a national conference for professors of preventive medicine.

THE SUMMARY STATEMENT

This document, a quarter the length of the statement of principles Trussell prepared in 1950, describes the reality of objectives, the structure to implement them and the reasoning behind them. Although unsigned, it could only have been written by him. This was the definitive version of the document referred to above as "Considerations Governing Hunterdon Medical Center Staff Appointments and Organization." The statement, approved by the Board 11 January 1952, exists in two versions. An edited version, dated 1 February 1952 makes few, but telling changes. A provision that the Board would set specialist fees was deleted and the discussion of "integration" of the voluntary agencies was modified to read "coordination and where possible integration." Records do not indicate whether this resulted from complaints by the agencies or fear about costs by the Board.[24] The three objectives are (1) maintenance and promotion of high standards of care with special emphasis on the role of the family physician; (2) community-wide application of health promotion, preventive and rehabilitative medicine; and (3) integration of community health services.

The most impressive feature of this document is how closely it adheres to the advanced spirit of the time. The open staff for family physicians was defined, as was their participation on the professional governing body, the Medical Board. Benefits of staff membership were listed. The term "family physician" is consistently used, although Board documents for a number of years later were inconsistent—the terms "general practitioner" or "generalist" being interchangeable. Programs in preventive health, integration of public and voluntary health organizations, school health, mental health and research were specified. Principles of affiliation with NYU-Bellevue Medical Center were defined. Services to the chronically ill, the prepayment insurance plan, program evaluation and research were deferred. Research, prepayment and evaluation were never fully realized.

The one major research project was the Chronic Illness Survey conducted by Trussell and Jack Elinson, an epidemiologist on loan from Columbia University. This will be discussed in greater detail later. Research was never a real option at Hunterdon, except for a modest flirtation via a grant from Seward Johnson. This was a major difference between Hunterdon and Bassett, where a research program on organ transplantation resulted in a Nobel prize. Trussell (and, separately, Board member Seward Johnson) had many ideas, including longitudinal studies of community residents' health, evaluation of services rendered, and measurements of resource utilization compared to health status, among others; after Trussell left nothing further was done. A School of Health was later established with money from Seward Johnson, but this venture accomplished nothing; Johnson withdrew his support and the School collapsed. Several efforts were made to develop a prepayment health plan. None succeeded.

Specialist staff, appointed jointly with the medical school, were to be responsible for providing specialist services, serving as department heads, supplementing,[k] supervising[l] and guiding the family physicians, medical education, and coordinating referral for services not obtainable locally. Financial policies for specialist staff clarified that they were fiscally separate from the operating account of the Medical Center. Payment of malpractice insurance, journals and dues, travel to meetings, retirement and moneys to bring in new staff were all designated as optional expenses, if funds were available. The salaries and expenses of residents and students, in contrast, were required expenses to be charged against the moneys

[k] This word was inserted in the final draft of the document. I could not obtain information indicating why. In the light of desires of the specialist staff to see patients without family physician referral, evident within a very few years, it might signify tacit recognition of such practice.

[l] In a letter to G Smith, 17 September 1952, Trussell makes plain he had concerns about variability in the quality of care delivered by family physicians. One of the important specialist functions would be assuring that all care was of highest attainable quality. Some of the family physicians obviously did a splendid job; for others he had little positive to say. He may have been influenced by Wescott's strong views on the topic.

earned by specialists from their practices. Thus the costs of the
teaching program were to be borne by the specialist staff, not by
the Medical Center, certainly atypical by any standards of the past
few decades. The Board was fearful that the resources needed for
the specialists could not be met from their earnings. It was hoped
that the arrangement would serve as an incentive for the specialists to work harder and thereby provide for their own ultimate
retirement with some sort of self-funded annuity. Despite the Board's
uncertainty, the first specialists to arrive at HMC had considerable
faith in the viability of this arrangement.

BUDGET FOR COMMONWEALTH FUND CONSIDERATION

Accompanying the Statement of Objectives was an Explanation
for Funds to Initiate Integrated Community Health Program, i.e.,
a budget for Commonwealth's consideration.[25] If the early 1952
date is correct, this is a remarkable description of a comprehensive
approach to individual health care at a time when there were no
clinicians on staff, or even the prospect of them. Although Trussell
came from a public health background, this document speaks of
the

> rights of the individual in the community to expect his Cen-
> ter to foster comprehensive personal health protection and
> medical care [and] the right of the community to compre-
> hensive group health protection through the medium of orga-
> nized group action and services on either a voluntary
> or official basis. Each person has unique health needs for
> treatment or advice that transcend the structural and finan-
> cial barriers erected by the health care delivery system of that
> day—*or any other day!* [emphasis added] . . . There must be
> no sharp geographic distinctions in the management of the
> patient. He is the individual who needs help for a given ill-
> ness whether he is home, in the family physician's office, in
> the ambulatory service of the Center or in the hospital wing.[26]

The family physician is a mandatory element of the health care
system and should

> retain continuous contact with the problem, either solely re-
> sponsible or sharing responsibility . . . There shall be a uni-
> versally applied humaneness to the practice of medicine based

on the dynamics of emotional development and the impact of illness and ill-considered handling on patients and their families—both for the present and for the future. Such a simple procedure as giving a child who is to have surgery a rectal anesthetic in his room with his mother present and having her present when he awakens is an isolated example.

An "across-the-board" understanding and application of principles governing healthy personal growth and inter-personal relationships throughout the Center staff is a prerequisite to its successfully fulfilling its role as a true health center and not just a scientifically accurate machine treating organic illness and disability.

These principles were a prerequisite to the Medical Center's success. Certain staff members were to be dedicated to teaching this humane and comprehensive approach. These ideals, I believe, distill all the influences shaping HMC up to this time: the Board's ideals, consultants involved, the background Trussell brought to his position[m] and the intense ongoing dialog that had been unceasing since February 1946, when the idea of a hospital had first been developed.

Finally, the document provided brief job descriptions for every major player on HMC's staff-to-be, with comments on the type of individual who could best fill that job. A proposed budget covering several years identifies how funds would be used. This masterful summary represents Trussell's work at its best: organized, clear, compelling, untainted by doubt, but also realistic in recognizing that not everything could be accomplished. The prepayment plan was placed on a back burner, along with a program of care for the chronically ill. He said later: "We just had too much to do."[27]

---

[m] Trussell had married a psychiatrist, Mary Mercer, who had experience at Cornell–New York Hospital in integration of psychiatric and pediatric medicine, under the guidance of, and later in succession to, Milton Senn.

CHAPTER 9

Organizing the Medical Staff

Family Medicine

At the same time HMC's pioneers were concerned with the programmatic, structural and financial aspects of the Medical Center, they also had to plan the medical staff in all its complexity: family physicians, specialists, the staff structure within which they worked and their interactions. What is most important is that those engaged in this process were twenty years ahead of the curve, recognizing that the primary locus of health care occurs in the family physician's office, negotiating with a patient "who is ill or believes himself to be ill"[1] and serving as a gatekeeper, agent for health promotion and medical home,[a] providing access to the entire health care system. This chapter describes family practice staff structure and function, recruitment, inter- and intrastaff relationships and their effects on health care delivery and resource utilization.

THE OPEN STAFF

From the first, the Board believed that HMC should provide a venue within which family physicians would not only work, but also improve their skills, to the betterment of the health of county residents. Corwin called for all family physicians to be on the staff, and the Board agreed. Physicians would receive technological, professional and educational support to enable them to maintain and improve the quality of service in hospital and in ambulant care. If

---

[a] A medical home is the place from which all of a person's health records may be accessed—typically the primary care physician's office. The term was coined by the American Academy of Pediatrics' Council on Pediatric Practice in a booklet titled *Looking Ahead*. Dr. Calvin Hsia, a pediatrician in Honolulu, Hawaii, wrote extensively on the subject, helping place the term in the medical vocabulary.

a practitioner were unable to provide care of acceptable quality, he would still do a better job on the Medical Center staff rather than if isolated in the community. The choice was impelled by a belief that doctors' skills would grow better in soil fertilized by the efforts of all. Could that choice be made today, in the world of the inspections by the Joint Commission, managed care, malpractice, the state Board of Medical Examiners? Probably not. Community and public health may be defended more vigorously today, but this alternative might even yet be debated.

The Board recognized even before engaging administrative or professional staff that the primary care physician (a term not yet invented) was central as adviser to the patient. Trussell called the Board "amateurs who had picked up a few words," but I believe they understood and agreed with this concept. The proposed hospital with its associated facilities was seen as ancillary and supportive. Patients would not be divorced from their personal physician in order to receive consulting or in-hospital care.[b] Not all Board members shared this view. One is said to have advocated a staff entirely of specialists, as at Bassett; another strongly believed that the public should be able to seek consultation on demand with the specialists.

When the Medical Center was under construction, staff membership was offered to all members of the Hunterdon County Medical Society. One physician declined, Dr. Junius Lemmon, owner and operator of the Lemmon Clinic, an unapproved hospital of ten beds in Glen Gardner borough in the north of Hunterdon County.[2] When Lemmon eventually applied for privileges, the Board of Trustees, based on the recommendation of the Medical Board, voted not to offer him a position. Lemmon and his hospital were not well regarded. "Loo" Looloian, a family physician in Whitehouse, remembered being "invited to come up there for a little snack at night and coffee to try to encourage us to send patients there. We never did, at least I never did . . . [Lemmon's clinic went out of business] before the Medical Center opened."[3] Lloyd Wescott in a talk some years later,[4] said the physician could "con" his patients

[b] Of course, at this time, the family physician was seen as the one who examined the patient, diagnosed the state of health or disease, and ordered treatment. I very much doubt whether any of those involved in the genesis of the Medical Center would today see the doctor in such authoritarian roles. Today, physicians negotiate beliefs about states of health and recommendations for actions.

into believing anything. Wescott blamed Lemmon for the death of a farm employee after surgery, and I heard him speak in very derogatory terms of the small private hospital. The Lemmon hospital was not used by the Welfare Department, and was not mentioned by the first study committee.

INITIAL INVOLVEMENT OF THE FAMILY PHYSICIANS

When plans for the Medical Center began, there were 27 general practitioners or family physicians in the county.[c] Of these, eight had graduated from medical school more than 20 years before Ray Trussell's arrival in Flemington. Some had appointments in nearby hospitals, usually on the courtesy staff. Some performed surgical procedures or assisted in surgery at nearby hospitals. For example, John Bambara, Ray Fidellow, John Fuhrmann and "Loo" Looloian delivered obstetrical patients in Somerville; Leonard Rosenfeld in Trenton. A staff appointment at a hospital indicates that the physician is entitled to perform certain actions, incurs certain responsibilities and is obligated to certain duties. For example, a physician may have admitting privileges for particular groups of conditions, say obstetrics, or ear nose and throat surgery or certain ages, as pediatrics. A physician is responsible for the care of that patient while in hospital as well as for proper planning at discharge. A physician may be required to offer unpaid time to work in the public clinic at the hospital, or for certain weeks or months to be available for indigent patients who have no doctor. A member of the consulting staff may only do consultations, or may also care for special patients. A member of the courtesy staff usually has a more peripheral involvement. Senior, honorary, or emeritus staff may no longer be active.

Ray Germain, a family physician, was influential in the Hunterdon County Medical Society. He said: "At first I was cold to the idea. The standards of care in small hospitals are questionable at best. But I got fired up when I saw the chance of getting a first-class medical center that would be linked with a big city teaching institution." Germain became a pioneer member of the Board of Trustees, before the institution was built and served as a vital link between community physicians and the Board. However, he was the object of suspicion from both sides: "I took it at both ends. I argued,

[c] Corwin noted 32, but I believe the Medical Society register lists the smaller number.

This Is What County Doctors Say -- What Do You Say?

The Hunterdon County
Component Medical Society

EXECUTIVE OFFICE
5 MAIN ST., FLEMINGTON, N. J.

There is no question that our county needs a hospital. Through this offer from New York University, the people of the County have a great opportunity knocking at their door. We, the undersigned, doctors of Hunterdon County, sincerely hope they will open that door wide through their generous contributions to the campaign to make this Center a reality.

[28 signatures]

Above, over their signatures, 28 Hunterdon County physicians attest to the fact that the 38,000 residents of this community vitally need the services that a modern hospital affords. On these grounds and on behalf of each of those residents they are appealing to the County at large to respond to the current drive for funrs which will make the Medical Center a reality. Names of the 28 subscribing physicians follow: George Henry, M. D., Samuel Felder, M. D., John F. Fritz, Jr., M. D., Arthur M. Jenkins, M. D., L. A. Hamilton, M. D., Edwin D. Merrill, M. D., G. B. Tompkins, M. D., Frank G. Clark, M. D., Alex. Christensen, M. D., C. G. Boyer, M. D., M. W. Looloian, M. D., E. W. Lane, M. D., Henry K. Davidson, M. D., Hannah J. Beatty, M. D., Barclay S. Fuhrmann, M. D., P. W. Baker, M. D., R. J. Germain, M. D., A. J. Bambara, M. D., John D. Fuhrmann, M. D., W. E. McCorkle, M. D., Vladimir F. Ctibor M. D., Joseph A. Smith, M. D., H. Andrew Knox, M. D., F. C. Simon, M. D., James A. Harps, M. D., M. H. Leaver, M. D., Paul H. Fluck, M. D., Henry Dantzig, M. D.

Resolution of Hunterdon County Medical Society (all family physicians) in support of the Medical Center.

pleaded, cajoled, and temporized."[5] Conservative, somewhat sus-
picious family physicians, worried about their future, nevertheless
acting through the Medical Society, endorsed the idea of the new
hospital early on. Corwin expressed some surprise at the lack of
enthusiasm from the family physicians, attributing it to their fears
about changes in their practice habits imposed on them, but he
noted that they came around before publication of his report, that
is, prior to January, 1948.[6]

A few were never in agreement, primarily because they wanted
surgical privileges. The majority, however, told their patients about
the project, and contributed, in some instances, up to $1,000. Al-
though Clifford Snyder "remained at a loss" to understand why
the members of "organized medicine" raised so many questions,[7]
by 21 April 1949 the Medical Society was ready to issue a joint
press statement with the HMC planning group over the names of
Snyder and E. D. Merrill, the Society's President and signed by all
of the Society's members. This show of support, obtained at an
early stage, before even a Director was appointed, rested on the
Medical Center's unequivocal declaration of the principle that the
family physician, "your doctor and mine,"[8] would be on the staff
of the hospital-to-be and serve on the Medical Board. That the
primary care physician should serve as the kernel around whom to
organize health care was recognized decades before the term came
into common use. Principles that a quarter century later were touted
as fundamental to the concept of the HMO were already common
currency in Hunterdon County even before the hospital towards
which they worked was in existence.

Trussell Further Involves
the Family Physicians

In correspondence prior to accepting the Medical Center position,
Trussell emphasized that his first and most vital step, despite all
that had been done previously, was to incorporate the family physicians into the fabric of the developing institution.[9] He regarded
them as independent. "Each of them was sort of The Man in his
town."[10] Within a week after Trussell began work as Director, he
made contact with many family physicians in the community. He
attended monthly meetings of the Medical Society, and encouraged the family physicians' attendance by subsidizing the dinners.
Trussell obtained a grant from Commonwealth for educational pro-

grams for the family physician staff. A local restaurant was reserved; the time of 9:15–10:15 p.m. was set. (The practitioner in
those days, as today, displayed endurance and willingness to work
long hours.) Speakers included the Chairman of Internal Medicine at Cornell–New York Hospital on physician–patient relationships and a professor from the same institution on the Cornell
Medical Index, an epidemiological tool of the time.

After four years, Trussell to his amazement was elected President of the County Medical Society. Perhaps he should not have
been, for his guiding principle was that "the success or failure of
the present Medical Center concept rests with the usefulness of
the Center to family physicians in rendering services to the most
people."[11] Trussell refers to Ray Germain and also Jack Fritz, another family physician, as particularly helpful,[d] but also points to
the special circumstances existing in Hunterdon County: "The only
reason this was at all possible was the fact that in Hunterdon County
there were no specialists and no hospital. You could never establish that approach in another existing situation. The profession
would never stand for it . . . because they would have been too
threatened."[12] Three family physicians interviewed (Bambara,
Fidellow and Looloian) already in practice when the hospital opened,
reported little contact with Trussell, and none of them was involved in project planning. Bambara saw Trussell as "an administrator. His M.D. was an aside . . . So I didn't expect much medically
from him. He was in the public health field and he was more or
less a contact man . . . He was approachable, nice to talk to."[13]
Trussell found Andrew Hunt and Morris Parmet, who arrived a
year before HMC opened, and Edmund Pellegrino six months later,
each highly qualified, personable and interested in the community
aspects of their work, and extraordinarily helpful. They built an
intimate relationship with the family physicians, forming a channel to administration on topics related to staffing, policies and
medical care.[14]

Evolution of a Department of Family Medicine

When HMC opened, there was no department of family medicine
within the structure of the medical staff. Such a department would
not have been a novelty at the time. The Council on Medical

---

[d] Other sources indicate that family physicians were, by and large, won over long before
Trussell arrived in part by Corwin and in part by the efforts of Ray Germain.

Education of the American Medical Association conducted a survey that showed 35 percent of hospitals nationwide had organized departments of general practice and the majority offered general practitioners positions in specialty departments as well.[15] The reason why a department was not immediately created at Hunterdon had nothing to do with the idea's novelty, but rather active resistance by Wescott and some specialists until such time as there was no choice. Even after my arrival, Wescott still resisted this idea. In 1961 I wrote him suggesting that full-time family physicians be hired to supervise a separate Department of Family Medicine. He found no merit in the proposal, writing, "To inaugurate this now would be a grave mistake."[16] The Summary Statement of Objectives of 1952, developed by Trussell and approved by the Board, made clear specialists would head all departments and be responsible for inpatient care.

Eleven years later, Wescott's opinion was unchanged: "It has often been suggested that we should establish with the hospital a separate "service" [a code word for department] for the family physician . . . This has never seemed to make sense to us. We want the family physician on a man-to-man relationship with all the in-house services . . . not off by himself."[17] Pellegrino bragged,

> There is no general practice department because it is felt that the organizational philosophy is such that the prerogatives and privileges of the general practitioner can be served without such a department. Indeed, he has an equal representation with the specialist in every aspect of the hospital's function, administrative and clinical, so that he enjoys a genuine sense of participation.[18]

What went unrecognized was the importance of autonomy, identification, and sense of independence, howsoever qualified by hospital rules and regulations. A medical specialty (what family medicine became) sets its own rules.

Although I cannot speak to early attitudes since my arrival in 1959 occurred almost six years after HMC opened, I believe there was something of a two-tier system. Concern about quality of care was real. Some bickering took place over how patients were handled. Obviously Wescott and Pellegrino were overt in their attitudes about a separate department; others less so. This may seem hypocritical, but was not. All the Board and the Staff felt—and still felt during my tenure—that the family physician was the primary source of health care for most citizens. The notions expressed about a family practice department relate to concern about support, supervision, and quality of care. This concern was real, and I also believe in some instances justified. Today, management of a hospital department is different; responsibilities are laid out much more rigorously; the Family Practice Department must document and demonstrate to the satisfaction of the Medical Board and external examiners how quality of care is maintained.

In the planning and construction phases, the general physicians in the area were known as "general practitioners." This term fell out of use, and "family physician" became the common denotation. The Board Statement of Objectives of 1952 codified the term at Hunterdon. On more than one occasion Board members asked whether specialists could see patients without referral. Until mid-1970s the Hunterdon structure with the family physician as gatekeeper was maintained. In 1939 recommendations to raise the status of general physicians by some sort of extra qualification began nationwide. A higher qualification for general practitioners ("Fellow of the National Board of Medical Examiners") was proposed but did not succeed.[19] After World War II, efforts resumed via the American Medical Association. In 1969 a certifying Board of Family Medicine was finally approved, ranked on a par with the existing medical specialties, the last of which had been created in 1948.

In 1965, Hunterdon was one of a few advanced programs to offer coordinated two-year training for family practice residents (see below on development of House Staff program). At first, the Director of Medical Education, also chairman of the Medical Staff Committee on Medical Education, was consistently one of the specialists. In 1971, when the Residency Review Committee specified a three-year residency for the new certification in Family Medicine, Hunterdon was one of the first dozen programs in the United States.[20] Family physicians, all trained at Hunterdon, routinely held the Directorship of Medical Education. Many left to take distinguished positions elsewhere. One, John Zapp, said that the family physicians had "a pretty good partnership and did not appreciate it."[21]

The final step in the evolution of a family practice department came in 1975 when the Joint Commission on Accreditation of Hospitals required a Department of Family Medicine. HMC opened its department on 8 February 1977, with Bernard Schapiro, a practicing family physician, as Chairman. The creation of a department and the concomitant assigning of responsibility for training new physicians in family medicine were critical in freeing the family physician from a sense of dependency and raising self-esteem. Family physicians now began to see themselves as specialists comparable to any other, a sea change in image. In addition to establishing a residency and a Department of Family Medicine, HMC opened ambulant care practices to train residents so that the bulk of their experience would be in the office, as well as offer care in underserved portions of the county (one of these will be discussed in the final section of this chapter on the Phillips–Barber Family Health Center).

The Concept of the "Family Physician" at HMC

Hunterdon anticipated and exemplified the role of the primary care physician in the larger context of the medical culture, as Means succinctly summarized: "The surgeon is interested primarily in the operation, the specialist is interested in the disease, but the generalist, the nonspecialized physician, is interested primarily in the person."[22] Yet despite all the statements and professed beliefs, initially neither the Board nor the specialist staff at Hunterdon were prepared to think of the "nonspecialized" physicians as members of a specialty. It was two decades before that opinion began to change. At first physicians moved delicately at the interface between specialist and family physician. Every opportunity was seized to support and improve the quality of service and sustain informal and formal educational programs. For example, surgeon Carl Roessel scheduled Looloian's non-urgent surgeries on Loo's day off so he could scrub. Family physician John Bambara, pediatrician Andy Hunt and psychiatrist Morris Parmet worked together on challenging cases. Internist Pellegrino made house calls to perform tracheostomies and he even read electrocardiograms in the restroom (more on this later). This is not at all bizarre or ludicrous. A group of peers created an atmosphere of informality to discuss important topics with each other when and where the occasion indicated.

Establishing a Department of Family Medicine enabled family physicians to assume power over their own work and, most importantly, to set their own standards for quality. The department now held regular meetings, reviewed quality of care, set standards, managed the training program for residents, and defined the privileges of its members, consistent with Freidson's definition:

> It is useful to think of a profession as an occupation which has assumed a dominant position in a division of labor, so that it gains control over the determination of the substance of its own work. Unlike most occupations it is autonomous or self-directing. The occupation sustains this special status by its persuasive profession of the extraordinary trustworthiness of its members. The trustworthiness it professes naturally includes ethicality and also knowledgeable skill . . . the profession claims to be the most reliable authority on the nature of the reality it deals with.[23]

At Hunterdon the culmination of these changes endowed family physicians with a feeling of autonomy—with favorable and unfavorable consequences. They met the specialty staff more as equals, negotiating patient care eyeball to eyeball in a marketplace. Paternalistic relationships, described elsewhere, were less frequent. A more collegial atmosphere existed. However, opportunities for mutual education, informal consulting and the camaraderie of early years have all diminished. In the early years, Hunterdon was an exciting place to work. The staff and families went on picnics together. Christmas parties were held for the children. As the staff grew in number, relationships became more distant. The opening of a Department of Family Medicine coincided with other changes in the status of the specialist staff, described later, resulting in bitterness among specialists, family physicians and the Board. Societal and fiscal pressures on physicians took their toll. It would be difficult to say how much of the change in relationships should be attributed to the formation of the Department.

Emphasis on family medicine and a conservative approach to medical care, which is characteristic of HMC's entire medical staff, has helped maintain a relatively smaller number of physicians in Hunterdon County without compromising the health of the population.[24] Data for 1997–98 show the total number of physicians in Hunterdon County per 1000 population to be 1.22 compared to 1.99 for New Jersey and 2.59 for the United States. Comparable data for family physicians show 0.5 per thousand for Hunterdon County, 0.19 for New Jersey, 0.24 for the United States. This suggests that the Hunterdon system has been successful at enabling residents of the county to have access to a family physician without inflating the total number of physicians.

DEVELOPING A MODEL PRACTICE—
PHILLIPS–BARBER FAMILY HEALTH CENTER

An early chapter described unsuccessful efforts led by attorney Edgar "Ned" Hunt to start a hospital in Lambertville. Despairing of ever finding sufficient funds, Hunt and the Phillips Memorial Board on 31 May 1934 obtained a *cy pres* ruling from the court allowing the estate greater discretion. Money was then given for an ambulance service, to neighboring hospitals for support of indigent care and other health services. Hunt's son, William, an architect, succeeded him to the Board, and also came on the HMC Board. Meanwhile, the leading practicing physician in Lambertville, Lloyd Hamilton, was aging. Another physician was cutting back. Concerns about the availability of health care arose, although there were physicians in nearby communities. The Phillips Memorial Board then moved in 1966 to ask Robert R. Henderson, at that time Medical Director of HMC, to prepare a report on unmet needs and ways to meet them.[e] Henderson reviewed current legislation, the economic and demographic characteristics of the community, and proposed that Phillips construct a modern ambulant care health center, that this be leased to HMC for a nominal sum, that HMC undertake the costs of operating that center and provide family physicians with privileges at HMC to be the staff, with HMC specialists to visit at regular intervals. Finally, building upon a suggestion Trussell had made,[25] Henderson suggested the health center be used as a training site in continuity of care for family practice residents.

The Boards jointly agreed to set this plan in motion: Phillips to construct a Health Center and Hunterdon to staff and maintain it. The Phillips–Barber Health Center was opened in Lloyd Hamilton's former home and office in August, 1970, staffed by John Lincoln, who left his practice in Flemington, and Kirk Seaton, who had finished his residency at HMC. Within two years a fully

---

[e] Henderson RR. Letter to Phillips Memorial Board. Letter is undated, but probably 1966 or 1967. Refers to Board motion of 9 September, 1966, requesting a report, which is enclosed with letter. Phillips-Barber file, HMCA.

equipped primary care center was established, which has since thrived as the site of a model practice staffed by family practice attending staff and HMC residents. The program includes specialists in behavioral health, an outreach service, nutrition, school health, industrial health, social service, rehabilitation, and other special services. A second similar model practice was established in an underserved riverfront town, Milford, in the northwest of the county. Both practices have continued to be staffed and operated by HMC.

In general, the work at Phillips–Barber has gone well. Problems arose in the first few years as family physicians strove to establish themselves as a genuine medical specialty and endeavored to mold the community's health habits. Because they wished to avoid offense to privately practicing colleagues in family medicine in the area, efforts were made to encourage patients whose family doctor was not on the health center staff to use that doctor. This produced anger in the community. Local individuals who sought care for an emergency, or because their own doctor was away, felt treated shabbily and complained to the Phillips Board. In addition, the professional staff was keenly aware that the practice was a model practice, designed to teach residents ideal guidelines in family medicine. The community was accustomed to walk-in hours at any time. The Phillips–Barber Family Health Center staff set up a policy of seeing patients by appointment, with delays of no more than 15–30 minutes. Patients who walked in without appointments were kept waiting up to two hours or more. Bitterness increased.

Finally the trustees of Phillips, led by Board President William Hunt, sent a strongly worded memorandum to Henry Simmons, then President of HMC, Wescott (it was just before he resigned), and the Phillips–Barber staff.[26] The memorandum complained about rejection of potential patients, asked for longer office hours, particularly evenings, to accommodate employed patients, and said, "We're no longer interested in being educated. What we want to know now is, how can the community get what *it* wants (rather than what the system thinks it should want)?" Hunt added, from his vantage point as a member of both HMC and Phillips Boards, that he was aware that the Health Center operated at a deficit, and suggested part of the reason was an unofficial boycott by members of the community. Subsequently the community and the Health Center have come to a more satisfying meeting of minds.

CHAPTER 10

Organizing the Medical Staff
The Specialist Staff

THE CLOSED STAFF CONCEPT

There was a striking contrast between the Board's early attitudes toward the specialist staff at Hunterdon and the patrician attitudes reported contemporaneously by Means, then Chief of the Medical Service at Massachusetts General Hospital:

> Full-timers are nearly always permitted to care for a restricted number of private patients. The agreement is usually that the amount of time consumed for private patients shall not materially interfere with a conscientious job of full-time work [read: teaching and research]. My chief, the late David Linn Edsall, introduced full time clinical work at the Massachusetts General Hospital . . . He asked the trustees . . . what portion of his time they would think it fair for him to spend on private patients. All the answer they would make was that they considered him a gentleman and they hoped he thought they were.[1]

When HMC opened, the specialist staff arrangements were quite different. At Hunterdon, the specialist staff was not permitted to care for "a restricted number of private patients" because it was expected that they would be engaged in consulting and follow-up care on patients whose primary source of care was the family physician. The educational program was a primary activity, but research, as noted earlier, was of very limited importance. The specialist staff rules, as promulgated by the Board, and enforced by the Director, were very specific. The structure of practice for specialist and family practice staff differed in three ways: method of appointment, circumstances of pay and employment restrictions.

1. *Method of appointment:* Specialists were hired by the Board after debate on the need for the position. The Board was concerned—more than that, frightened—about costs. Opening of a position, interviews and appointments were carefully recorded in minutes. Family physicians were financially autonomous; if they opened a practice within the county, they were eligible for appointment to the staff. Records do not indicate how carefully in the early years family physicians were vetted.

2. *Circumstances of pay:* Specialists, as employees, received a salary with possible raises over time, depending upon the total income of the specialist staff. (See below in the section on Professional Service Fund for more details.) Family physicians were in private practice on a conventional fee-for-service basis.

3. *Restrictions of employment:* The closed specialist staff structure approved by the Board specified duties of consulting, teaching, support and supervision. On the family physicians were placed requirements for attendance on inpatients and presence at staff meetings.

The closed specialist staff structure was soon challenged, as noted in the section on shaping plans into a program. In late 1950 a physician in training for surgery bought a home in the county, announced entry into surgical practice, and applied for staff privileges. This led to consideration by the Board and Director of what HMC was about. Notes of conversations at that time show that "medical care must rest on the shoulders of the general practitioner," and that "the prestige and income of the general physician must be protected against the possible competition of the senior staff of the hospital *at the same time* that the patient is being protected against incompetence in medical care."[2] Trussell and the Board offered the physician privileges in general practice but not surgery, appealed to the lack of university affiliation, and after a troubled time with the local community won their point.[3]

A report by Commonwealth early in 1951 illustrates the thinking about the elements of the staff structure. Read carefully, it reveals good understanding of concepts—note the terms—of "gatekeeper," "medical home," the importance of preventing illness and the primacy of the care of the individual. However, it does not yet show an understanding of health maintenance, as opposed to illness care or prevention:

The patient is the key to the whole program of comprehensive medical care in Hunterdon County. The citizen who feels
the need of such care will turn first to his family physician,
on whom responsibility for medical care is firmly based, or to
the nurse or social worker. If he needs more skill or a different kind of skill than the family physician can offer, his doctor will take him or send him (but every convenience will be
offered to induce the doctor to *take* him) to the Medical Center where diagnostic facilities are amply available and where
consultation . . . can be easily secured . . . The trustees have
indicated their willingness to protect his interests by seeing to
it that surgery is performed only by a full-time member of
the hospital staff, and to this end will bar the competition of
surgical newcomers who might seek to exploit the advantages
which the hospital offers. From the patient's side, therefore,
the services he needs will flow together naturally and he will
never be out of touch with the person to whom he has committed the continuing health care of his family.

The Medical Center will be as much interested in preventing sickness as in curing it when it occurs. The consultants . . .
will be as accessible to the walking patient as to the bed patient (at home or in hospital) and with the house officers will
carry their share of responsibility for the preventive and clinical services ordinarily associated with a health department.
What is usually called the hospital and what is usually called
the health department will be under unified direction. Home
visitors and sanitary engineers will work out of a common
center.[4]

Trussell, in 1952, initially called for five specialists, with salaries
backed by the grant from the Kress Foundation: internist, surgeon, pathologist, radiologist, and obstetrician plus a pediatrician
involved with mental health, school health and public health activities. He made no mention of four specialists plus residents from
the University in a particular specialty field, with on-site consulting backup from New York, as originally suggested by Corwin.
This idea was not brought up at any time after his arrival.[5]

Obstetrician Herman Rannels pointed out that it was not unique
for specialists to practice in rural communities in 1950.[6] Data from
the u.s. Department of Commerce and the American Medical As-

sociation indicated that although there were almost no specialists in communities of fewer than 5,000 inhabitants, in a community of 25,000–49,999 inhabitants, approximately 40 percent of the physicians might have specialty qualifications. The real reason why there were no specialists in Hunterdon County before 1953 was that there was no hospital. At that time most specialists were surgeons or dealt with sick patients in hospital. Accordingly, they would group themselves closer to where much of their work was performed. The exception was the family physician who traveled considerable distances to provide obstetrical service or assist at surgery on his or her patients.

In June of 1952 Trussell, summarizing the Board's intentions and actions to date in appointing specialists to the staff, wrote to the family physicians.[a] He referred at great length to the structure and functions of a closed specialist staff and expressed concern about misunderstanding in the community and among the family physicians. Despite all he and others did, fear and misunderstanding was not readily erased. Where Trussell refers to community understanding below, read family physician understanding. Note how Trussell was much more cautious than the authoritarian leadership at Bassett Hospital, who said, in effect, freedom of choice be damned.

> I have repeatedly reassured groups and individuals that their own family physician can attend them in the Medical Center, providing he is a general practitioner in good professional standing who has been properly appointed to the Medical Center staff. [The community does] not understand the difference between an open staff and a closed staff . . . It is impossible to have specialists practicing medicine under two different economic arrangements . . . The project as presently conceived offers a middle-of-the-road approach to redefining the role of the specialist and the role of the general practitioner in rural medicine . . . The role of the specialist here is supportive rather than competitive . . . I view the family physician as a key man.
>
> It is my feeling that if an individual wishes to have a surgeon who does not operate in the Hunterdon Medical Center that the patient should by all means go to the place where

[a] Note that Trussell slipped into using the term "general practitioner."

that surgeon is most used to working . . . This concept in no
way impairs freedom of choice.[7]

RECRUITING THE STAFF

Pediatrician Andrew Hunt and psychiatrist Morris Parmet arrived
before the Medical Center opened, working out of makeshift offices on Main Street in Flemington. Internist Edmund Pellegrino,
arrived six months after them. Because Hunt was the first specialist to arrive, his appearance was carefully orchestrated so as not to
threaten the family physicians. He would be supportive rather than
competitive, offering "refresher" work in postgraduate training. From
the summer of 1952 till the hospital opened on 3 July 1953, Trussell,
Hunt, Parmet and Pellegrino worked together to create a functioning institution and a network of relationships that would launch
the Hunterdon Medical Center in smooth and effective fashion. It
is not clear when Corwin's original proposal[b] of four full-time
specialists augmented by residents and NYU consultants was changed
to the eight full-time specialists ultimately hired by the time HMC
opened.

In late 1952 and early 1953 others were added: surgeon Carl
Roessel, pathologist Edwin Olmstead, radiologist Stephen Dewing,
and two internists brought in as fellows for the chronic illness
screening program, Pauline Goger and Robert Henderson. The
Director of Nurses, Lela Greenwood, began work 1 April 1953.
The Board authorized a full-time position in anesthesiology after
some indecision caused by fear of problems with the American
Board of Anesthesia[c] and whether or not to rely on nurse anesthetists. Michael Colella was appointed to the position in May 1953.
Alexander Mitchell in urology and Walter Petryshyn in otolaryngology started on a per diem basis; they switched to full time soon
after. Several ophthalmologists came—and went.

In 1953, the hospital was about to open with no obstetrician
despite letters sent to training programs. On 7 May the Executive

---

[b] Lewinsky-Corwin EH. Proposed Medical Organization of Hunterdon Medical Center, 3
August 1948. Corwin file. HMCA. He recommended at that time specialists in medicine, surgery,
pathology and radiology.
[c] That organization required fee-for-service payments for its members; working on salary
was sternly forbidden. Apparently no conflict ensued.

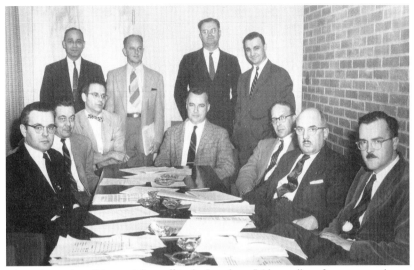

An early meeting of the specialist staff in the "penthouse" (the small conference room above the ambulant care wing). The photograph is undated but identity of those present indicates it was made before 1955. Seated, left to right, Walter Petryshyn, otolaryngologist, Carl Roessel, surgeon, Andrew Hunt, pediatrician, Ray Trussell, Director, Morris Parmet, psychiatrist, Herman Rannels, obstetrician, Steve Dewing, radiologist. Standing, left to right, Michael Colella, anesthesiologist, Edwin Olmstead, pathologist, Fred Knocke, orthopedic surgeon and Edmund Pellegrino, internist.

Committee discussed engaging a female obstetrician, but debated "How well a woman can supervise the work of the general practitioners who will be doing obstetrics is difficult to answer."[d] Two weeks later, the group interviewed Herman Rannels, but postponed action pending a response from another candidate. On 4 June Rannels was offered the position. W. Scheurman agreed to serve as consulting neurosurgeon on a fee-for-service basis, and Albert Accettola agreed to serve part-time as orthopedic surgeon. In August 1953, Fred Knocke was offered a position as orthopedic surgeon, effective as soon as sufficient beds were open. C. B. Katzenbach was approved as second surgeon. The two internist fellows, Pauline Goger and Robert Henderson, became full-time staff with Pellegrino. By January 1956 there were 12 full-time specialists; Henderson and Goger were listed separately; Bertram Bernstein in physical medicine and Katzenbach in surgery were part time.

[d] Minutes, Executive Committee, Board of Trustees, 7 and 28 May 1953. Board of Trustees file, HMCA. This may be indicative of concerns about gender discrimination forcefully expressed by internist Pauline Goger, the first female member of the specialist staff, in internal medicine.

PAYING THE SPECIALISTS:
THE PROFESSIONAL SERVICE FUND

EQUAL SALARIES

HMC's initial plans called for all specialists to be salaried employees paid identical salaries, dependent upon rank, unrelated to how much income the individual generated, as had been recommended in the final report of The Committee on the Costs of Medical Care.[8] Rufus Rorem, the report's author, believed salaried physicians in groups could maintain marketplace incomes. Corwin, however, had not addressed the topic. Trussell says, "The only full-time people I recruited had equal rank and responsibility and received equal salaries."[9] Fringe benefits included funds for travel to meetings or the medical school.

Behind this idealistic plan was a complex mixture of tradeoffs. Specialists in some instances initially earned less than elsewhere; for others, salaries were competitive. Specialists were expected to teach, which took time away from seeing patients. This educational part of their work, for the benefit of the family physician and the house staff, was not explicitly recognized, but was real. The complementary tradeoff was that they were provided with practice management services, collections, support staff, and office space in the Medical Center—a very convenient work setting. All of these services were paid for from the reserves earned by specialists' fees. Specialists had to step nimbly between competing obligations: teaching versus earning money to provide for their leisure in an idyllic country setting. Specialist staff distress gradually mounted.

In August 1953, just after HMC opened, Trussell and Seward Johnson exchanged revealing letters. Johnson sent a handwritten letter from his summer home in Chatham, Massachusetts, raising two questions: First, "Recognition of the earning capacity of individuals on the Medical Staff. It is on this point that most group medicine has failed." Second, "Should we operate our kitchen, restaurant and/or our laundry, or should we farm this out to private business, that is, to call established private operators?" Or, in the corporate buzzword of the 90s, outsourcing.[10]

Whether or not to recognize the differences in earning capacity of different physicians brought a detailed response from Trussell:

> Ours is not a conventional group practice, namely it was not formed by a group of doctors who were primarily interested in their earning capacity. [Doctors who practice primarily to earn a large amount of money] we have studiously avoided . . . The ideal goal in medicine is to have it served by physicians who are primarily interested in the good practice of medicine, and who, because they do such a good job, receive adequate compensation both in personal gratification and material income.
>
> Your entire staff here has been recruited solely and exclusively on the basis that every man of equal rank would have equal income and that this would be made possible through a true group practice . . . the unrestricted pooling of income earned by all . . .
>
> If the system ever breaks down to the point that we reimburse doctors on the basis of what they earn, we will have arrived at a complete circle of having started with an ordinary community hospital, having developed something far superior, and then having returned to an ordinary community hospital.

Trussell was not unrealistic, despite this idealistic statement. He went on "it would be quite dangerous . . . to open up the question with the group as to compensation on the basis of earning power."[11]

HMC's egalitarian system seemed to work well initially, fortified by the idealism many specialists brought with them, notably Hunt, Parmet, Pellegrino, Knocke, Roessel, Katzenbach, and Goger among others. These specialists believed they were engaged with a new system representing a departure from traditional forms of health care organization and several had given up larger incomes in more conventional environments. They developed an esprit that spread to include the family physicians, administrators, and most of the hospital's employees. Kate Tantum, a laboratory technician hired in 1956, voiced this sentiment: "It was very much like an extended family."[e]

Idealism was soon trumped by feelings about income, and certain doctors opened up this question within a few years. Several

[e] Tantum C. Interview by author, 16 October 1996. She describes how they all drove "old muddy cars, carried lunch in pails and ate together"—a memory perhaps gilded by nostalgia, but nevertheless suggestive of the atmosphere that existed and still to some extent exists today, especially among the more senior employees.

ophthalmologists left, and the otolaryngologist was openly distressed about his income. Within five years, when Hunt and Pellegrino left (for academic posts), dissatisfaction mounted. As will be described in another chapter, the end result was that most specialists became independent practitioners, in effect being reimbursed on the basis of what they earned. Whether or not Hunterdon has become "an ordinary community hospital," in Trussell's words, should be judged on its current status.

FINANCIAL SUPPORT

Certain specialists' salaries were guaranteed by a commitment of $150,000 from the Kress Foundation, dispersible as needed over a five-year period

> in connection with any deficit applicable to the establishing of five full-time heads of departments, namely, Radiology, Pathology, Medicine, Surgery, Obstetrics and Gynecology and/ or Pediatrics . . . This is an experimental program in connection with our post-graduate education in which our Foundation is so much interested and we will expect it to become the model for similar future progressive accomplishments throughout the entire United States.[12]

In the spring of the second year, according to Trussell, Kress was "sufficiently pleased with everything that he just gave us the whole thing."[13]

Early thinking about specialist staff finances was fuzzy; there was no plan for allocating income from services beyond that required for salaries, nor whence would come funds for departments, such as psychiatry or pediatrics, that might not earn enough to pay their salaries. How would fee income in excess of salaries be utilized—for specialists' overhead, fringe benefits, larger salaries, or to support general hospital services? Early in 1950 Robert Jordan of Commonwealth thought that specialists' salaries and full costs, including house staff, would "be borne by the center as part of the operating costs."[14] In late 1950 Wescott is quoted as saying that the specialists (then referred to as "the senior men") might be organized as a group practice, which, he thought, would operate at a profit to support the hospital's educational and administrative needs, but would not be asked to make up the patient bed deficit.[15]

In mid-1951, as reflected in Board minutes, NYU Medical School staff raised objections to Wescott's proposed financial relationship between the specialist staff and HMC. "The chief concern was whether the hospital would be practicing medicine in the sense that the money earned by the physicians over and above their salary and overhead would be used for other hospital purposes." The minutes go on to state, "It is believed that the Board policy, whereby money earned for physician services will be handled for professional purposes only, will avoid such a criticism."[16] With that assurance, NYU agreed to cooperate in a general practice internship program and assign a surgical resident as needed.

None of HMC's voluminous early records refer to Bassett Hospital, whose salaried physicians were integrated into the hospital financial structure, with cost of their offices and activities allocated from general funds. Why there was so much concern about that in Flemington and New York, and so little in Cooperstown, is unclear. It may reflect different local climates in general medical affairs, or it may be related to the mode of support, with Bassett subsidized by a wealthy family and controlled by specialists. A half century later it is also unclear what led the Board and Commonwealth to assume that specialists would agree to provide the financial support for operating a community hospital or to work without fringe benefits. In the event, a device was created to allocate the use of money earned by specialists.

A PROFESSIONAL SERVICE PLAN AND FUND

The earliest mention of a Professional Service Fund is found in paragraph 3 of the "Summary Statement of the Objectives" (see Chapter 8), which sets forth policy governing income from services rendered by the salaried specialist staff. To avoid applying specialists' income to other hospital departments and to allocate it to specialists' salaries, overhead and travel, the moneys were isolated from the general hospital budget. If sufficient moneys were earned, they were to be used for other purposes to the benefit of the specialists.

Andrew Hunt was appointed as Director of Pediatrics on 6 June 1952 and started work on 1 July. Although he did not as yet have a license to practice medicine in New Jersey, the Board, anticipating that he would soon be seeing patients, set forth the following policies that were to govern specialist activities for many years. Hunt would not see patients directly, only those referred to him by general practitioners. When he saw a patient, the patient would pay a reasonable fee. Moneys so collected would go into a Professional Service Fund and would be deducted from the latest Commonwealth Grant since this grant was paying all of his salary. Hunt's consultation should be a teaching experience for the general practitioner and was a form of postgraduate education.[17]

The origin of the Professional Service Fund is disputed, but it was born in 1952, with the business affairs of the specialist staff carefully separated from those of the Medical Center. There is some question who devised this. Trussell says he modeled the Fund on a plan that had come into being at the University of Iowa Medical School, his alma mater. After World War II, junior faculty at Iowa newly returned from military service and feeling a greater sense of freedom and maturity, led a rebellion against the prior pattern of unlimited private practice by departmental chairmen and limited salaries by everyone below them. Asked to produce a proposal, they did so, in the form of a professional service plan including a basic salary that was the responsibility of the institution combined with private practice privileges for all. The accumulated fees were divided up and used for agreed-upon purposes. Trussell says that he prepared HMC's Professional Service Plan based upon his knowledge of the Iowa plan. He said what he wrote "in its original form" was more or less a standard professional service plan and that other members of the specialist staff had nothing to do with it. The Summary Statement of January 1952 is the initial description of a Professional Service Fund. "In later years other staff members contributed changes . . . This was approved by Hunt, and by a financial group sought out by Lamont (Board Treasurer) before any of the specialists arrived."[18] On the other hand, Parmet stated that he had "devised the personnel practices for the medical group."[19] In contrast, several specialists—none on the staff initially—believe obstetrician Herman Rannels, who arrived just shortly before HMC opened, designed the Professional Service Fund. Rannels told them that he had. Some specialists wanted to believe the plan was produced by one of them. Whether uncertainty about parentage is due to memory lapses after more than 40 years or wishful thinking is not important. What counts is that the form worked, at least for the first few years, until issues of money and managerial control began to surface.

In December 1953, the Board approved a Professional Service Plan, including a contract for specialist staff defining job descriptions and financial terms. The contract followed the model created by Trussell and the Board. All the physicians on the specialist staff signed it that month. Before and after December 1953 Board Minutes reveal varying attitudes about the position of the specialists. In August 1953, the Executive Committee was still investigating how doctors set their charges.[20] Rufus Rorem, the distinguished student of group practice and health care delivery, visited 16 November 1954, as an interested spectator as well as eminent guru. He exhorted the Board to reduce all barriers between lay and medical affairs by lumping all income together—presumably as was done at Bassett. "[Specialist] services rendered should be considered as rendered by Hunterdon Medical Center."[f] Such a policy might have resulted in a storm of opposition not only from the doctors, but from many outside powers.

The Board was quite concerned about this issue, and about the fate of specialists' earnings from practice. Was this the "corporate practice of medicine"? At that time these code words excited strong emotion, comparable to terms such as "right to life," or "freedom of choice" today. The New Jersey Legislature had banned corporate practice of medicine, although it is not clear how well the term was defined. The American Board of Anesthesiology refused certification to salaried anesthesiologists. There is no evidence that anesthesiologist Mike Colella was affected by this policy. Trussell explained to the Board: "Medical Societies watch the activities of hospitals with great diligence, and attack vigorously any attempt on the part of trustees to practice medicine through salaried physicians who have no control over the money which is received for their services."[21] In general the Board did not seem to wish to exert managerial control, except for Louise Leicester. Leicester and the rest of the Board shared concerns about quality and whether these distinguished and powerful physicians they introduced into

---

[f] See minutes, Board of Trustees, 16 November 1954. Board of Trustees file. HMCA. Actually the Board went the opposite direction. Ray Germain, a very influential figure in the Medical Society in energizing the entire hospital movement, had been on the Board for some years. However, in September 1950, the Steering Committee (the forerunner of the Executive Committee) voted to accept his resignation because they felt it unwise for a physician to occupy a Board position. This policy continued until the dramatic change in staff organization in 1977; since then, physicians have served on the Board. Rorem also attempted to stir the pot by predicting that in five years HMC would need 500 beds and 50 specialists. The former prediction has not happened yet.

the community would follow the Hunterdon plan. But she was the only one who fussed about their fees. In 1955 she complained charges were too high and stated that HMC should set the specialists' fees.[g] With this concept she was felt by the others to be too close to the unspeakable "corporate practice of medicine,"[h] which had been an issue with NYU several years earlier. It was pointed out to Leicester that specialists' charges were less than in nearby cities, and there was little chance physicians would accept such action by the Board.

As mentioned earlier, Kress Foundation eventually turned over the balance of its large grant to HMC. Trussell recommended to the Board that the funds be used "to clear up whatever negative balance might be in the doctors' account and to buy them health insurance and to start a retirement program." Trussell said he announced this to the specialist group in a private meeting that they had, and the specialists thought it "very, very fair. Just about that time, they asked Herman Rannels to sort of think about their business affairs and Herman had grabbed the bull by the horns and had gone off to some commercial insurance company to talk to them about retirement."[22] Ultimately, Trussell said, he arranged admission to TIAA-CREF, the huge money management firm serving nonprofit educational organizations. The Kress grant provided reassurance and backing for the specialists' income for the first two years and the seed money to initiate a program of fringe benefits.

Murray Rubin, who came in 1954 to audit the hospital and was then hired to be HMC's chief financial officer,[i] recalled the retirement issue differently. He said that he recommended TIAA-CREF after looking into a number of choices: "Herm Rannels was strongly in favor of TIAA-CREF from its inception and convinced other people likewise. Everyone voted their approval to join TIAA-CREF."[23] Board

---

[g] In a handwritten note on a draft of this document, Trussell wrote: "Wow! The fees were Blue Shield fees agreed to in a meeting of specialists and GPs—certainly not high."

[h] In 1949, the AMA's Committee on Hospitals and the Practice of Medicine issued the "Hess Report" on employment of physicians. Following the advice of a comparable committee in Massachusetts headed by Leland S. McKittrick, it recommended that when hospitals hire physicians on salary, each side, hospital and physician, should be self-supporting and not exploit the other, that fees should be established by the physician, and invoices issued in his name. This helped assuage the anguish felt by the AMA as well as many political figures on this question.

[i] Both Grant and Trussell claim to have hired him—the difference appears to be one of hired to what position. Rubin arrived first as an employee of an accounting firm to perform an audit, then was hired to straighten out the business office and finally given a title.

minutes show that disability and malpractice insurance were offered on 28 May 1954, and the first allocation of money for retirement consisted of the purchase of annuities for this purpose in December 1956.

CLEARING THE DECK

The Professional Service Fund was designed to separate financing of the specialist staff from the Medical Center, thereby avoiding charges of corporate practice of medicine and simplifying income tax considerations. All income from physician activities, except royalties and honoraria, was turned over to the Professional Service Fund (PSF). Earnings from professional writing, malpractice consulting, and activities at the medical school were to be turned over to the PSF. HMC charged the PSF for support services, such as salaries of nurses and clerical help, supplies, space utilized, accounting and fiscal services, including billing and collection—all expenses that a group practice might sustain as overhead. Expenses for salary, room, board and uniforms for residents, and all but salaries for medical students, were paid by the PSF until 25 June 1954, when those expenses—$13,500 per year—were transferred to the hospital account. At the same time, the hospital agreed to contribute $5,000 each from pathology and radiology department income to the PSF for supervision of staff by the physicians.

Each year hospital auditors prepared a separate study allocating expenses and costs. Murray Rubin said that the PSF was accounted for as a separate business within HMC. "The PSF would have assets (primarily cash and accounts receivable) and its liabilities (for payroll and other expenses)."[24] Rubin was accountable for the finances of the PSF to the Director. Ed Grant, who came as administrator when Trussell left in 1995 and Pellegrino became Medical Director, was enormously enthusiastic about this system:

> I remember going before a meeting with the American College of Surgeons, and nobody could understand how everybody could work in a communal sort of fashion, not knowing what other members of the staff were contributing in the line of income and I made it clear to them that this was probably one of the purest forms of medicine that I had ever encountered. I was absolutely thrilled with it . . . I went before the

National Institutes of Health. I traveled all over the country just sold on this thing . . . and it just was a thing that I was happy to be associated with.[25]

There were problems with third-party payers and with the Internal Revenue Service. For example, the Blue Cross and Blue Shield plans could not understand that the physicians, employees of the hospital, did not retain their fees. Because the Kress Foundation agreed to underwrite possible losses in the specialist finances, the Blues also felt there was no reason to pay for physician care. Six months before the hospital opened Trussell met with the Blue Shield administrator to discuss these and related issues. The issues were resolved, and Blue Shield agreed to cooperate.[26]

However, Blue Shield refused to make payment directly to salaried physicians. Instead, fee reimbursement was paid to the patient, who was to turn it over to the physician. Human nature being what it is, all too often the money was never seen again. Ultimately, HMC built accounting programs that clarified the separation of specialists' earnings from the hospital budget. The third-party payers then dutifully reported to the IRS money paid the physicians as personal income. The IRS decided to tax both physicians' salaries and fees for service, which they had turned over to the institution. Serious audits of individual physicians occurred until Grant and Rubin demonstrated that there was no hanky-panky; physicians did not retain fee-for-service money. The specialists underwent repeated IRS audits. The IRS audited the hospital seven or eight times specifically with reference to the PSF, to establish that it was a separate fund and not part of the hospital, which would enable them to tax the doctors on fees even if they did not personally receive the money. Resolution hinged in part on demonstrating that no physician had any interest in the PSF assets or accounts receivable. If a physician chose to leave, he could not take any of it with him.

One abortive effort to blur the distinction between HMC and PSF funds occurred in 1965, when it was proposed that HMC establish a risk fund for two years to underwrite opening new medical specialties, notably neurology. At the time, the PSF was just breaking even. Specialists differed over what to do. Younger men wanted to work harder; some of their seniors were uninterested. The situation was resolved by discussion. The risk fund concept did not fly.

CHAPTER II

Building Relationships and Opening the Doors

SPECIALIST–FAMILY PHYSICIAN–BOARD RELATIONS

The initial staff developed an intimacy looked back on with great satisfaction as specialists bonded with family physicians. As Pellegrino said:

> It takes good people in the first place to build something like Hunterdon. An interesting group of people came together. The interactions between us brought out some of the better features of our individual characters . . . that brought out the best in us, the "best" being defined in this case as trying to achieve the vision and goal that was Hunterdon. We had the unusual situation of people really united for an ideal . . . People wouldn't have come to Hunterdon unless first they were interested in the idea . . . unless they were willing to take the chances that went with the idea, to make a personal, emotional and intellectual investment in the ideal.

The memories of those early years are articulated by the pioneering wives of Hunterdon's staff. Within the specialist staff, and between specialists and family physicians, close friendships, supportive relationships, and much warmth marked those early days. When queried, Elise Fidellow, the wife of Raymond Fidellow, sighed, thought for a moment, a dreamy expression on her face, and said, "We were all young together."[2] Belle Parmet, widow of Morris Parmet, said, "I have never had a better time in my life. I had never met more interesting people . . . Those were golden times." She added:

> We . . . bought a farm like every other member of the staff . . . the idea of living on a farm scared me . . . we had a chicken house equipped with electricity and so as part of [our son's] character building experiences he raised chickens for his 4-H membership. Being naive, we did not know that chickens drank

huge amounts of water and we didn't know that the pipes could
freeze and so every morning before anyone went to school or
work, we were lugging buckets of water out to the chicken
house. Morris had an egg route at the Medical Center.[3]
Marylu Katzenbach, wife of C. Buckman Katzenbach, said: "It
was all new to everyone and you had to be sort of like a family or
it wouldn't have worked."[4] Staff and Board children came to parties, picnics, and Christmas gatherings. Favors were exchanged;
old-timers helped newcomers.

Surgeons often crossed over specialty lines. Katzenbach and Roessel
treated patients with fractures, urological, otolaryngological or even
neurosurgical problems if the appropriate specialist was unavailable. Other specialists in turn recognized the contributions that
each made. Even the secretarial staff recognized this atmosphere of
good will. Cathy Timerman (Rosswag), Trussell's secretary during
his later tenure, said: "It really was like a family. Everybody got
along with one another. It was a good time in my life . . . It was
new, we were all in there together. Everything was new. The concept was new, the building was new . . . everybody worked together."[5]

Staff and spouses interviewed describe warm and involved relations with the Board, comparable to those among the members of
the staff. Wescott, Johnson, Klopfer, Schley and others on the Board
opened their homes. Board members signed guarantees on mortgages for new homes or even took back the mortgages themselves.
In 1958, when I was a candidate for appointment, Board members
were deeply involved with the recruiting process. All members projected joint agreement on goals combined with much interpersonal warmth. There was no doubt that on the Board, Wescott
was in charge then, earlier, and later, but there was also a personal
commitment on the part of many other Board members. After the
first decade such intimacy became the exception, rather than the
rule.

STRUCTURE OF THE SPECIALIST–FAMILY PHYSICIAN RELATIONSHIP

The Board Statement of Objectives of 1952 says specialists were to
"supplement, supervise and guide within the scope of their de-

partments the work *within the Center* [emphasis added] of the family physicians (general physicians) on the staff." In addition they were to supervise the house staff program, and serve as heads of departments, all for "the maintenance and promotion of high standards of medical care and other health services for individuals and families, with special emphasis on the role of the family physician in serving rural people."[6]

Trussell had drafted a memorandum of considerations governing staff appointments, organization and relationships for the Board to approve. In keeping with the guiding principles, he emphasized: teamwork among all professional personnel; the primary role of the family physician, backed up by the specialist who only saw patients on referral; a strong educational program for the staff and residents of the community; integration through HMC of all organizational activities related to health and welfare; acceptance that hospital care was but a small fraction of overall care of the individual, and that a comprehensive approach taking into account emotional and social factors was important. This relationship encompassed several elements: the position of the family physician as fully qualified member of the staff with privileges commensurate with ability; the position of the specialist as full-time consultant and educator; that sensibility, which has been commented on elsewhere, of being in a new venture together; and the unvoiced, unspoken element which underlies all—trust and respect.[7]

Between family physician and specialist exists a relationship that mirrors that between patient and family physician. That relationship is based on trust—trust in competence, trust in purpose, trust in kindness. An extensive literature indicates the extent to which patient agendas dominate these relationships as well as the processes of referral and consultation.[8] Communication between patient and physician is more hazardous because the two tend to speak different languages. One language is that of illness, the patient who says, "I do not feel good. I feel sick." Another is that of disease, the physician says, "The heart muscle is weakened by limited blood supply due to narrowing of the arteries." Yet another is that of diagnoses, such as, "Viremia due to influenza virus, or basal cell carcinoma of the cheek." The language of illness tells how the patient feels about him- or herself. The language of disease tells about what the physician believes exists in nature. The language of diagnosis tells what label the physician has placed upon the process.[a] Physicians hope that they correctly understand the language of disease, and deal practically with the language of diagnosis as a conceptual entity providing a basis for scientific thought and interaction, and a rationale for therapy. On the shoulders of the physician lies the obligation to translate among these languages. In the consulting relationship, that obligation is shared between the family physician and the consulting specialist.

Recently Fisher and Welch have emphasized untoward consequences of regarding a diagnosis as identical with a disease—more diagnosis leads to identifying patients who have a "pseudodisease" that would never become manifest in their lifetime without modern diagnostic testing. A good example is cancer of the prostate, present in 50–75 percent of men over the age of 75. The vast majority will die of something else. At the moment physicians do not know how to tell the difference between men for whom this is a serious condition, and those for whom it is present but will cause no harm in their lifetime.[9]

A very important staff structural element was and is the relationship between the full-time staff and the family physicians. Limiting the full-time staff to practice in the hospital was a necessity so that they would not compete with the family practice staff, as well as assure their availability to provide formal and informal consultation. Nonetheless, the system was breaking down months before the hospital opened. Board minutes of 24 April 1953 report that already 10 percent of patients seen by the specialists were self-referred. Many community residents felt, "we have contributed our money to create our fine new hospital and bring these wonderful doctors here, now we want to have access to them. We will go to our family doctor for ordinary illness."

Informal consultation, casual contact and discussion of patients were critically important elements in the equation of relationships that made up the new hospital's staff. Just how informal such consultation could be was reported by internist Ed Pellegrino. Pellegrino found some family physicians running after him in the hallway with an electrocardiogram to interpret. One might ask, "Are those ventricular ectopic beats?" Pellegrino emphasized that this did not

---

[a] No effort will be made to discuss the issue of the language of disease versus the language of diagnosis, which has been repeatedly, forcefully, but unavailingly put forth by Thomas Szasz; see, for example, *Lancet* 338:1574–1576, 1991. Szasz argues that diseases exist in nature.

irritate him. Some of his colleagues wanted to know why he let the practitioners do this. Other specialists felt that he was being taken advantage of. Pellegrino says, "This is what it's all about."[10] He felt very strongly that being available in informal consultation on a full-time basis was critical to the clinical success of the specialist staff. True enough, but it was also indicative of interactions that eventually led to undoing the bonds between family physicians and specialists.

Far ahead of its time, HMC's staff system was not automatically accepted by local citizens. John Lincoln, a family physician, recalls that early on the people in the community had a variety of expectations.

> It was a little bit like a family that is expecting a new baby, in which all of the members of the family have some kind of a concept of what the baby is going to look like and what the baby is going to do in the family, but once the baby actually comes the family members realize that their expectations may not be met.

He recalls one local who growled "You had to have written permission from Christ to see anybody at the hospital."[11] In 1952, community attitudes reported by a questionnaire and analyzed by Belle (Mrs. Morris) Parmet and Mrs. Richard de Rochemont revealed residents' idealistic and unrealistic expectations. The community would have to learn to live and work within the new system. (See Trussell's Chapter 5 on community attitudes in *The Hunterdon Medical Center* for more details.)

QUALITY OF CARE

What did not exist in 1953, or at any time thereafter, was a means, other than house calls and informal exchanges, to support quality of care in the family physician's office. It was hoped that interactions within the hospital would have an educational effect resulting in better care everywhere. Mechanisms to deal with quality of ambulant care remained informal, haphazard and unsystematic.

Trussell said that during his stay at Hunterdon he had never been able to do justice to the issue of quality of care. He met with Corwin to discuss the issue:

> There was just one thing that I wanted to get very straight with Dr. Corwin. I wanted his agreement and made my

position clear. If I was going to bring a group of specialists
out there with faculty appointments and responsibility for working with the general practitioners, in the final analysis they
had to be in charge in the hospital and had to be responsible
for the quality of care in their departments . . . I just didn't
like the idea that local doctors could come in and have a
consultation but still go ahead and do anything they wanted
to. You may have noticed in my book [*The Hunterdon Medical Center*] . . . two areas I didn't talk about. One was the
quality of medical care being provided in the county at the
time that I went there . . . The medical care in the county . . .
was, to put it mildly, highly variable . . . The role of the
specialist here is supportive rather than competitive . . . A
failure [of the project to succeed] will result in one of two
alternatives . . . The first will be to move to a Cooperstown
type of organization [hospital closed to all but the specialist
staff]; the second would be to move towards a completely
open hospital . . . In either event I see the role of the family
physician jeopardized. This . . . would be unfortunate because I view the family physician as a key man."[12]

Trussell added in a later interview: "You have to have a chief of a
department and you hold him responsible for what happens in
that department on behalf of the Board of Trustees who are legally responsible."[13] Concern on the part of new salaried specialists about the quality of care available from the family physicians
was real, but it never really came into the open.

Pellegrino believes that Trussell, coming from a public health
background and having left clinical medicine, "did not do justice
to the practitioners." Most, Pellegrino felt, provided care of very
good quality. The difficulties they faced were brought home to
him with his first consultation in the home. John Bambara had
asked him to see a patient with him because he wasn't quite sure
what was going on with her. She turned out to have aplastic ane-
mia and had ulcerations on her larynx. "While we were talking
with her, she shut down [went into respiratory arrest, ceased to
breathe] and we had to get an emergency tracheostomy. That's
when I realized how protected I had been in the hospital setting
and how different it was to confront medical care in the world
outside the hospital."[14]

Pellegrino's presence saved the woman, illustrating how the new Medical Center in its original, idealistic state improved health care.[15] He understood that as

> chief of service I would have responsibility for the overall quality of care of all the patients on that service . . . no matter who the attending [the doctor actually in charge of the patient] was . . . It was my task to work out an arrangement cooperatively. But, if things went badly, I was responsible. I was trained at Bellevue Hospital in the days when the chief resident was *the* responsible person. When you got to be the chief resident (it is elitist and people don't like it today) it was a tremendous vote of confidence . . . You had to respond in kind . . . At Hunterdon I made rounds twice a day on every patient on the service . . . Now it was never written down anywhere saying I had to do this.[16]

Herman Rannels, HMC's first obstetrician, wrote about the relationship with family physicians. He noted that "responsibility for the provision of medical care in rural areas rests on the general physician at the present time [with] no indication that present methods in the field of medical education will change this in the foreseeable future." He spelled out the objective of HMC: "to provide the physician with a medical environment which will stimulate him to improve the quality of both private office and hospital practice."[17]

Family physician John Bambara and pediatrician Andrew Hunt jointly described their experiences.[18] Bambara spoke of intellectual stimulation from interchange with the specialist staff:

> I have found myself going back to my books more often than before . . . by the desire to be able to hold up my side of a medical discussion . . . The interns also are a source of education for me. The questions they ask, the things they do, the need for explaining my attitude.[19]

Controversy arose from time to time about inclusion of all family physicians in the community on staff. In 1956, when Pellegrino was Medical Director, the Board developed deep reservations about staff positions for practitioners whose work was judged to be subpar. Pellegrino insisted that care would be better by maintaining them on staff to educate them through communication with peers, and attendance at staff meetings, journal clubs, and committees.

He describes the debates over the issue as a "knock-down, drag-out battle," but the Board finally adopted Pellegrino's view.[20]

As to the quality of the specialists, Aaron Rausen, who was HMC's first medical student, in July 1953, said that he would attend almost every conference that went on because

> it was like open doors and I was very, very impressed . . .
> with the people who were there. I look back at it now—they
> were all kids. Then, of course, I thought they were old men
> . . . [I] was not conscious of the fact that I was basically being
> exposed to people who were in fact giants in their fields.[21]

My perception from my interviews is that each staff specialist felt it necessary to reaffirm responsibility for quality of care in the hospital, but my initial orientation on arrival at Hunterdon in 1959 did not clearly delineate the structure of responsibility. Emphasis was placed on collaboration with family physicians. When I was interviewed by family physicians, Board members and specialists, interpersonal relationships and quality of care were dominant topics. Specialists often discussed quality among themselves. The clear principles outlined in Trussell's memorandum and proposed rules and regulations for the staff (discussed below) were not provided for me.[22] All physicians felt keenly the rising threat of malpractice actions. Specialists felt trapped as they considered how they could preserve good working relations with the family physicians, offer consulting help without intruding into the existing physician–patient relationship, ensure quality of care, and protect themselves in the event of a poor outcome. Overt supervision of family physicians changed to reliance on an informal network of nurses, residents, students, and on indirect methods of communication. My personal experience found serious missteps by family physicians to be uncommon. When they did occur, it was incumbent upon me to reach a decision on dealing with the problem in a way that first, safeguarded the patient, second, was acceptable and understood by the family, and third, was helpful to the physician. I did not always succeed. Persuasion and reason have limits. Rarely did I feel it necessary to go over the head of the family physician—twice in more than 25 years as chief of pediatrics, each time with misgivings, whether or not the same result could not have been accomplished in a less blunt fashion. In each instance I did my best.

OPENING THE ACTIVE STAFF

Questions about staff relations arose when By-Laws were prepared for the Medical Staff structure. The *Hunterdon Democrat* reported that 26 local general practitioners, members of the Medical Society, were formally inducted into the Medical Staff on 22 January 1953, along with six specialists (Dewing, Hunt, Olmstead, Parmet, Pellegrino, Roessel). The Medical Board met with the entire Medical Staff in February to deal with potential medical issues. Members of the Medical Board included family physicians Baker, Bambara, Jenkins and Hamilton, plus Hunt, Parmet, Pellegrino, Roessel, Trussell and NYU's Clarence de la Chapelle.

The Medical Staff met as a group for the first time on 3 March and the second time on 24 March 1953. John Fritz of Flemington was elected President, Arthur Jenkins of Frenchtown President-Elect, and Morris Parmet Secretary. The minutes of these meetings are extraordinarily instructive. Physicians struggled to come to grips with a hospital structure then novel to the entire country. Parmet carefully recorded a series of questions and potential controversies arising at the first meeting.[b] When a patient was admitted, who was responsible, the attending family physician or the consulting specialist? How was this to be determined? If the specialist detects unusual events on rounds, when do these observations become a consultation? What about patients who want to be seen or treated by the specialist? How are fees determined under these varying circumstances? What happens to a patient when the family physician is not available? Clearly regulations were needed to define responsibility for quality of care, authority to deliver care, processes of interaction between specialist, family physician and patient, problems arising from competition, charges by physicians and costs resulting from physicians' orders and ways to provide the public with satisfaction.[23]

At the second meeting proposed rules and regulations for the staff were circulated and discussed. Coverage for absent physicians was felt to be a Medical Society, not a Staff problem. (This, of course, is no longer true for inpatients, and malpractice litigation has focused on the issue of patient abandonment.) The problem of

[b] At this time, and henceforth, in the records the term "general practitioner" was finally abandoned in favor of "family physician."

patients seeking direct access to specialists was talked around, but no specific conclusion was reached. Hunt, representing the then-embryonic specialist staff, spoke reassuringly and the family physicians muttered but did nothing else. Defining every patient as a teaching patient produced another chorus of growls: "Some private patients would not want to be pawed over by the intern." As before, the specialists were reassuring, and "the discussion boiled down to the fine art of medicine which concerns the sensitive handling of each patient."[24]

One family physician commented that he did not see why every surgical tissue needed to be sent to the laboratory—the diagnosis was often obvious and it only added to the patient's hospital expense. There followed a discussion of quality and standards in a teaching hospital. Issues were dealt with seriously and carefully. Extensive documentation records the efforts to reach consensus. The results were transient. Chapter 16 shows how many differences recurred. It is rather appalling how few of the controversies were resolved until the titanic struggles of the 1970s, which altered the fabric of the institution. It is rather impressive how clearly this first group, arguing from first principles, identified just what those controversies would be.

At the same time as these meetings Ray Trussell prepared and promulgated a memorandum and proposed rules and regulations for the staff. He covered most of the ground debated at the first two staff meetings. A Medical Board was defined and provided with duties, primarily to recommend medical policies and oversee quality of care on behalf of the HMC Board. The work of the family physician both in the hospital and outside was defined. The work of the specialists, and their ultimate responsibility for inpatient and consulting quality of care—to "university standards"[25]—was defined. Neither interviews nor documents indicate if Trussell's memorandum and subsequent Board actions were in response to issues raised at the staff meetings. Trussell's prior accomplishments suggest that he had been working on this earlier—specialists had been on board for almost a year at that time. After the rules and regulations were reviewed by the Staff, the Medical Board and HMC's executive committee the full Board adopted them.[26]

A brief digression on consulting relationships might be helpful.

CONSULTING PROCESS

A consultation is an interchange between colleagues, one seeking information, an opinion or an advanced treatment from one perceived able to provide the same. In medical practice, prior to the rise of managed care, consultation was traditionally formal, involving a patient's out-of-pocket fee. Also, traditionally, informal exchanges take place, often without the patient's knowledge, between referring and consulting physicians who know each other well. Such informality was encouraged by Pellegrino, Hunt and Parmet prior to the hospital's opening. On the one hand, this can be interpreted as open exchange of collegiality and camaraderie between peers, each of whom supplements the work of the other; on the other hand, it could also be interpreted as encouraging dependency.

The practice produced varying responses from staff members. Hostile staff encounters occurred between a physician seeking a prompt answer to a query from another physician who was very uncomfortable providing an answer without sufficient information about the patient to assure that the problem was correctly formulated and the answer relevant. Consultants resented this informal process because it lowered income, distracted from other duties, and laid the consultant open to charges of malpractice should something go awry. Internists complained about surgeons who wanted electrocardiograms inspected before general anesthesia on patients already prepared for surgery, thus spreading responsibility should an untoward cardiac event take place.

Willingness to help out under any and all circumstances may not always be in the best interest of either patient or practitioner. Consider, for example, the electrocardiogram inspected in the hallway to determine whether there were ventricular ectopic beats. Under some circumstances, these may be a normal finding; it is the context in which they arise and the patient's general condition which that determines whether one is dealing with a major or minor disorder or a variation of normal function. It might be difficult to decide from viewing an electrocardiogram standing in the hall.

Why did a practitioner find it necessary to pursue the consultant? Was the matter of such urgency that it could not wait for a few minutes? What was the real source of practitioner anxiety?

What kind of practitioner behavior is being encouraged? Pellegrino stated what he wanted to accomplish:

> My view was genuinely to be accessible to the general practi-
> tioners, to make available to them what I knew . . . It wasn't
> so much a question of dependence on me. Rather, I wanted
> the GPs to be confident that they would be helped when they
> needed it . . . I could teach them some things and some they
> would do for themselves. They could teach me too—as they
> did . . . There is no way that I could have taught them how
> to read EKGs in that kind of informal approach. What I wanted
> them to appreciate was that the patient might need an EKG
> and they could get it easily . . . helping the GPs to recognize
> when they needed help and how to get help. I don't think
> that forced a dependence on me. Rather it gave them an ease
> of dealing with their own clinical situations.[27]

No value is added to this discussion by a polar viewpoint. Any social relationship may involve learning elements wherein one may teach another; skill is required to perform teaching to foster independence rather than dependence. Pellegrino's position on informal consultation is supported with evidence summarized by Felch and Scanlon[28] on the wide range of learning styles of physicians as well as the difficulties of producing changes in physician understanding and behavior, even when demonstrably efficacious. They emphasize how many different forces may alter physician behavior. Peer communication ranging from a chat in the hall to a formal consultation, a change in reimbursement rates, administrative actions, and evidence from literature or observed results may all stimulate change. The collegiality expressed by Pellegrino's comments is harder to attain when structural barriers arise from specialists working only in hospitals and generalists only in offices. Systems of peer communication may be impaired, as in several European countries.[29] These findings may be relevant for the rapidly growing number of hospitalists in the United States, whose function, in contrast to the specialists at Hunterdon, is exclusively care for sick inpatients.

NEEDS OF THE INDIVIDUAL VERSUS NEEDS OF THE COMMUNITY

Is the welfare of the individual, or the welfare of the community primary? This was not often overly discussed during HMC's early years. When the total resources available for health care are finite, it becomes more of an issue. Some have misinterpreted the function of HMC and its staff during its first three decades of existence. Anne Somers, for example, in the back-to-back epitaphs she and Wescott[30] wrote about Hunterdon when the staff structure changed, said: Two [concepts] were never explicitly stated but taken for granted: the first criterion in determining allocation of health care resources or organization of services is community need—not individual patient demand or individual physician preference; and the most health-effective, as well as cost-effective, way to meet this need is on the basis of health care planning with the community hospital assuming primary responsibility for assuring high-quality primary and secondary, but not tertiary care.[c]

As to Somers' first point, from the beginning the Board considered the needs of the community and did its best to provide resources to meet them. Both Board and staff recognized that the unit of medical care is the encounter between individual and physician (or nonphysician provider) and that decisions on resource allocation for individuals are made with their best interests in mind. Some ethicists are adamant on this issue, even in the face of the current climate for financing health care. The entire staff at Hunterdon, family physicians and specialists, practiced conservative medicine, recommending actions as deemed appropriate in light of what was known about the patient and his or her environment and available therapies. This was done because it was seen as good medical practice, not because it was seen as good resource conservation. (In contrast, see anecdotes about practice elsewhere by Buck Katzenbach, the second general surgeon at Hunterdon.)

Somers' second point reflects how Ray Trussell felt. He arrived at Hunterdon believing in the ambulant care portion of the entire

---

[c] Somers AR. "Hunterdon – 'may it never be forgot!'." *N Engl J Med* 1979 Apr 26; 300(17): 977–9. In context Somers refers to primary care—that managed by a primary care physician—and secondary care—that provided by a local specialist. Tertiary care would be offered at a large teaching institute.

Hunterdon complex as one of the novel features. Recall his comment quoted earlier that he thought of the inpatient hospital as a conventional structure. Despite his efforts, the voters rejected a county health department in a referendum and the Board, seriously concerned with finances, could not support a physical plant large enough to incorporate, as had been hoped, the public and private agencies concerned with health and welfare. Trussell's planning was as Somers described, but reality constrained implementation. The responsibility for planning referred to by Somers was not, when she wrote, a central part of HMC's program. In more recent years serious efforts have been made to work closely with local agencies in exactly this direction, of which more later. But early on, there was no way for the institution either to monitor or modify most medical care given, which was in the offices of the family physician or in the home by the patient and family. Health education was the one tool thought about seriously, but the only major effort, the "School of Health" that Seward Johnson hoped to finance (and which he saw as focusing on what the individual could do, not the community—in other words it was not a school of *public* health) collapsed because it accomplished nothing. Later, health education became a major activity of the Medical Center.

THE COUNTDOWN

OPENING THE HOSPITAL

Opening day had been set for 1 July 1953, but Hunterdon Medical Center did not open until 3 July 1953. The delay was not attributable to the administration but to supplier snafus: the emergency generator was sent to the wrong institution. Other supplies, stored in warehouses all over the county, did not arrive in time to prepare the floors for opening. Miss Lela Greenwood, the Director of Nursing, had assembled a staff of 34 registered nurses and 19 practical nurses, nurse's aides and nursing clerks. The Board of Trustees, on the recommendation of Ray Trussell approved her opening only those beds she felt she could staff well. Accordingly, the fourth floor was opened for obstetrics and the third floor for medical, surgical and pediatric patients.

No one showed up until 2 p.m., when 11-year-old Henry Potopowitz of rural Annandale arrived with acute appendicitis.

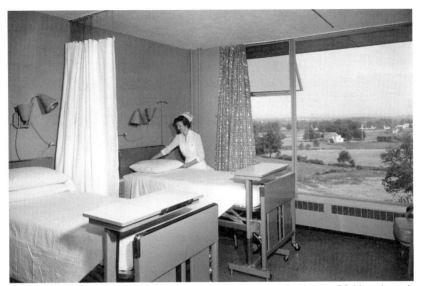

A typical patient room, on third floor surgery, looking out on a landscape of fields and woods with a few houses and a plentitude of deer. Hot water heat, no air conditioning, two hand-cranked beds to a room and few amenities. Nurse Barbara Livingston readies for admissions.

Miss Greenwood had to invent an admission procedure on the spot. When it was discovered that no pre-operative medication was available on the floor, she went off to the storeroom to obtain it.[31] The second patient had a strangulated hernia, the third a ruptured lumbar disc. On 4 July, the first baby, Rose Marie Kessell, of Stockton, was born: her mother's ninth child. The first death occurred on Sunday, 5 July, Mahlon T. Otto had a fatal heart attack. By that day there was a census of 12.

Gradually, as equipment, supplies and nursing staff were made available and as patient load increased, additional floors were opened. At the end of the month, a baby was being delivered every day. Two patients with poliomyelitis were admitted, and Ray Trussell warned the community about the possibility of an epidemic.[32] The entire hospital was open by 1 October.

OTHER PROBLEMS

The initial financial situation was dismal. In the first four months of operation the deficit was $75,000. On 4 October 1953 auditors reported that the situation was fiscally out of control. Earlier meetings in September and later meetings in 1953 found many similar com-

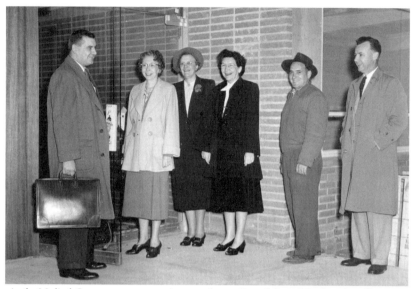

At the Medical Center entrance as patient care began. From left to right, Joseph Williamson, administrator, Miss Lela Greenwood, Director of Nursing, Marguerite Moore, Secretary to the Board, Beatrice "Bea" Walters, assistant to Mrs. Moore for finances, Frank Navarro, chief of maintenance and facilities, Ray Trussell, Director.

ments. Several changes of staff and auditors were made, including asking for the resignation of Joseph Williamson, the administrator. Auditors reported lack of controls in the business office. Murray Rubin, who came the next year, told the author that soon after his arrival, he discovered that bills for hospital care, instead of being sent out, were stored in a closet in the business office.[33] Six years later, when the author commenced work as pediatrician, he repeatedly heard complaints from patients about inefficiencies in the business office: bills were not sent out until many months after discharge, insurance was never notified or billed and bills were inaccurate. It was many more years until community and physicians were more confident about business office efficiency. Worries about fiscal viability led the Board into adopting attitudes towards the specialist staff, described elsewhere, that were not always constructive.

Managing HMC required delicate balancing of the relationship between the Board (read that as Lloyd Wescott) and administration. What is most remarkable is how Wescott and Trussell, another imposing figure, managed to work together during Trussell's

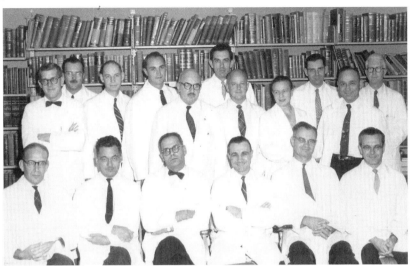

Within a few years the specialist staff expanded dramatically. This photograph was taken in late 1957 or 1958, perhaps a year before I arrived at HMC. Seated, from left to right, Morris Parmet, psychiatrist, Carl Roessel, senior surgeon, Andrew Hunt (my predecessor), Edmund Pellegrino, chief of internal medicine and Medical Director, Fred Knocke, orthopedic surgeon, Walter Petryshyn, otolaryngologist. Standing, Robert Henderson, internal medicine, Steve Dewing, senior radiologist, Buck Katzenbach, second surgeon, Edward Slomka, ophthalmologist, Herman Rannels, senior obstetrician, Gerald Barad, junior obstetrician, Ed Olmstead, pathologist, Pauline Goger, internal medicine and first woman on staff, Fred Woodruff, radiologist, Mike Colella, anesthesiology, Alexander Mitchell, urologist.

five years at Hunterdon. While in subsequent correspondence Wescott wrote tartly about Trussell and Trussell, in conversations with me, made equally tart comments about Wescott, during the time they worked together they collaborated with remarkable facility, as far as I can determine from interviews and documents.

Ray Trussell left in 1955. HMC changed. Only two others were thought able to serve as a leader and counterweight to Wescott. Ed Pellegrino, Chief of Internal Medicine, was a clinical inspiration, a shining star. He explicitly acknowledged that he did not know how to run a hospital, demanding that an administrator (who turned out to be Ed Grant) be hired if he were to accept the position. In addition, he asked the title be changed to Medical Director to show that he was not the chief executive officer. Pellegrino left in 1958 for an academic position. Andy Hunt, Chief of Pediatrics, was offered the position but he also entered academia. Pellegrino had recommended Robert Henderson, also an internist, to succeed him. Henderson was followed by Fred Knocke, an orthopedic surgeon, Eleanor Claus, a nurse (in a brief role as acting) and then in 1977, Henry Simmons, a physician and administrator. All of these Medical Directors served more as caretakers. Simmons, the last, became a lightning rod that attracted specialist staff anger. Subsequently, the chief has always been a distinguished hospital administrator. After Trussell left there was always a trained administrator (for much of this period Ed Grant) who actually managed the hospital. More of this later. None of the Medical Directors had much opportunity to display vision or administrative expertise they might have possessed, because now HMC was Lloyd Wescott. Grant and other administrators might debate, suggest or manipulate, but it was the by-then perennial Chairman of the Board, Wescott, who ultimately made decisions. Knocke was the most respected of all the Medical Directors; from what I could see, Wescott would listen most carefully to him. Lloyd Wescott left the Board in 1976, about the same time as Knocke. Cowles Herr, a Board member from 1964 to 1987 said:

> It didn't seem to me there was too much direction. It didn't seem that the institution was run with a business purpose in mind . . . I didn't think any of the administrators [I knew] had any experience of the larger problems that must have been present in any academic hospital even though this was a JV academic hospital . . . There were problems with the budget. There was no long-range plan. Lloyd Wescott carried all the long-range plans around in his head, and it was probably a lulu . . . It seemed to change with the flow. That came with the mentality that allowed this doctor compensation problem to reach such cataclysmic proportions . . . Today I think it is an A number 1 operation. I think it has a marvelous staff. I think the doctors have the best interests of the community in mind.[34]

PART II

Evolution of Programs

MAJOR PROGRAMS BEGAN before and after the hospital itself opened. Some succeeded; some did not. One of the earliest, the regional affiliation with NYU, thrived initially, was succeeded by an affiliation with Rutgers Medical School (now Robert Wood Johnson Medical School), and finally died. Although today there is no formal affiliation with a medical school, Hunterdon still accepts second year students from Robert Wood Johnson for training in physical diagnosis. The relationship between the open family practice staff and the specialist staff altered dramatically. An early prepayment program never got off the ground; subsequent efforts failed; current efforts are along related but not identical lines. A mental health program has been greatly enlarged, and, after a restrictive and introspective period, once again reaches out into the community. Care of the indigent was, and remains, a responsibility for county residents, subject to steadily increasing fiscal stress. Educational programs have continued and grown in training for family medicine; medical students, who once worked on several services, are present only for training in physical diagnosis. Innovative pediatric and obstetrical programs have continued and expanded. HMC's roles in the public health department and in school health have changed; a small social services department continues. The groundbreaking Chronic Illness Survey did not lead to an organized program in chronic illness or geriatrics; however, individual specialists serving such patients have worked at HMC since its opening. A Department of Senior Services is now staffed by geriatricians. Structural affiliations with private and public community agencies, except for a dental clinic, never developed. In the last decade, several new ventures have begun; more about them in Chapter 17.

CHAPTER 12

Affiliation with a Medical School

ORIGIN OF REGIONAL MEDICAL PROGRAMS

Regional hospital relationships were not novel. As far back as 1920 Lord Dawson, in Great Britain, led a commission that reported to the Ministry of Health on the future organization of health services, including creation of regional relationships.[1] One of the first regional programs in the United States evolved from an agreement in 1929 for the Boston Dispensary, the Floating Hospital for Children, and Tufts University Medical and Dental Schools to unite in offering care for the poor, and teaching, research and "health care programs for the benefit of all New England citizens."[2] The Bingham program, created in 1932, described in Chapter 4, took advantage of this consortium. Commonwealth Fund in 1927 had built upon its program of rural hospital construction by offering fellowships for study to physicians staffing rural medical centers.

Commonwealth encouraged regionalization in 1945 with the Rochester, New York, Regional Hospital Council. The Council held to a very broad-scale regional viewpoint and linked even small entities. Area hospitals simultaneously began educational programs for primary care physicians (many had previously been unaffiliated) and encouraged them to join their staffs.[3] By 1945 the concept of regional programs was circulating widely.[a] It is well described as "the new system of medical care which we now see developing sporadically on all sides."[4]

Within this context, NYU crafted a program, supported in part by the Kress Foundation, to affiliate with hospitals within 100 miles

---

[a] Herrick WW. "In the future: centralization, more group practice, more insurance and better teaching." *Hospitals* 1945; 19: 88–94. Herrick was President of the New York Academy of Medicine; there he and Corwin shared common experience and thought.

of the Nyu Medical Center. Clarence de la Chapelle describes how during World War II the faculty of the Nyu College of Medicine "under the inspired leadership of an acting dean, Donal Sheehan, evolved plans for a new Medical Center and subsequently published these under the title of The Mission of a Medical School. These plans [related] to newer concepts [including] regional responsibilities."[5] The earliest mention at Hunterdon in connection with nyu is on 1 March 1946, when Louise Leicester met with Lester Evans at Commonwealth. Soon plans for an affiliation with Nyu College of Medicine were well advanced.[6] An agreement was reached in 1949. De la Chapelle described Hunterdon as an attempt to "fulfill the standards of a university hospital type of medical care in a rural community . . . [It] integrates care of patients with teaching and research and thereby renders optimal medical care!"[7] He added that no other institution in the United States had achieved the features found at Hunterdon.

Although affiliation was approved on paper, Trussell was disconcerted on his arrival by the attitudes he found at the university. In the postwar era, Nyu Medical Center, like many others, had a huge surplus of physicians flowing back from the armed services. Therefore, comprehensive regional affiliations not only met this challenge but the presumed need for regionalization of health care. Although extensive discussions had taken place among Hunterdon, Commonwealth, and Nyu Medical Center, nyu staff reaction to Trussell's first visit was upsetting to all. Trussell wrote to Lester Evans:

> The meeting fell to pieces rather badly because not all were briefed on what they were there for and many controversies arose . . . I came into a roomful of faculty and they acted like they didn't know what I was talking about. The Professor of Medicine was particularly negative. The Vice President of the University could see this meeting was getting nowhere and he adjourned it. I went back out to Flemington and wrote them a letter to end all letters . . . I pointed out to them that on the basis of their promise the people of a rural county had gone out and raised a million dollars. As a result they then appointed Dr. Clarence de la Chapelle to represent them. From then on, the university relationship was just marvelous.[8]

CLARENCE DE LA CHAPELLE

Clarence de la Chapelle was, along with Lester Evans of Commonwealth Fund, revered by the group at Hunterdon. After graduating from Fordham in 1921, de la Chapelle worked his way through NYU medical school using his skills as a medical illustrator, often doing drawings in color in the operating room. He performed distinguished work in pathology, cardiology and health care administration at NYU School of Medicine and Bellevue Hospital. He was deeply involved in medical education, supported the libraries at the Medical School, and "was the force behind the establishment, in 1947, of the Regional Hospital Plan of NYU. He instituted a program . . . which lasted nearly two decades. The system enabled 20 hospitals in 4 states to become affiliated with NYU for postgraduate physician training."[9]

De la Chapelle was devoted to his duties at Hunterdon, regularly attending Medical Board meetings despite the long drive from his home on Long Island. He was a constant source of support from an early stage. He worked closely with the Board of Trustees before Trussell arrived. It was typical of the man and his work that having made a commitment, he set about fulfilling it in every possible way. De la Chapelle recruited Pellegrino, Edward Grant in administration, Lela Greenwood as Director of Nursing and Walter Petryshyn as chief of otolaryngology. Trussell summarizes what all who knew him said: "one of the most helpful, considerate, warm, friendly, uncritical people I have ever known in my life."[10]

Only his passion for excellence led to critical comments, typically to a junior who had not looked into a patient's pathophysiology, diagnosis or management needs in the most careful manner possible. His son described him as "devoted to providing high quality care to all who needed it—regardless of their ability to pay." The high standards he exemplified attracted a large following of young physicians who became in turn friends and colleagues, and who remember de la Chapelle with great affection. The son adds: "Father was always 'collecting' brilliant young students, so my brother and I were always surrounded by one or two 'adopted' big brothers around the house."[11]

172 ◆ EVOLUTION OF PROGRAMS

SUBSEQUENT DEVELOPMENTS

The affiliation with NYU continued for over 15 years. After the first 10, it became honored as much in the breach as in the observance. Some of the specialist staff devotedly worked at research, clinics or teaching at NYU; others took to playing golf on what they called "their day off." Wescott and Medical Director Henderson attempted, unsuccessfully, to deal with this by coercing the specialist group to agree to a change in personnel practices. This was done; one golfer resigned to practice in a nearby town; no one was pleased. University faculty showed a comparable range of responses. In the early 1970s, New Jersey established a medical school at Rutgers. Wescott moved quickly to work with it, recognizing that an in-state affiliation would benefit more from rapidly advancing regionalization of care, that geographic proximity might improve the flagging quality of the affiliations and a new, bare-bones institution might value Hunterdon more highly. Wescott pushed through a contract with Rutgers, signed 6 March 1972, providing for students in medicine, obstetrics, surgery, psychiatry and pediatrics, and a Department of Family Medicine in the new Medical School designed by HMC, with a graduate of the Hunterdon program, Frank Snope, named Chairman.

As the affiliation with Rutgers Medical School was in negotiation, Wescott gave a talk on Hunterdon before the Association for Hospital Medical Education. With respect to NYU he said: "Our affiliation . . . failed for the simple reason that we did not provide them with something they thought they needed. No medical school can continue in a relationship that to them represents all 'giving' and no 'getting.'" Of the proposed affiliation with Rutgers, he said: "As of now we are important to the Rutgers school because they need our full-time staff, organized and competent to teach, as they expand to a four-year program. Over the long haul, however, we must recognize that an affiliation will continue only if it makes what the Medical School feels are important contributions.[12]

Indeed, affiliation with a medical school has faded away. For some time, Rutgers students came in Surgery, Medicine, Ob–Gyn and Pediatrics, and occasionally in other departments. Residents in surgery from Lenox Hill Hospital attended for a time. Stimulated by a grant from Robert Wood Johnson Foundation, Rutgers

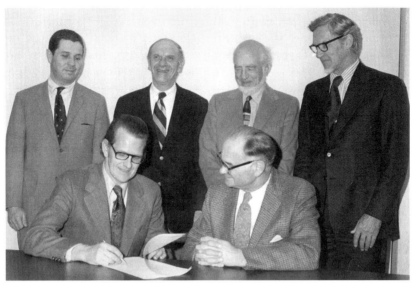

Signing the affiliation with Rutgers Medical School. From left to right, seated, Rutgers Medical School President Stanley Bergen, HMC Medical Director Fred Knocke. Standing, Rutgers Professor of Surgery James McKenzie, Herman "Red" Somers, Rutgers Board of Trustees, J. Seward Johnson and Lloyd Wescott, HMC Board.

changed its name to Robert Wood Johnson Medical School, moved to New Brunswick and administratively became part of New Jersey College of Medicine and Dentistry. As other regional affiliations were established, the need for Hunterdon as a teaching affiliate decreased. Exactly as Wescott had predicted, the affiliation fell apart, since the Medical School had no reason to send students or residents to HMC. Progressive increases in faculty at the Medical School meant competition with rather than need of the Hunterdon staff. One department at a time ceased to send students. The last to do so was the Department of Pediatrics, in 1995, after my retirement, by mutual agreement: Robert Wood Johnson felt it could no longer afford to pay for teaching; the Pediatric Department at the Medical Center felt it could no longer afford to teach without pay.[b] Although today there is no formal affiliation with a medical school, Hunterdon still accepts second year students from Robert Wood Johnson for training in physical diagnosis.

[b] At the same time, the Department of Pediatrics at Robert Wood Johnson was paying staff salaries of at least two other community hospitals where medical students rotated. I believe other reasons for discontinuing the program were primary.

When Hunterdon ended the era of salaried, geographic, full-time specialists in 1978, Robert Haggerty, Chairman of Pediatrics at Rochester, warned that this meant the end of HMC's quasi-academic atmosphere, although it might take ten years before the changes would be observed.[13] In my view, in the intervening 20 years HMC's Board, Staff and Administration should be proud of maintaining a highly sought-after Family Practice Residency program and a staff that performs its work of patient care in a conservative,[c] efficient and thoughtful manner that would meet with the approval of the founding staff.

---

[c] Conservative in this context means using costly resources as needed, rather than for medical adventuring. It means treating people with care, but not throwing prescriptions, knives or hospital care at patients unless they are likely to help them.

CHAPTER 13

Innovation in Mental Health, Pediatric and House Staff Teaching Programs

Three areas of creative planning and execution by the staff and administration of a small community hospital are worth special emphasis. This chapter will describe the formation of the mental health program, the pediatric program and the house staff teaching program. I describe how these evolved and what has happened over the years. Close attention may prove useful to others desiring to encourage novelty in health care organizations.

MENTAL HEALTH PROGRAMS

The history of the mental health program is instructive for understanding the challenge of providing mental health services for a population a large portion of which cannot afford to pay for them. Hunterdon's Board recognized and wrestled with the challenge. They knew the idealistic approach they took might not be sustainable without outside funds, which carried its own risk. If the injection of extramural support eventually ended, it would have an unfavorable impact on the institution's credibility. (Mental health was not the only arena in which this struggle occurred, but it is representative.) Initially the Board erected a program of outreach service heavily dependent on surrogates; later a more intensive, restrictive program with limited goals was devised. Today the program seeks a middle position, offering the most for the greatest number consistent with available resources.

EARLY DEVELOPMENTS

In the mental health field, as in so many others, HMC adapted and combined ideas from many sources to create an exemplary program.

In the decade before World War II, humanistic observers recognized that the personal and social qualities of an individual related to his or her health and treatment. In 1940 Canby Robinson, in magisterial fashion, summarized progressive opinion of the time: "Each patient needs to be treated . . . as a unique individual, and the unity of the human being must be constantly borne in mind . . . The study of the social problems of hospital patients is essential in order to determine factors causing illness, to evaluate and relieve the effects of illness, and to complete restoration of health."[1]

At the same time, various exploratory programs demonstrated the value of psychiatric liaison, consultation and collaboration in the general hospital.[2] Just after the war, Commonwealth, stimulated by Lester Evans, began programs to bring psychiatric teaching into medical education. One grant went to Cornell, which later, through Mary Mercer, was to influence Hunterdon's program. In 1950, Evans wrote Trussell about what he envisioned: "Not . . . a special Mental Health or psychiatric program but rather what can be drawn from those fields to make the whole health and medical activity of Hunterdon County concerned with the patient's welfare."[3] Trussell's letter to Evans later that summer indicated that they had discussed "integration of the psychiatric and psychologic techniques throughout the services given by physicians and nurses and social workers."[4] How satisfying this exchange must have been to Evans and others at Commonwealth, seeing how the Fund's work in pioneering the application of psychiatric knowledge to other medical services bore fruit. Evans encouraged Trussell to take advantage of social work consulting services of Commonwealth's Mildred Scoville, and Ethyl Ginsburg.[a] By November of 1950 Ginsburg was visiting Hunterdon one day a week to obtain data for developing a program.

Commonwealth's Harry Handley noted that he met with John Bambara, a family physician in Flemington since before World War II: "[Bambara] talked at some length about the need for psychiatric consultation in the community and . . . [stated] that at least 60 percent of the people he saw in his practice had problems

[a] Ginsburg, an experienced social worker and administrator, was the Director of Mental Health Services for the National Association for Mental Health. Mary Mercer, a child psychiatrist on the faculty at Cornell–New York Hospital, described Ginsburg as a "powerful person" associated with all of the new leadership in psychiatry who were influential in the Group for the Advancement of Psychiatry.

relating to their emotional life, in addition to purely physical conditions." Bambara went on to say that it was difficult to devote the necessary time because

> individuals generally are unwilling to pay him for therapy which involves only discussion . . . They were willing to pay just as much for two minutes' discussion with a prescription as they were for a half hour discussion without a prescription . . . The only possibility of getting them to pay the cost in time for psychotherapy was to have this therapy given by persons trained in this specialty.[5]

Bambara had always been more interested in behavioral and emotional aspects of health care than any other physician in the community. A television special on him, his practice and the Medical Center, made some years later highlighted his interviews with patients. In 1959, finding himself overburdened and burned out, he left family medicine, took a residency, and entered the practice of psychiatry.

COMMONWEALTH CONSULTING

In Trussell's words, Mildred Scoville "next to Lester Evans . . . was the second most influential person . . . on the staff . . . She was a social worker . . . very fond of using Ethyl Ginsburg[6] as a consultant. Ethyl was a psychiatric social worker who was the widow of a psychiatrist named Sol Ginsburg. She helped write up the application to Commonwealth for the grant that made it possible to bring in Parmet."[7] Ginsburg's report was issued in draft form at the end of February 1951 and presented to Hunterdon's Board on 2 May 1951. She laid out community resources, recommended immediate appointment of a consultant in psychiatry to work a day a week, to be followed promptly by a full-time psychiatrist. The psychiatrist would lead a team including social workers oriented to a community approach. The team would work with key individuals in agencies, schools, voluntary and health care groups, all assumed to be in touch with those with personal or social difficulties. Her report, although broad and nonspecific, defined community mental health and encouraged prevention as more likely to yield long-term results than curative efforts.[8]

Using earlier programs financed by Commonwealth as a model,

mental health would be sewn into HMC's fabric of inpatient and ambulant care and interaction with other community agencies. From the beginning, the Board was concerned about the program's financial viability. Could it continue without outside support, which must some day be withdrawn? Perhaps they should proceed one step at a time? But they endorsed Ginsburg's recommendations and applied for, and received, a grant from Commonwealth. In June 1952, in a report to the family physicians, Trussell described the Commonwealth grant. It would bring in specialists in mental health who, in addition to coordinating services, would "develop a training and consultation program with those people in the community who wish to participate."[9]

Louise Leicester, who had been away on an extended trip, launched one of her missiles at the Board, expressing her dismay at how the grant was put together. The bluntness of her assessment makes clear the difficulties of negotiating with her. Her legitimate concerns were on the budget: Did it underestimate in a major way expenditures? If so, the program could not be executed as planned, leading to community loss of confidence in the institution. "We shall for the third time [the first two concerned Hill–Burton plans and the architect's underestimate of the construction bids] be forced to retract figures vital to our plans, because they are inaccurate. This may sorely test the faith of the Community, which is one of our most valuable assets."[10] No response from the Board (i.e., Wescott) was found in the archives.

In June 1952, psychiatrist Mary Mercer, head of the division of Child Development at Cornell–New York Medical School, was engaged as a day-a-week consultant to HMC's Mental Health program, underwritten by Commonwealth. Mercer had an extensive background consulting with pediatricians. After completing her training, first in pediatrics and then in psychiatry, as a Commonwealth Fund Fellow at Cornell, she succeeded Milton Senn at Cornell–New York Medical School, who had left to replace the late Arnold Gesell at Yale. She brought to Hunterdon her conviction that the best mental health programs should reach out to all groups: "Physicians, public health nurses, school teachers, P.T.A. leaders, 4-H club leaders, the clergy, judges and probation officers."[11]

At that time there was considerable impetus in preventive medicine and mental health to get beyond traditional public health concerns. Trussell had learned a great deal from his colleagues at the New York State Health Department in Albany, where staff relied on public health nurses and health officers as contributors to mental health. Its distinguished Commissioner, Herman Hilleboe, arranged a weeklong program in mental health for his staff; one of the instructors was Mercer. She and Trussell met briefly. When Trussell moved across town from the Health Department to become the first professor of Preventive Medicine at Albany Medical College, he initiated a health council "and got exposed to a lot of issues right away, alcoholism and so on . . . I was around a lot of very good people and a lot of ideas were floating around."[12] Shortly after Trussell's appointment at Hunterdon, Commonwealth suggested that he seek Mercer as an adviser on mental health. When they met again, she says, "I decided I was going to marry him, and I did."[13] Their collaboration was productive though stressful since she maintained her work at Cornell, necessitating a four-hour round trip from their home in Hunterdon County.

In the spring of 1952, around the time of Mercer's appointment, Morris Parmet of Children's Hospital in Philadelphia was recommended to the Board as psychiatrist. Mercer for a time saw private patients at the Trussell–Mercer residence. Wescott became concerned that she would be competing with Parmet. Mercer replied that she was primarily Professor of Pediatrics in Psychiatry at Cornell–New York Medical Center and that the patients she was seeing in New Jersey traveled from New York to see her. On weekends, Mercer played the role of "Director's Wife."[14] Competitive fears allayed, by September of 1952, she, Hunt and Parmet were attending meetings with local groups to learn the public perception of mental health problems in children and how HMC could assist.

FLESHING OUT THE PROGRAM

Parmet brought a depth of wisdom mixed with pragmatism. He was aware of the difficult position of a psychiatrist in a general medical group, "as he represents an unstable investment in an economic partnership."[15] For Parmet the most intriguing aspect was the absence of an inpatient segregated psychiatric service. Every bed in HMC was potentially a psychiatric bed, whether on pediatrics or obstetrics or dermatology. The entire hospital would be imbued with a mental health attitude. This was not a new idea.[16] Parmet believed that

> psychiatry functions more effectively and provides a more constructive influence when it is not segregated physically and functionally, but rather when it relates itself to the many psychological needs within the framework of other existing departments. A roving psychiatrist found many opportunities to carry on informal discussions [with other professionals], patients and their families . . . The psychiatrist is here, as everywhere, under pressures to treat seriously disturbed patients, but he must be willing to devote considerable effort to the development of other resources for prevention and education.[17]

The Board of Trustees, already sensitized to the issues by Corwin, Mildred Scoville, Ethyl Ginsburg and other Commonwealth consultants, backed the program fully. As Trussell said, "[Parmet] was practicing community psychiatry before the term was invented."[b] A mental health committee of the Board interpreted the program to the community in the hope of avoiding unrealistic expectations. The committee recommended that newspaper reports of public meetings avoid emphasizing mental health. School referrals should include parent involvement. Board members testified. One related his experiences as a patient in a New York hospital. He observed, "The patient is the forgotten man of hospitals, with the patient considered as a case instead of as a whole human being."[18] Parmet's task was aided by the inherent idealism of the atmosphere at HMC. Along with Trussell he was concerned how mental health personnel would be able to charge for services and earn their salary.

The open approach of Parmet extended to ambulant care. He was proud of the common waiting room which served all the specialists, because this demonstrated that the psychiatrist functioned as a part of a mixed medical group. As administrator Ed Grant said, "These were patients whose illness happened to be one of an emotional kind."[19] These innovations occurred in the midst of national debates about the importance of privacy of psychiatric encounters. Some psychiatrists aimed to be a physician–scientist who saw the psychiatric disorder as comparable in principle to other

---

[b] Trussell RE. Interview by author, 9 December 1995. The term "community psychiatry" was probably invented by Kurt Deuschle, who was with Pellegrino at Kentucky and later went to Mt. Sinai in New York.

disorders of other bodily systems. This permitted openness and candor as required in any health encounter. Others felt that absolute secrecy was necessary to encourage the patient to share innermost thoughts. Parmet was devoted to the rightness of his approach, to meet with those to whom he might offer help under conditions where privacy was not even an option. Thus he encountered conflict between his ideals of practice and the approach of many, perhaps most in the field. The conflict was not resolved during his stay at Hunterdon.

Trussell prepared a long report to the Board that demonstrated how well the entire mental health staff had been absorbed.[20] By 1953 Parmet's collaborators included Margaret Wiles as Associate Director of Nursing,[c] Beatrice Tileston in social work and a psychologist. Trussell emphasized multiple roles for each team member to influence community members constructively and avoid physical and functional segregation in a separate department. The mental health group worked together intimately to uncover problems that bedevil community-wide mental health programs to this day. The Trussell report, a masterpiece of organization and exposition, outlines their efforts in detail. A sensitive topic, repeatedly raised, was what to do for community members thought to be in need of help, but who did not see themselves as such. No solution appeared other than to hope that a light bulb might go on over the individual's head as a result of consciousness-raising efforts.

The goal of Trussell's report was to convince the Board to support this extraordinarily complex project as Commonwealth grants were time-limited and would diminish. Most of what was accomplished was on a nonfee basis. Such an apparatus of community mental health could not support itself. The federal funds used years later to build and help support a Community Mental Health Center were not then available. The Board discussed future support of mental health services in late 1954.[21] Contrasting approaches were considered. Mental health could be conceived as the province of a special interest group responsible to raise funds as needed. Alternatively, "The mental health program [could] be considered as it was originally conceived as an integral part of Hunterdon Medical Center and not be singled out for separate support with the possibility of failure."[22] The Board unequivocally chose the second alternative.

[c] Wiles had a background in public health nursing and came initially to work on the Chronic Illness Survey.

SUBSEQUENT EVOLUTION OF MENTAL HEALTH SERVICES

In 1954 Trussell sent Evans a brief outline of possible programs, including "a generalized case-work service, . . . another bridge to community health and welfare [to meet] an almost unbelievable number of difficult family situations [uncovered by the Chronic Illness Survey] . . . about which nothing is being done due to the lack of any resource."[d] Morris Parmet prepared a follow-up report in 1956 for internal consumption.[23] After restating and emphasizing the program's original premises—integrating prevention and treatment; integrating the entire program with all areas of HMC; working actively to influence community agents who worked with people—he summed up its achievements. Staff also published articles about HMC's unique psychiatric program.[24] Integration was an important aspect of the program from whence Parmet and Hunt came, at the Philadelphia Child Guidance Clinic and Children's Hospital, where for years a major goal of the Department of Psychiatry had been to achieve just such integration.

Ed Grant, who came in 1955 as administrator, said "I learned the fact that one of the greatest things that you could do was to admit psychiatric patients to an open medical floor. Now that never took place in the traditional hospitals."[25] There was a progressive increase in utilization of services by the adult public. On the other hand, use of such services by children remained static despite extensive efforts to educate the community. In 1956 support from Commonwealth Fund had already begun to taper off; it was not known how the enormous effort would be supported.

Parmet left in 1959, soon after Hunt. Demands on the Department of Psychiatry expanded progressively, overwhelming available resources. The Department came under attack from Pellegrino's successor as Medical Director, Robert Henderson, who believed that it was too heavily oriented toward working with children. Henderson expressed in strong terms his opinion that this focus accomplished little. In general, he approached mental health from the disease-oriented viewpoint of the internist; therefore, he believed that the department should devote itself more to problems

---

[d] Trussell RE to LJ Evans, 24 June 1954. Commonwealth 1954 file, HMCA. This letter included half a dozen ideas for research programs, including a much-needed follow-up of the Chronic Illness Survey, a study of market penetration by HMC, and studies of resource utilization by patients. Trussell, as usual, was throwing out ideas as an oak throws out acorns. Some might grow.

such as schizophrenia. He seemed not to recognize the importance of either developmental or environmental issues to a comprehensive program or their interplay with neurobiologic factors nor did he mention depression, which is more common than schizophrenia. Wescott felt that neither large institutions or private physicians nor most general hospitals were assuming responsibility for mental health problems.[26] For over two decades a series of changes facilitated but also held back the Department's work. Several working groups developed plans for expansion, under the leadership of Parmet's successors, Richard Oliver-Smith and then Colin Fox. A federal grant for a comprehensive Mental Health Center was obtained.

The most significant consequence of the opening of the inpatient unit was a dramatic 180-degree turn in the orientation of the Mental Health program. Hunterdon now treated mentally ill patients in a segregated inpatient unit. It became closed off, turned inwards, and cut off all contact with the rest of HMC and much of the community. HMC's Joint Conference Committee, composed of specialists, family physicians and the Board of Trustees met to consider this issue on 2 July 1973, just 20 years after HMC opened. Someone stated that the Department had drawn an Iron Curtain around itself. Family physicians bitterly objected that they were cut off completely from the care of patients hospitalized with mental health problems. Robert Adams, Chief of Psychiatry, presented a lengthy memorandum at that meeting. Adams makes plain it "would be destructive" to his work to have patients seen by anyone not on his staff. He could not "in any stretch of my imagination" visualize how family physicians could admit patients.[27] This completed the reversal of the integrative program and philosophy developed by Morris Parmet, shut the mental health program off from all communication with every other part of HMC, and commenced a period of isolation comparable to that of North Korea in the community of nations today. So adamant was the Department in its stance that staff psychiatrists refused to release any information to other HMC physicians, of any kind, even at the written request of the patient or guardian—not even that the patient had been seen there.[28] One possible reason is that record-keeping was not up to the task. When the N.J. Division of Mental Health and Hospitals performed a survey in September 1982, every aspect of the Mental Health Center's record keeping was found inadequate.

In the last few years, partly because of a change of leadership, partly because of the gradual loss of federal funds and partly with recognition of dramatic changes in mental health care, the Department has adopted a different stance. A new name, HMC Behavioral Health, signals a new approach. Emphasis has been placed on outreach. Satellite offices are open; more are planned. Large new grants from the state and county provide money for crisis intervention, a screening center, improved access to outpatient therapy, partial hospitalization and addiction therapies. The greatest need, child and adolescent service, is not yet fully met. Ambulant care is offered at new locations outside of HMC, serving the more affluent population who prefer privacy. Staff continues to serve the less affluent population at the Louise B. Leicester Community Mental Health Center on the Medical Center campus. The staff looks toward preventive behavioral health, concern with community attitudes, the persisting stigma of mental sickness and how these perceptions may be altered.

Pediatric Innovation

Andrew Hunt, HMC's first pediatrician, came from a distinguished academic career at Children's Hospital of Philadelphia. Dissatisfaction with a traditional disease-oriented focus and experience with the visionary psychiatrist John Rose led Hunt to study behavioral and environmental factors in child health.[29] At Hunterdon, pediatric nurses became sophisticated observers of parents, children, and their interactions. Developmental histories were done on all patients admitted, regardless of reason. Children with complex problems thought to represent somatic and behavioral interaction that could not be resolved in outpatient settings were admitted for study.[e] The approach was based on a clear consensus of experts in pediatric hospital care and maternity–newborn care of the time.[30] Today inpatient care for children is less frequent at a community hospital of this size; sick children are transferred, less sick children are treated at home.

Pediatric and mental-health personnel interacted in multiple

[e] Hunt AD, Parmet M. "Collaboration between pediatrician and child psychiatrist in a rural medical center." *Pediatrics* 1957; 19: 462–6. The administrative and financial climate of the time made this approach possible. It is almost unheard of today except where supported by research funds and approved by the Institutional Research Board.

ways. Joint rounds occurred weekly. Cross consultation was a frequent occurrence. Hunt and Trussell write:

> Weekly rounds with [the child guidance team] are devoted to a discussion which interprets to the pediatric, medical and nursing staffs the emotional implications of the parent–child relationships . . . Thus the program was launched under the supervision of a pediatrician who is "psychiatrically oriented," but without formal experience in psychiatry, and with graduate nurses of average training. The relationship with child psychiatry is collaborative . . . The core of the successful hospitalization of the child is the maintenance of continuity in the parent–child relationship . . . [The child] will continue to sense the nearness and participation of his parents during a trying and often necessarily unpleasant experience; the mother retains her identity, and the nurse does not succumb to the temptation to become a substitute parent.[31]

PARENT VISITING

Background: In the West modern notions of hospitals developed in the 19th century. Initially, sick children requiring hospitalization were deemed to need care by physicians and nurses—parents were superfluous if not deleterious. Sir James Spence, professor of child health at the University of Durham, England, originated and encouraged parent visiting for the care of the sick child in the late 1920s. Spence also believed that care of sick children in the hospital by the mother was a necessary step to alleviate a shortage of nurses and to improve nursing care quality:

> It is an advantage to the child. It is an advantage to the mother, for to have undergone this experience and to have felt that she has been responsible for her own child's recovery establishes a relationship with her child and confidence in herself . . . It is an advantage to the nurses who learn much by contact with the best of these women, not only about the handling of a child but about life itself. It is an advantage to the other children on the ward for whose care more nursing time is liberated. In teaching hospitals it is of further advantage to the students, who gain a practical experience of the form of nursing they will depend on in their practices and learn to recognize the anxieties and courage which bind the mothers to

their children during illness; a lesson which fosters the courtesy on which the practice of medicine depends. I advocate
this method of nursing, not on sentimental grounds but on
the practical grounds of efficiency and necessity.[32]

In the mid-20th century, it was demonstrated that separating a
child from his or her parent could lead to serious and sometimes
disastrous physical and psychological consequences. Advanced hospitals opened visiting for sick children by parents in the belief that
care by parent was more than suitable, it was highly desirable.[33]

HMC's Inpatient Program: When HMC's first Chief of Pediatrics
Andrew Hunt began training at Children's Hospital of Philadelphia in 1945, visiting hours on the children's wards were once every two weeks, while parents of private patients could visit and
stay as they wished. When Hunt was chief resident, visiting hours
on the wards were liberalized. The nursing staff was opposed, but
Hunt, a strong advocate, helped all to accept change. Care of very
sick children, particularly the psychosomatic aspects, was much
easier when parents were there helping to care for the child and
interacting with the professional staff.

At HMC Hunt proposed that parents have unlimited visiting
hours. Ray Trussell, sensitized by his prior exposure to mental
health programs, strongly endorsed the program. The Board voted
on 26 June 1953 that mothers could stay with their sick children,
infants in the nursery might room-in, and only fathers could visit
on the maternity floor. The Pediatric Nursing staff objected strongly.
The Pediatric Supervisor, Barbara Lloyd, had been trained and
qualified in pediatric nursing in a hospital with traditional visiting
policies. Hunt described her as

a placid . . . very competent nurse and her staff felt the way
that pediatric nurses traditionally were, that the worst thing
for a hospitalized child is the parents. They were a toxic
influence. When I announced that we were going to have free
parent visiting, they were horrified. We agreed that they would
give it a try for a few months and see what happened. Actually, they became real converts. If there was a toddler in there
who was suffering some sort of hospitalism or whatever, they
would call that mother and say "you get in here and be with
this child, she needs you." It became a total change and it
was great fun . . . [We] were one of the first to do it as an
administratively established role.[34]

In their article, Hunt and Trussell spoke of the vital importance of "strong support and encouragement" from administration and nursing. "Maintenance of continuity in the parent–child relationship" was central to their task. They recognized (and wrote about this as novel) that children live embedded in the social context of family, community and culture. The child is not a separate entity. Great credit for the success of this program goes to Miss Lela Greenwood, HMC's first Director of Nursing, who provided day-to-day support for the nursing staff, firm backing for Hunt and his policies and a willingness to innovate in patterns of care as new to her as they were to the Pediatrics nursing staff. Family physicians did not object—they enjoyed visiting their patients as a family. Psychiatrist Morris Parmet was immensely supportive, writing with Hunt that the arrangement permitted specialist and family physician to come closer together, understand each other better, and therefore provide better care for children.[35]

Hunterdon was widely known for this policy. Lay and professional workers often visited to see the program in action.[36] Today, of course, visiting everywhere is open, not only for parents but for other family members, so it is difficult to realize just how jolting the introduction of open visiting was in an era when family exclusion was the norm in both academic and community hospitals. Despite the work of pioneering institutions like Hunterdon, 10 years after the Medical Center opened Wolf wrote with passion about hospitals, and in particular children's hospitals, which did not allow parents to stay with children, nor prepare them for the experience. Wolf states that in 1954, the year after the Medical Center opened, just 25 percent of the hospitals in New York City allowed daily visits. No mention was made of parents staying with the sick child.[37]

ROOMING-IN PROGRAM FOR MATERNITY

Background: Rooming-in programs, like parents visiting with sick children, became accepted in the mid- and later 20th century, a reaction to the isolation and "we-know-best" attitudes of "scientific" child and newborn care practices in the West. The scientific approach altered centuries-old traditions, which assumed that the mother cared for a newborn helped by women from family and social group, and those who knew the sick child provided care.

Spence drew a graphic picture of the depression and isolation in a typical maternity hospital unit under rigid rules and contrasted it with units with rooming-in:

> Throughout the puerperium night and day mothers and babies are kept within reach of each other, where the mother may pick up her baby when she desires, where everything that is done for the child is done within sight of the mother at her bedside, and experience shows that with simple precautions not only is the danger of neonatal infection less than it otherwise would be, but breast feeding and the relationship between mother and child is firmly and safely established in a physiologically natural manner.[38]

Widespread awareness of the importance of rooming-in appeared after World War II and an innovative program at Yale.[39] Moloney summarized the advantages of rooming-in, relating the practice to the enhancement of breastfeeding, and advocated mother and newborn sharing a room as much as possible so long as the mother is comfortable. Several hospitals in Detroit offered 24-hour-a-day rooming-in; fathers were encouraged to spend time with the family.[40] Montgomery reviewed the literature and his own experience with hundreds of patients who roomed in.[41] He and others noted increased rates of breastfeeding. Richardson brought these findings up to date in 1951.[42]

Hunterdon Program: As with other innovations Hunterdon combined idealism with the spirit of the time. Rooming-in on maternity, mentioned by the Corwin report of 1949, was not difficult to implement. Much credit belongs to Clara Anthony, HMC's first Maternity–Newborn Supervisor. She came from Geisinger Memorial Hospital, where she was converted to liberal visiting as a result of encounters with the group from Yale. Permissive rooming-in became the practice at HMC. With nursing support, most babies roomed-in most of the time. David Sanders, a resident in Pediatrics from July through December of 1953 and experienced with a rooming-in program in the military, was comfortable and supportive. Sanders describes Hunt as having "a fervor" about rooming-in.[43] Hunt is less definite.

> What we did as I remember it was to try to see to it just that they took the babies in to the mothers and that they kept them there as long as possible. I don't think I made a big issue of that rooming-in . . . We tried to be sure that if the

mother wanted to keep the baby all the time she could. A lot
did but a lot didn't. The obstetricians were indifferent and it
never was a big issue. I was more interested, I think, in the
issue of the sick children and using the hospital [for psychosomatic problems].[44]

Even though there was less written about the topic, HMC soon
became known for its maternity policies. Obstetricians Herman
Rannels and Gerald Barad were quite comfortable with them, and,
again, Mental Health provided support. In those days, before intensive care units, mothers were invited in from birth to interact
and care for premature infants, offer feedings, help with procedures, and to be a part of the caregiving efforts. Barad was strongly
motivated towards family-centered obstetrical care, giving further
impetus towards noninterventional obstetrics, participation of family
members and breastfeeding. I initiated a lactation consulting service. By 1998 Hunterdon was a "baby friendly" hospital for staff
support of breastfeeding.

Visiting for the father in the newborn nursery came by the
tenth anniversary of the hospital. I can remember around that time
a lesson in complementary medicine. By then routine, a father (in
this instance a local chiropractor) was present in the operating
room when his infant was delivered by Caesarean section. He was
there to work with me to stabilize the newborn. When we brought
the baby to the newborn nursery, he asked whether he could give
the baby a chiropractic treatment, promising that it would be soothing, not risky. He felt that the baby would benefit because he had
been shaken up by the stresses of delivery and asked me to watch
what he did in case I had any questions. It was not at all clear
what he proposed to do, but I could not imagine what harm would
come as long as I remained to observe. It was a lesson for me, as I
observed the father give the baby the most soothing back rub I
have ever seen, gently, warmly. The baby calmed, became peaceful
and looked around as he entered first a state of quiet alertness and
then drowsiness. The infant literally glowed. I wanted to ask for a
treatment myself!

During the first six years after HMC opened, newborn infants
on maternity were registered as patients of the delivering physician. The obstetrician was attending physician of record for those
newborn infants who had not been delivered by a family physician. This was true even though the pediatrician carried medical

responsibility. Hunt was unable to recall his attitude to this practice, nor whether it had an influence on his care in the nursery. When I arrived, in 1959, I asked to change this practice, so that newborn infants were on the pediatric service, and, if the pediatrician were the attending, this would be so listed. Obstetrician Rannels objected, and a tussle followed. For a number of reasons, including administrative clarity, aligning administrative policy with medical responsibility, and avoiding unnecessary malpractice exposure, the administrative officials put the change into effect.

Subsequent Developments: These programs have been expanded and refined in cooperation with HMC nursing and administrative staff. Nurses assume the role of educator and work to support parents while maintaining high standards of technological nursing care. Emphasis on cost containment and shorter lengths of stay have made it impossible to admit, study and treat children with psychosocial problems, except for the few whose long-term health or life are at risk. Programs of family support have been sustained. On the Pediatric unit, visiting is freely available to all family members, including siblings. Parents routinely remain overnight if they wish. On the maternity floor entire families visit, and family-centered childbirth and neonatal care is routine for all. Only those parents who specifically do not desire rooming-in do not do so. Through zealous efforts of the nursing staff, lactation consultants and pediatricians, Hunterdon is rated as a "baby friendly" hospital for the breastfeeding mother and her infant. Approximately 80 percent of new mothers breastfeed. Martell emphasizes that at least some of the problems initiating rooming-in and baby-friendly breast feeding policies in many hospitals stem from reluctance on the part of nurses to change familiar systems.[45] In Chapter 20, Hunt has described how this reluctance in adopting new policies for parent visiting was overcome. The issues are the same as for lactation.

The first lactation consulting service in New Jersey for the pregnant woman and new mother was begun in 1980, supported by a grant from the Hunterdon Health Fund.[f] The program offers public education on breastfeeding, education for physicians and nurses, a

[f] The Hunterdon Health Fund was created by Rutgers Medical School with funds provided by J. Seward Johnson. The monies were transferred from the expiring Hunterdon School of Health that he had established at HMC, but which was moribund from birth. Failure of the School of Health signaled the end of Johnson's work with HMC.

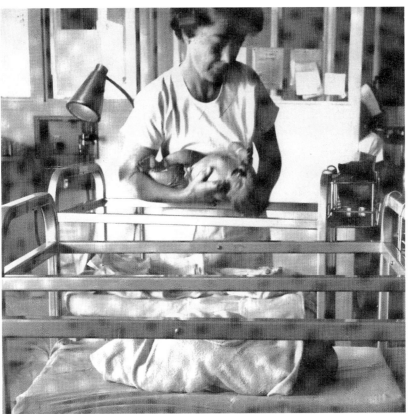

Helen Neid was for many years an attendant in the newborn nursery. Despite the handicap of an early life injury, which interfered with function of one arm and leg, she provided thoughtful, devoted and exemplary care to the neonates and advice to their mothers. Her work was typical then and now of nursing care at the Medical Center.

breastfeeding consultation service, and collaboration with interested groups. A private room with refrigeration was provided for breastfeeding HMC employees who return to work.[46] After the first three years, the breastfeeding consultation service was supported by the Department of Pediatrics. Later, it was amalgamated with HMC's education program and the Maternity/Newborn unit.

A service for developmentally disabled children was spurred by Elks Lodge 1928, located a few yards from the Medical Center. In 1969 they sent a committee headed by Dennis Compton to ask about equipment they might purchase for "crippled children." I proposed instead that the Elks fund an early intervention program for children with handicapping conditions. A multidisciplinary team of professionals would meet with parents and young children, evaluate child and family function, and offer therapy, stimulation and training for parents on what they could do at home. Directed at infants and toddlers, this was soon expanded to preschoolers. Sara Carlton, an occupational therapist, headed the combined program. The preschool program was eventually transferred to the local school districts, but the early intervention program continues to this day, combined with a Child Evaluation Center to offer comprehensive study and treatment for children with disabling or chronic illness. Approximately 450 children in the Early Intervention and Special Child Health programs are served each year. An additional 500 children are served in the Evaluation and Pediatric Rehabilitation program.

Teaching Program House Staff

"House Staff" refers to resident physicians who have graduated from medical school and who are employed for one to as many as five or six years in a hospital. These physicians seek to further their education in a field of medicine preparatory to entering private practice or joining the faculty of a medical school. They earn salaries, room and board—a pittance when HMC opened—now more generous, though well below the earnings of a practitioner. House Staff may be assisted by medical students, also working in the hospital in their third and fourth year, not as employed physicians but rather as clinical clerks, to learn while helping out. For both these groups, there is the tug of a certain tension between activities from which they learn and activities which primarily further patient care or enable the hospital to function more successfully. House Staff contribute more than they receive, not only in service, but also by providing the learning and teaching atmosphere influential on practicing physicians to maintain their own standards, to do work of exemplary quality and serve as a role model for their juniors.

Ray Trussell was actively developing an educational program for at least a year before HMC opened. In a lengthy memorandum to the Executive Committee of the Board, he described his efforts, arranging temporary approval for a residency program and medical school assignment of students. He complained about issues related to the small size of the hospital and problems of salary.[47] From the time HMC opened, students and residents were present, not only from NYU, but also from Albany Medical College, University of Pennsylvania, Jefferson Medical College and Lenox Hill Hospital. Corwin's recommendation, that residents, supervised from NYU, lead several services, was never implemented.

Within a year after HMC opened, the goal of a house staff program had been formulated: to train family physicians who would practice in the community. Trussell wrote a perceptive letter to Commonwealth's Lester Evans:

> We have not yet established any mechanism whereby a man can actually get the kind of experience which he will encounter when he opens an office in the community and we recognize this as a serious lack. The question is beginning to be raised by some of the staff here [to establish] a selected group of families for whom they would serve as the family physician, in a setting of specialist–family physician relationship which exists nowhere else in the country.[48]

Trussell was as usual clairvoyant. By the 1970s this sort of training—now known as a "model practice"—was the standard for family physicians. Two such practices now serve Hunterdon County.

House staff initially lived at one end of the adult medical floor in a suite of rooms set aside for them. For at least 10 years after HMC opened, the refrigerator there was kept stocked with beer, a custom discontinued when it became more widely known. Later Seward Johnson provided a grant for Hillside House staff apartments overlooking HMC. Residents buy their own beer.

Issues of consultation, in one form or another, became inextricably bound up with issues of education of House Staff. House

Staff provided care and, if needed, prompt action for patients in hospital, inserting a layer between the practitioner and the patient. Teaching occurred on daily rounds with the specialist having an opportunity to influence the family physician. Pellegrino said: "It was a teaching setting so that without being obtrusive, we could reach each practitioner with daily clinical teaching in the care of their own patients. It was also the most painless teaching."[49]

Specialist and nursing staff tacitly agreed that all patient care would be monitored, and if care seemed of questionable quality, a specialist would be called. Jeannette Ash, a nurse in the Emergency Room, said she felt free to call a specialist whenever a resident or student seemed to be in deep water, and that the senior physician responded at once. In the early years, the family practice residents provided exemplary care, recognizing disease and pathophysiologic processes, and serving as junior attending physicians. However, within a few years, as inpatient care became more and more technological, residents were receiving training to treat patients they would not be seeing as family physicians. There was implicit tension in the training program between the need for the service to care for sick inpatients and the educational needs to train physicians for the actual work they would be doing later in life. In part this was resolved with the creation of model practices, within which the resident worked in ambulant care. Today service has become more subordinate to education for our residents, who interact less with other specialists and more with family physicians. Hmc's popular, high quality residency program in Family Practice continues filling its quota each year with graduates of u.s. medical schools.

Exigencies of practice also influence teaching relationships. Hardworking family physicians often make early hospital rounds. As a pediatrician, when I arrived at 8:00 a.m. to round with residents and students, the family physician had been and gone, typically to be in the office the rest of the day. Although the family physician managed inpatients for routine matters, when urgent situations arose, the resident on duty, supervised by the appropriate staff specialist, provided care. Again and again this led to some degree of hard feelings. On one side, "You didn't call me or tell me"; on the other, "You weren't there when the patient needed you." In other words, the very problems outlined in the initial meetings of the Medical Staff in March 1953, before hmc had opened.

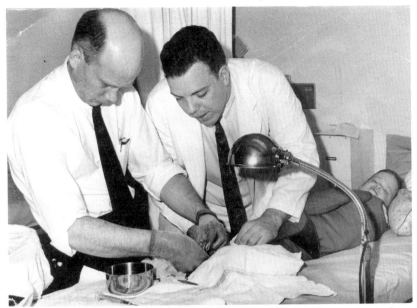

Family physician Frank Snope, a graduate of the HMC residency, treating a patient in the Emergency Department, assisted by resident David Sharp.

Inevitably the resident, caught in the middle, was forced to take sides between one kind of role model, the family physician whom he was training to emulate, and another kind of model, the specialist physician who was his academic mentor. The ameliorating factor was the desire of both specialists and family physicians to make the system work. During the early years, the specialists simply made themselves available. After the first decade greater stresses emerged, as the specialists and family physicians both became more vocal about the difficulty their defined roles imposed. By the end of the second decade, roles were redefined into a more traditional relationship. A Family Practice Department and service emerged. The specialists, not without some grumbling about quality of care, turned over patients to the family physicians and did not participate in care unless asked, or in case of dire emergency. From the residents' point of view this resulted in clearing the air with respect to role models and mentorship. It made plain to them who they were, and what they would grow to be.

CHAPTER 14

Efforts to Offer Health and Sickness Care to Those Who Lack Money to Pay

This chapter describes separate efforts to make health and sickness care available to persons with limited means in the time before Medicare and Medicaid. Before HMC appeared, when the only physicians in the county were family physicians, they offered care without charge to patients on welfare or thought to be of limited means. Patients sometimes paid in garden produce, other items or services. As noted in Chapter 2, neighboring hospitals offered care for which payments were made by the Board of Freeholders based on recommendation of the Welfare Department. While HMC attempted to increase these payments, Board and administration, eventually in collaboration with medical staff, made several efforts, ultimately unsuccessful, to establish a prepayment program.

CARE OF THE INDIGENT

EARLY POLICY

Ray Trussell, the Medical Center's first Director, said that during his tenure policy for care of the indigent was never clearly spelled out. The *Hunterdon Democrat* reported on 28 May 1953, just before HMC opened, that Trussell met with the Board of Chosen Freeholders to discuss payment for indigent hospital care. One difficulty was determining just who was unable to pay for services. Usually the County Welfare Department certified indigence. In 1952 the county paid a total of $12,505.26 for 50 patients hospitalized in neighboring areas. The next month Mrs. Walker, the new head of the Hunterdon County Welfare Board, met with HMC's

Board to discuss the issue. HMC agreed to provide care at the pre-vious rate: $9.00 per day plus extras. The Freeholders' hospital plan was pointed to as a model: Welfare certified eligible patients, including not only those on public assistance, but also employed persons unable to meet costs, with Welfare staff providing case-work services to those needing personal or social help but who did not fit administratively specified categories.[1]

In 1954 the Freeholders paid a flat sum of $40,000 for indigent care. Wescott then convinced them to increase payments to over $100,000 for the following year. He then suggested they pay ac-tual costs instead of a flat sum, with a still greater increase in their payments. In 1957 a prominent local attorney, Judge George K. Large, endowed the Large Foundation to help, among other ac-tivities, with costs of care for indigent residents of Raritan Township.[a] Several HMC representatives served on its Board, including Pellegrino, administrator Ed Grant[b] and George Hanks and Wescott from the HMC Board. The documents of incorporation said that income from the fund Large donated would be used

> to establish or maintain in whole or in part charitable, scientific, literary or educational activities, agencies, institutions or cor-porations already established. To provide medical surgical and hospital care for persons in need of assistance; to provide funds for the erection of additional hospital buildings or facilities and the purchase of equipment therefore; to offer training for doctors and nurses in special problems connected with the aging, and to establish endowment funds to help maintain the services to be rendered by said hospitals, provided said hospitals and the services rendered thereby are supported in whole or in part by private charities.[2]

The Large Foundation has not only been most generous to HMC, but has provided a grant for part of the expenses of producing this

[a] Large, like many other leaders in the community, was prominent in local Republican politics and also served in the state Senate. In the 1930s he assisted the prosecution in the trial of Bruno Richard Hauptmann for the notorious kidnapping and murder of the infant son of Charles Lindbergh. Large's law practice was greatly aided by state tax law at the time; Flemington, and in particular his office, became the official headquarters of a number of large corporations.

[b] Grant always maintained that Large asked him to serve on the Board because he was a good storyteller. A favorite told of an HMC patient who arrived late in labor and delivered her infant on the grounds. When she received a bill for delivery room services, she complained and was told by the clerk, "Well then, we'll call it a Greens Fee." According to Grant, "Judge Large took a fit of laughing at that . . . and he asked me to join his Large Foundation." Grant E. Interview by author, 6 February 1996.

book. Attorney and HMC Board member Wesley Lance reported that Judge Large had been initially skeptical about the need for, and success of, the Medical Center.[3] However, Judge Large became enthusiastic enough to write (unsuccessfully) to John D. Rockefeller to solicit funds for HMC on the strength of the belief that the Rockefeller ancestors had first settled in Hunterdon County, and that a gravestone existed.[4]

HMC By-Laws as adopted 26 June 1953 stated that the attending medical staff (this term includes both family physicians and specialists) shall have the direct care of all charity patients in the hospital.[5] No other reference to the medically indigent is contained in the document. When I arrived at HMC in 1959 I saw a memorandum of agreement between the Hunterdon County Medical Society and HMC on the care of the indigent. The agreement said physicians and hospital would care for every resident of Hunterdon County in the same way, regardless of financial status or ability to pay. It was to be a one-class system—no public clinics or public wards for the poor. Selection of patients for clinical or case teaching by physicians would not be influenced by social status or financial factors. Everyone made appointments the same way; everyone was cared for in the same beds. The mental health program relied on this approach as it sought to make the Medical Center an example of mental-health-oriented health care. The memorandum predated Medicare and Medicaid laws by some years.

None of the early specialists or other physicians with whom I spoke recalled other documents that formalized this policy. All agree, however, that a policy reflecting the substance of the memo existed. There apparently was no structured discussion by staff or Board. *Patients were simply taken care of. Everyone would be treated alike.* On admission, a patient received care from a family physician or specialist, according to the nature of the medical problem, not according to the ability to pay. When Pellegrino was Medical Director, he spoke to community groups about the deficit, offering to show them hospital accounting records to demonstrate that the deficit was not from inefficiency or poor management, but from care for members of the community who could not afford care. Pellegrino said that when he became Medical Director, "we did find shoe boxes filled with accounts receivable—bills which had not been sent out."[6] Lou Doyle, a family physician, recalled that on his arrival at Hunterdon in 1958, he was told that

you would do your share in the office, which [family doctors]
did gracefully, never billed these people, never bothered with
collection, and as a result the hospital would not open . . .
clinics . . . They would not deny seeing people in the emergency room and again at no charge if there were money problems . . . There was not a welfare clinic . . . It never would
be.[7]

DIFFICULTIES IN THE SECOND DECADE

After a decade differences arose between specialists and family physicians about responsibility for the indigent and/or patients who
came to attention at inconvenient hours. Some specialists believed
that poor patients, without a source of payment or with a very
limited source such as Medicaid, were being referred in dispropor-
tionate numbers by the family physicians to the specialist, and
similarly with respect to patients who called for help at night or
on weekends. On the other hand, some family physicians felt that
specialists were difficult to recruit for help under the same circumstances. The intensity of such feelings was low, in part because
there were few pockets of poverty in the county. Those of limited
or no income were scattered throughout the county. However,
low-level irritations were part of a larger series of differences described in Chapter 16. With the inauguration of an Integrated Delivery System in the 1990s, formal arrangements between physicians
and HMC have been made, including care for all the indigent in
same manner as paying patients. HMC receives some state funds
for this purpose, shared with physicians.

PREPAYMENT HEALTH CARE INSURANCE

EARLY NATIONAL EFFORTS

During the second decade of the 20th century fraternal or benevo-
lent societies whose members were bound together by a common
tie began to offer insurance for sickness care for their members. A
Special Bulletin from the American Association for Labor Legislation, February 1919, was devoted to the "Three fears: the fear of
ill-health, the fear of unemployment and the fear of want in old
age . . . The greatest of these will be banished by universal health

insurance."[8] Health insurance and prepayment plans were not unknown prior to the founding of Hunterdon Medical Center. In
1916, the distinguished Boston physician Richard Cabot, who had
pioneered the development of hospital social work departments to
help patients obtain the care they needed, called for a system of
health care insurance centered on the hospital or group practice.
Such a plan, he believed, would offer better care for less money.[9]

Blue Cross plans arose with the Great Depression. According
to Rothman, the first was started in 1929 by Baylor University in
Texas: up to 21 days of free hospital care a year for a premium of
$3 a semester was offered to schoolteachers.[10] By the time Ann
Stevenson organized the Blue Cross group for the Hunterdon County
Board of Agriculture, during and just after World War II, national membership was close to two million. By 1950, half the
population had some sort of hospital coverage.[11]

Rothman contends that the Blue plans grew to provide protection for the middle class against catastrophic hospital bills; provide financial security for the hospital system to which they were
principally responsive; and prevent creation of a national health
program. He points out that Rorem, ostensibly the fire-breathing
leader of the movement to offer protection for everyone and also
the first head of the Blue Cross system, "was indefatigable in making known that supporting Blue Cross was the best way to fore-
stall a compulsory national health insurance system." These plans
offered private, voluntary, nongovernmental protection for middle
class employed or self-employed families. They did not attend to
the poor, nor did they offer encouragement for health care and
preventive medicine.[12] Rothman pointedly contrasts the advertise-
ments by Metropolitan Life for its group insurance program in
the 1950s, featuring preventive health care and early consultation
with a family physician.

PLANS AT HUNTERDON

Four attempts were made to establish a prepayment or managed
care program (terminology has changed through the years). None
succeeded. In 1950 Trussell and Commonwealth's Lester Evans considered an insurance mechanism a matter of high priority.[13] Trussell
recalled no specifics of those early discussions but added: "To do
so without an enormous amount of advance planning about how

to get primary care taken care of by the family doctors and how to make them part of an integrated insurer arrangement—it just simply never came to fruition."[c]

The Health Insurance Plan of Greater New York (HIP) was founded 1 March 1947. By 1951 it had over a quarter million subscribers. HIP was a capitation program offering physician care by groups of primary care and specialist physicians, with particular emphasis on health education, preventive examinations and early recognition and cure of disease. HIP included older persons, demonstrating that their care was financially feasible to incorporate into a general health insurance plan. In a published description of the plan, George Baehr, the President and Medical Director, presciently wrote:

> If voluntary hospitals and voluntary insurance plans cannot evolve ways and means of including [the aging population] governmental institutions will have to be provided and the cost met . . . through taxation . . . The point at which the insurance dollar and the public . . . dollar meet has to be carefully fixed, but both must be there. The point at which these two forces meet in our free society is determined in large part by our theories, preconceptions, practical experiences of the past, and hopes for the future.[14]

By 1951, the Health Insurance Plan of Greater New York was well established.

Late in 1950, Wescott, Evans and Geddes Smith discussed group prepayment or group practice. Smith noted: "Wescott is clearly disinclined to suggest an inclusive prepayment plan on the general basis of HIP, which would cover both general and special services."[15]

Despite Smith's note, Trussell recalls he had received a deputation of labor representatives from Riegel Paper Company in Milford (which had made the largest pledge to HMC's fund drive—$50,000) who were interested in a prepayment program of insurance of some sort:

> These people were particularly interested in three things. The idea of an annual checkup done by a general practitioner supplemented by a package of laboratory and x-ray tests in the Medical

---

[c] Trussell also recalled his embarrassment at being elected to the Society of Scholars of Johns Hopkins University in 1975 for starting the first HMO in the United States, since the Kaiser plan was already well established when Hunterdon was being created. Trussell's memory was not always perfect. See material in Chapter 7. Trussell RE. Interview by author, 5 December 1955.

> Center, all-inclusive voluntary health insurance and a blood
> bank . . . The meeting was very constructive and indicates the
> pressures which a man on salary finds himself when it comes
> to medical care.[16]

Trussell and I agree that this was a measure of public interest in the idea, particularly since it came from a labor group, perhaps not particularly sophisticated in health delivery affairs, but responding to the climate of the times.

HMC's Summary Statement of Objectives, of January–February, 1952, mentions prepayment insurance, along with services to the chronically ill and evaluation of services, as "yet to be studied and developed in detail, if feasible."[17] On 27 June 1952, the Board appointed a Committee on Third Party Payments chaired by R. Carter Nicholas[d] and Bill Lamont, the Board's Treasurer. Nicholas explored relations with a number of different entities and plans. Inevitably, Louise Leicester was intensely involved, providing the Committee with "leads, and with a considerable, if not formidable bibliography."[18] Nicholas commented: "Since it became apparent that the scope of this committee's investigation was enormous, and that the apparent boundaries were merely curtains which parted at the slightest touch, I called Dr. Evans of the Commonwealth Fund to ask for advice and assistance."[19] Evans worked his usual magic to provide an introduction to Kenneth Williamson, the Executive Secretary, and Odin Anderson, the Research Director of the Health Insurance Foundation of New York (HIF). Williamson, of course, knew Louise Leicester. HIF was eager to initiate a national series of prepayment insurance plans for entire countywide populations, including public assistance recipients. In March 1953, Anderson met with Trussell. Ever skeptical, Trussell wrote Evans:

> Hunterdon Medical Center is not in a position to undertake
> an insurance program at the time it opens next July 1. The
> amount of study, negotiation, legal proceeding, and so forth,
> required to establish a medical care insurance program in New
> Jersey is considerable, and we have never given any serious
> thought to attempting to start out with a combined service
> and insurance program on the day of opening . . . We are . . .
> definitely looking forward to the possibility.[20]

[d] Nicholas RC. Report of Committee on Third Party Payments, 4 June 1953. Prepayment Insurance file, HMCA. Nicholas, an attorney, was not a member of the Board at that time, but had participated in the incorporation of the Blue Cross hospital plan in New York City. He was an uncle of J. Seward Johnson, an influential early Board member.

Trussell and Wescott discussed with Evans the timing of such a venture. Anderson and the Health Insurance Foundation wanted to conduct a utilization study in Hunterdon County, paid for by a Commonwealth grant. The entire population of the county would be enrolled as a "laboratory to test" marketing techniques and to study managing a health insurance program.[e] HIF would have jurisdiction over the entire venture, and Commonwealth was to underwrite a health insurance program if created. Trussell was wary of any study conducted by an outside group "in which the Medical Center did not have a direct professional participation."[21] Besides lack of control, he was concerned about conflicting goals because financing came from two different foundations. Trussell was never interested in ventures when he did not exert direct control.[f]

Nicholas told the Executive Committee on 12 February 1953 that they were looking at a countywide insurance group. In April he and others from Hunterdon, Commonwealth and HIF discussed this further.[22] Wescott reported on 1 May that Commonwealth was interested "in financing any studies which need to be done on developing an insurance program [and] the underwriting of an insurance program should we elect to do one. This is a project which will take two or three years to develop."[23] The final recommendations of the Nicholas Committee were that HMC contract with the Blues, honor patients' private plans, form an employee Blue Cross group, consider publicizing the fact that all county residents could join the Board of Agriculture group started by Ann Stevenson, and proceed with the contemplated prepayment study.

Nothing ever came of it all. Trussell and Pellegrino framed the issue as just too much to do. I would also add to this serious concerns about how the venture would turn out and the impact it might have on other, more central programs. Contemporaneous records indicate political infighting played a role, along with concerns about hospital or corporate practice of medicine, a major issue of the day on which the AMA regularly erupted. Memories of President Truman's unsuccessful efforts to obtain a national health insurance system, and the intensity of opposition to this form of "socialism" probably also played a role in diminishing enthusiasm at Hunterdon.[24] Wescott, however, did not give up. The topic was

[e] This was very reminiscent of the goals for the second such venture, in the 1970s, in which I was a participant.

[f] The matter of control—this time related to the executive rather than the Board—was exactly the same issue as that raised by Louise Leicester earlier.

raised in a letter to Evans at Commonwealth devoted to other more pressing matters[25] and yet again in a letter six months later mentioning "a beginning study of the potential for an insurance program with the Medical Center as the focus."[26] As for the involvement of the specialists, pediatrician Andrew Hunt states that insurance was discussed only in casual conversation, not at meetings of the specialist group. In 1962 an administrative resident from the Columbia School of Public Health, Steven Sieverts, again raised the issue. The Medical Director recommended giving it serious consideration or dropping the idea permanently.[27] It appears the latter was the decision.

In 1950, a different insurance issue opened when Wescott met representatives of the Blues about a reimbursement rate for hospital care. Trussell reported: "They tried to give him the brush-off. They said we were financed by a foundation and they weren't going to pay. He really took them head-on. I wasn't there but he told me about it. You know how he could be. So they included us into Blue Cross."[28] Despite favorable evidence from various sources,[29] HMC did not adopt an inclusive rate structure for inpatient care until it was mandated by state regulators. An inclusive rate structure means a fixed dollar amount per patient day in the hospital to cover all care. The hospital loses money if the patient needs unusually intensive care and makes money if the patient's care requirements are minimal. Trussell said, "The only other insurance issue was at the County Medical Society meeting in which we discussed what our people in the hospital would use as a basis for charges. It was agreed that our full-time people would use the New Jersey Blue Shield fee schedule. Certainly such fees were modest enough."[30]

LATER DEVELOPMENTS: THE 1970S TO THE 1990S

Prepayment came to the forefront from 1970 to 1972, with a strenuous effort to create a program in HMO form, the Hunterdon Health Plan. After prolonged and regrettably acrimonious debate, the specialist staff voted against such an idea.

Lloyd Wescott, in typical fashion, adopted an idea from his experience: He had served on the Perloff Committee of the American Hospital Association. In 1970 the AHA published the Ameriplan concept, which was nothing less than a blueprint for national health insurance to which everyone who was able would contribute.[31] Service on this committee was for Wescott a major event, and I remember his often referring to what he learned at the meetings. The Committee was formed predominantly of hospital executives; the report was of, by and for the hospitals of the United States. In retrospect, one sees that the report accomplished little or nothing to further the concept except to fuel Wescott's enthusiasm for another go at a prepayment program. He found an ally in William Kissick, of the faculty at the Wharton School of the University of Pennsylvania. Wescott also brought in the Prudential Insurance Company, at that time interested in testing the HMO waters. Prudential agreed to help with initial financing.

Kissick, an enthusiastic soul, saw opportunity at Hunterdon. Financed in part by Prudential, he and his associates of the Leonard Davis Institute of Health Economics at Wharton made preliminary investigations. They found a low ratio of patient days to population at HMC.[g] Since insurance premiums for Hunterdon County residents were similar to those charged elsewhere in the state and expensive inpatient utilization was low, the third-party payers were pocketing quite a profit. To the Leonard Davis group this differential offered the possibility of enormous savings, comparable to those obtained at the Kaiser plans. If HMC and Medical Staff joined to create an HMO, they could offer significantly lower premiums with financial security by keeping the difference between predicted (by the insurance companies) and actual community inpatient utilization.

The concept was certainly realistic. Implementation required capitation. This means payment to primary care physicians at a fixed sum per year per patient cared for plus a lump sum per patient per year to be dispersed for specialty care. This provided financial incentive for the physician to make conservative care decisions, particularly of expensive inpatient care. A bitter debate ensued. Felix Salerno, spokesperson for a majority of the specialists, said that "the HMO was felt by the physicians to be a threat . . . It was controlling . . . We were worried about how much external influence would come from the group at Penn . . . or from the

[g] Their data revealed that compared to the rest of New Jersey, HMC's average length of stay was a full day less, community admission rates a third less and per capita costs of care comparably lower. Planning and Implementation Recommendations for the Hunterdon Health Plan. 1970, W. Kissick et al., Leonard Davis Institute of Health Economics, University of Pennsylvania, Philadelphia, PA. Prepayment file, HMCA.

federal government?"[32] Other risks of capitation were too great—
potential loss of income, a structure (Hunterdon Health Plan, HHP)
to which physicians would be irrevocably tied and general fears of
the new and untried. At the time, the role of the University of
Pennsylvania group had not been fully defined. They had been
engaged, as noted, to perform a study. They hoped to have the
primary consulting and design role in the proposed HMO, the HHP.
Many felt the project was created by Wescott for his own glory
and personal advancement, although I saw and heard nothing to
suggest this. (Full disclosure: I served as professional leader of the
venture, the Executive Director.) In March 1972, the staff, by a
wide margin, voted down the plan. Ever since, relations between
staff and Board have been strained, at times quite difficult.

In hindsight, the plan might have failed not because of an in-
trinsic flaw, but because HMC and its Medical Staff were not intellectually or emotionally ready for capitation. Of the core concepts
of managed care,[33] some, such as the central position of primary
care, and coordination and interdependence among many professions, were already in place at Hunterdon. Others, such as acceptance of some sort of controlling influence and the need for extensive
information on patients and clinicians, were not. HMC physicians
were accustomed to advocate for the individual patient, rather than
the welfare of the health care organization. Perhaps staff could
have eventually worked in an HMO, but only with extensive and
prolonged educational efforts, including sensitive response to physician concerns.

The third major effort to create a prepayment system occurred
in 1987–1988 during Donald Davis's tenure as President (1979–
1990). He negotiated with the Blue plans for a prepayment health
care system, based on evidence that HMC's physicians continued to
practice conservative health care, with a low level of resource utilization. Ten years earlier McKinsey & Company[34] found that HMC's
inpatient days, and both outpatient and inpatient care costs, were
well below comparable New Jersey and U.S. figures. For example,
for the population served by HMC, inpatient days per 1,000 per
year were 768, compared to 1,262 for New Jersey as a whole, 1,212
for the United States, and 524 at Kaiser. Per capita inpatient costs
were $132, compared to $180 for New Jersey and $185 for the United
States. There were fewer hospital beds and fewer physicians in the
community. Davis felt Hunterdon could still produce comparable

conservative resource utilization. Although most physicians at Hunterdon were practicing independent fee-for-service medicine, they displayed the same careful approach to utilization of health care resources. Physicians do not, despite what economists think, always behave in a manner to maximize financial gain.[35] Davis was able to win from the Blue plans agreement that they would assume the "upside risk and split the downside risk with us, 50 percent to us and 50 percent to them."[36] By this he meant that the Blue plans would absorb losses, and split profits due to lower than predicted utilization half and half with the physicians. However, the Medical Staff would not agree to proceed.

I believe on an anecdotal basis working with many colleagues at HMC that population and physician attitudes remain conservative. However, the controversy over physician responsibility to the individual patient versus the responsibility to a given population in a world of limited resources appears to have been settled.[37] The marketplace now controls ethical medical choice—the degree to which the physician is able to do everything he or she perceives as needed by the patient. Now we can watch whether or not patient trust in the physician will survive this change and whether patients will accept this change and agree to give up the mantra of "spare no [insurance] expense."[38] If it is true that local utilization is conservative, and relatively low, it will be easier for local physicians to make this transition. They will have lost the opportunity to share in the savings, but they have preserved some degree of autonomy, at least for a few years. It may also be possible to avoid some of the ill effects of excessive medical care.[39] Since the rapid transition from capitation to discounted fee-for-service payments by insurers, risks have shifted back to the companies, but at the price of incentives for physicians to do less, work faster, and order more tests and procedures. Latest data on physician earnings suggest that in general physicians are not only not participating in any possible savings, but are earning less, and working harder to do it.[40]

The final effort to respond to the changing health care environment and to create some sort of prepayment plan began in 1993 with efforts to create a Medical Service Organization, including with the Medical Center sufficient members of the staff to provide a wide range of services. In 1990 Robert Wise, whose selection signaled the Board's concern about furthering transition into a new environment, succeeded Davis. Wise elected to create a joint planning process to refocus on HMC's original mission: "The large health care systems are not adding more value to the community per health care dollar other than what is accomplished locally. Adherence to the original premises—that is, conservative use of resources combined with education on healthy life-styles and preventive medicine would be the best approach to ensure a healthy community."[41]

Creation of a medical office building, which opened in 1989, had brought the Staff, Board and Administration together in a cooperative venture for the first time in many years. Wise built on this by pushing for joint ventures with physicians. HMC had given up, towards the end of the Davis's tenure, attempting to provide management services for medical practices. Hospital administrative expertise was a very different matter from outpatient and physician administrative expertise. Wise believes that "hospitals in general are notoriously poor at being service-responsive to the private practice of medicine."[42] He agrees that salaried physicians should obtain medical management expertise. An Integrated Delivery System (IDS) has been formed: a 50–50 partnership between the Hunterdon Health Care Systems and self-selected members of the medical staff. About two-thirds of the staff (120 physicians) have joined. There are contracts with most managed care organizations in place. The IDS provides services to patients through member physicians and hospital; financial arrangements are more favorable and overhead is reduced. The initial purchase of a family practice by the Medical Center produced a storm of medical staff opposition, arising from residual distrust of Board and administration from years of conflict, as well as the staff's perception it was not involved with or notified about the arrangement. Other purchases have since taken place. My perception of staff attitudes based on multiple casual communications is that some lack of trust persists. Larry Grand, Executive Vice President and Chief Operations Officer, states in contrast that there is a significant degree of trust, confidence and strength in multiple joint ventures of hospital and medical staff.[43] He feels relationships are open, honest, supportive and collaborative. If he is correct, this is a major change from what I witnessed for many years.

CHAPTER 15

Community and Ambulant Care Facility

To what extent was HMC to function beyond the bounds of the traditional community hospital—as an ambulant care center, to prevent sickness and promote health? In the early days, the Board and professional advisers pulled together the best wisdom of the day. The Committee on the Costs of Medical Care advocated for the community hospital to be engaged in the community.[1] Lester Evans wrote in 1938 about the importance of community hospital collaboration in traditional public health areas and spoke of the hospital's role in the health of the individual when not an inpatient. Health care (preventive medicine in the terminology of the day) rather than sickness care was a recognized goal. A hospital was not just a place to send the sick, but the central node for all efforts to maintain and enhance the health of every individual.[2] In the 1940s, many others were exploring these ideas. Walker enumerated many ways in which productive collaboration could take place.[3] Cody wrote: "We passed . . . from the time when the hospital was merely a remedial institution to the time when it is a positive, constructive apostle of health."[4] In the pediatric age range, Brown outlined a program at the Hospital for Sick Children in Toronto anticipating with uncanny prescience what Hunt and Parmet hoped to accomplish at HMC.[5]

At Hunterdon, plans for mental health, school health, public health, health education, and a home for community agencies fit such a concept. To fit this approach, the Board changed the name of the small ambulant care office building from the Clinic Building to the Diagnostic Center, which name it and its successor structure held for years.[a] It was the Diagnostic Center, not Treatment Center, because patients would be referred back to the family

---

[a] Because this was—and still is—a one class system, there were to be no clinics or hospital wards at HMC.

physician for treatment. Or, so the thinking was then. Trussell's request for funds to initiate an integrated health program was built on this, and on the integration of all community health and welfare services. It never came to be. Did the Board understand the implications? No one is now alive who can say so. Some think not. Ray Trussell said:

> If you go back to those Board of Agriculture minutes, you will find that they say that the project was going to be a Health Center. I think frankly that you had a group of laymen who were picking up words and had only the most general idea of what they were talking about. The preventive aspects were approached in part accidentally by our doing that Chronic Illness Survey. We did a lot of screening of people who normally would never have been screened.[6]

The Chronic Illness Survey

ORIGINS

Concern about the burden of chronic illness, particularly among older citizens, was voiced during HMC's earliest planning stages.[7] Rose Angell pointed to this area of need in her reports to the Welfare Board, and Louise Leicester raised unanswered questions. At the time Trussell arrived in Flemington, the National Commission on Chronic Illness, headed by former Surgeon General Thomas Parran, employed as Director Dr. Morton Levin, a well-known cancer epidemiologist, on loan from the New York State Health Department where he knew Trussell.[8] The Commission received a grant from Commonwealth to conduct a survey and asked Trussell if he would take on the rural section at Hunterdon.[b] Trussell agreed, although the drain on time and energy was far greater than he had anticipated. Levin and Trussell developed objectives: to determine for rural patients the prevalence of chronic disease, needs for care, and rehabilitative potential. The National Opinion Research Center was to conduct the survey. Jack Elinson, an employee of the Center, was placed in charge. Trussell described Elinson as a real

---

[b] Elinson believes it was Trussell who initiated arrangements to have the rural portion of the study done in Hunterdon County (Elinson J. Interview by author, 7 December 1995). However, a letter from Trussell to Evans seems to confirm that the arrangement originated with Evans and Commonwealth. Trussell RE to LJ Evans, 23 August 1950. RAC, CF. Commonwealth 1950 file, HMCA.

find, with marvelous insight and intuitive, accurate judgment on major questions relating to sampling methods, survey tools, statistics and other epidemiological issues.

JACK ELINSON, PH.D

Jack Elinson, raised in a slum, graduated from City College at 20, joined the War Department as a psychologist and performed pioneering work in large-scale testing, surveys, and statistics during and after World War II.[9] Little sociological work had been done on health surveys, according to Elinson: "That kind of work was given to people who were very junior because health was not an important sociological question—not like race relations, or morale or why we fight, questions which were given to the senior [researchers] . . . I learned my trade there . . . I regard that as really my graduate education."[10] To converse with Jack Elinson is to long to have taken courses with him. He speaks in complete, crystal clear, informative sentences, with enthusiasm and vigor and is a born storyteller. Trussell said he was one of the most popular and effective teachers on the faculty at Columbia. It is easy to see why.

Elinson was superb at working with other professionals. Trussell describes how: "When the social workers and the public health nurses were having trouble, he would say, 'Sit down and write out what it is you do.' He would get people to commit themselves."[11] He helped reconcile differences within the survey clinical team by focusing on what kind of care was needed based on clinical findings, rather than which professional should provide that care. Selection of a caretaker for a particular problem depended upon local features of the patient's community, available caretakers and their abilities. After completing field work on the Chronic Illness Survey, Elinson joined the Columbia University School of Public Health, where Trussell had become Dean, and where Elinson has remained in epidemiology, medical sociology and biostatistics.

PERFORMING THE SURVEY

There were five phases of data gathering:

1. Community Self-Survey: In 1952 volunteers delivered a 12-page demographic and health questionnaire to every household in

the county. Marguerite L. Moore, who led the volunteer portion for many phases of the study, describes this effort: "All this was done at a very busy season in the farmer's year and during the closing time for schools. Yet these time-consuming operations . . . were done with patience, understanding and good will by approximately six hundred persons."[12] Of 43,000 questionnaires, 56 percent were completed and returned. Although not sufficient for statistically rigorous study, it introduced a large portion of the county to the new hospital, scheduled to open a year later.

2. Family Interviews: A geographic-area sample of the population was interviewed for the purpose of encompassing a year's health history of the entire family within a single folder. Interviews were performed by schoolteachers trained to interview. Every municipality was mapped, and every residence on each map was identified. Mechanical drawing classes in the high schools created many maps, and students presented their results at assemblies.

3. Medical Verification: To check on conditions reported on interview as having been attended by the family physician, physician records were compared with interview reports. More than four-fifths of physicians approached provided information from their records. Most conditions mentioned by patients on interview were found in physician records. However, a third of the conditions found in the physician records had not been mentioned by the patients on interview.

4. Clinical evaluation was performed by examination of a random sample of patients by internists or pediatricians. Marguerite Moore, together with Helen de Rochemont arranged for examinations, follow-up tests, and consultations.[c] Moore often gave sales talks to rural people who never had a complete physical examination, and "who were not eager to find out that there might be something wrong . . . A very considerable number of those persons who first refused . . . said 'yes' when Mrs. de Rochemont or I reopened the subject . . . Since the county had come to consider the Medical Center and its projects as its own, it was felt a duty to

[c] Moore says of de Rochemont: "Her assistance was invaluable to the whole project. Her insight, friendly influence on people and her interpreting of the Medical Center to the people and the people to the Medical Center was an outstanding civic contribution done wholly on a non-paid basis" (Moore M. Records of Conduct of Chronic Illness Survey, n.d. Moore file, HMCA). De Rochemont was also very involved with the development of mental health services in the county. She and her husband Richard de Rochemont, who produced *The March of Time*, a pioneering news film shown in theaters, owned a large farm in Raritan Township and later built an unusual octagonal home (*Current Biography*, 1945).

say 'yes.'"[13] Margaret B. Wiles was the nurse on the survey team. She interviewed the patients selected for examinations, reviewed the clinical data obtained from them, and drew up recommendations for nursing needs.[14] A nurse who assisted in examinations reports that while some patients were grateful for the free and very complete examinations, others felt differently: "There were the old-timers who felt the examiners were being too nosey. The old-time farmers, you know—well, if there is something wrong with you and you don't know, what's the difference? You just keep on going."[15]

5. Multiple screening sought evidence of nonmanifest disease. Another volunteer effort was begun in the fall of 1953 to convince those persons found in good health at the time of the family interview to undergo screening tests. Barely a third agreed, perhaps because less effort was put into this phase. The concept of screening was then established, and for many years volunteers staffed a Multiple Screening program at HMC that offered, without charge, blood pressure, urine and other types of screening. With the passage of time, questions about the value of such screening tests appeared in the literature, and interest in the program decreased, It was eventually discontinued.

The specialist staff participated little in the survey, except for performing examinations. Hunt recalls no meeting to explain the project or its background. Trussell never took him or the others into his confidence. Most of the survey subjects examined were adults, and internists Pauline Goger and Robert Henderson, who were hired for the Chronic Illness Survey, did the evaluations. Physicians were instructed to proceed as if they were doing a consultation. They performed a medical history, physical examination, and requested laboratory tests, images, and consultations, as appropriate.

RESULTS

The results of the Chronic Illness Survey provided information not only about the principal goals, but also unexpected information about the methods used. The survey found:

1. High prevalence of chronic conditions or persons believed by the clinician to be at risk for chronic conditions (six out of seven examined). Elinson says: "We used to have a joke that if an

internist examined someone and didn't find a condition, the person had not been well examined."[16] On examination, 1.3 conditions per person were reported.

2. Many residents of the county were exposed to HMC even before the building was completed. Medical records were opened on all county residents who participated in any phase of the Survey. Many conditions not previously known were identified. Trussell said: "A large number of doctors got some useful information from the Medical Center in a nonthreatening way and it really had a jump start effect."[17]

3. Community expectations: Suggestions for services to be offered by HMC were solicited. Seven hundred persons replied. Mrs. Morris Parmet, a social worker, and Helen de Rochemont tabulated the answers.[18] Respondents revealed high, even idealistic expectations, and most felt the goals were attainable. A major source of future difficulty for HMC lay in these expectations, which probably were more than any medical center could have delivered. When staff and administration did not live up to those ideals, a backlash resulted when less than perfect care was provided.

4. Clinical examination of a randomly selected, geographically defined population: There was debate over whether to include people who described themselves well, rather than only those with a self-described chronic illness diagnosis on interview. On advice of Eli Marks, sampling statistician for the Bureau of the Census, everyone in the county was included in the sample.[d] This yielded a surprising result: a great deal of disease in people who reported none in the interview, either because they were unaware or had not been told. Of every four conditions found by clinicians only one was reported on interview.

5. Methodological comparisons of the work of the two internists: Their responsibilities were identical; patients were assigned at random, but examinations were not standardized. Productivity in terms of time per patient and diagnoses per patient were measured. One of them, "I forgot who," said Trussell, completed the examinations much faster. The other took more time but produced more diagnoses. I believe Trussell and Elinson avoided this issue during our interviews.

[d] Pellegrino felt that he had the definitive role in arranging for clinical evaluations: "My role in the Chronic Illness Survey was to provide the absolutely essential clinical input, to insist on actual examination of the patients."

6. Evaluation of various epidemiological approaches to measuring chronic illness: "[The survey] changed the views of many in the field of public health as to the validity, reliability and generalizability of methods of estimating morbidity in a population," according to Elinson.[19] This finding had a major influence on the National Health Survey, originally visualized as solely a household interview survey. Trussell and Elinson were invited to present their data at a meeting in Washington with the staff of the National Health Survey (which they described as "hostile"). The result was that the National Survey revised its plans and added health examinations.

7. Concepts of disease versus illness: For Elinson, this became a central concept that influenced his work for the remainder of his career—the difference between what people feel when they talk about themselves as being sick or ill (illness) and the results of a clinical evaluation (disease). Trussell and Elinson wrote: "We take note of a major deficiency in the Hunterdon County study, in its companion study in Baltimore, and in virtually all household or family interview surveys of 'morbidity' . . . The defect is the failure adequately to conceptualize, make clear, and take account of the distinction between disease and illness."[20] Elinson later said:

> Disease is a label which a medically trained person, a physician, gives to a set of observations that has been made, whether it is via test or whether it is a physical examination or whether it is reporting . . . an agreed-upon label so that the definition of these different diseases have more or less been systematized. Symptoms do not come with a disease label attached to them. The label has to be given to them; and it is given by medicine, by physicians. My subsequent career has been in recognizing differences between the way a physician looks at a person and finds a "disease" based on a set of observations—you can attach a number to it from the International Classification of Diseases and Causes of Death—and what people think about themselves . . . as to how they function, the way they expect to be functioning, and whether they are bothered by bodily conditions. Because of my work on the Hunterdon study, at a meeting . . . I came up with a classification of health care outcomes—there is death, disease, disability, discomfort and dissatisfaction. Physicians pay most attention to . . . disease as a cause of death (or disability). [Of those of which

survivors are concerned] people tend to pay attention more to disability, discomfort and dissatisfactions.[21]

What Elinson called disease, I would call diagnosis—a label or construct found empirically useful by clinicians and scientists. One cannot assume that a construct is grounded in truth. Both diagnoses and illnesses have fuzzy boundaries. What exists in nature, which we can know but imperfectly, I would call disease. In every instance, I argue that the central concept may be more or less clear, but the boundaries are soft. For example, an infant diagnosed with cystic fibrosis on the strength of DNA analysis was, and remains, clinically well.[22] Had the child been seen before availability of DNA studies, she would have been diagnosed as normal. The use of terms such as "disease" and "diagnosis" interchangeably, with lack of precision, unfortunately continues.

Study clinicians felt hampered by the need to use uniform classification schemes, with coding of all health conditions identified. Pellegrino, in particular, believed coding imposed mechanical rigidity on the relationship between patient and doctor, destructive to good medical care. He went on to say that "if medicine should get to be computerized like this, he would leave it . . . I am sure that from the statistical point of view our clinical thinking appears very muddled."[23] Many years later he said:

> Often we felt that we could not honestly fit patients or their signs and symptoms under the prescribed categories . . . The differences [are] the divergence between the individualized, personalized, clinician's approach and the statistician's population based approach—this is the same divide that separates us in managed care today when the economists want us to use population ethics as opposed to individual patient ethics in the interests of managed care.[24]

SURVEY FOLLOW-UP

As early as 1954, Trussell was thinking about following up on the data accumulated from the survey. He dreamed of studies to determine what became of the patients, the extent to which the problems were dealt with, what services were in place and continuing surveys of incidence and prevalence. The original survey included no plan to follow the individuals studied. Later, the notion of replicating the survey would surface, then disappear. Questions about the health care in Hunterdon County and whether a fresh survey would reveal changes in prevalence or appropriate care would be discussed. The School of Health supported by Seward Johnson was to do this, but never became organized or truly functional. Funding from other sources was not obtained.

Public Health Department

EARLY EFFORTS

Soon after World War II, interest in joint housing and administration of public health departments, community hospitals and laboratories appeared in many areas.[25] Commonwealth's Carolina Randolph conducted a survey in Hunterdon County in 1950 that revealed disparate and uncoordinated public health elements,[26] costing well over $50,000 a year.[27] HMC's Board, Commonwealth, local authorities, Trussell and Daniel Bergsma, the N.J. Commissioner of Public Health, envisioned a County Health Department as a unit of HMC. Important functions such as home health care, health education, sanitation and statistical analysis were to be added. By the end of 1950 plans were in place for these efforts, to be housed in a building designed for combined services.

HEALTH EDUCATION

In the mid 20th century the climate of ideas about health education for the public was quite well developed; realization was scanty. A program of health education in hospitals and outpatient departments was described as World War II ended.[28] Hunterdon plans included a position for a public health educator, as developed in an unsigned document, most likely written by Trussell.

> The goal of the public health educator would be to develop a local health education program as an integral part of the total community health program . . . [and] motivate people towards the development of positive health habits.
>
> The person . . . must have the ability to help create a well-informed public opinion and have exceptional ability to stimulate concerted action based on facts . . . He must operate on the basic belief that any problem can be worked out if people get the facts they need, think clearly about these facts and plan

together to do what needs to be done . . . He must also be
pleasing in appearance, have poise, tact and special ability to
meet and work with various segments of the population.[e]

The public educator position was never implemented. Ten years
later, in 1961, Seward Johnson wrote HMC's Medical Director about
the importance of health education and proposing that a School
of Public Health be created with the income from $10,000,000 in
Johnson & Johnson stock he made available.[29] Nothing came of
it. In 1986, Lloyd Wescott described to HMC's then President what
happened:

> Seward's interest, I am absolutely sure, was the interest of
> *individuals* in a community; not the community as a *group* of
> people with its own *group* needs. He was always bothered by
> the impersonal approach to health care. His concern was the
> individual in need . . . Seward's attempt [was] to establish
> what he hoped would be a school of health, not a school of
> *public* health, and which was so badly mishandled by the staff
> at Hunterdon . . . [that] the lawyer for Seward decided that
> the school had to be dissolved and the assets distributed, as
> years of gifts had been made and no school existed.[30]

Of the endowment, 40 percent of the funds went to the
Smithsonian, 20 percent to HMC, and 40 percent to Rutgers Medical School for programs in health. The latter was earmarked to
support programs related to the Hunterdon area. However, after
grants supporting early intervention for disabled children and lactation programs, and in 1974 to found a Department of Health
Education at HMC (a large and very vital division),[31] the remaining
funds were devoted to projects of the New Jersey College of Medicine and Dentistry. The conflict between the goal of the best of
care for the individual and the best of care for the community,
which remains one of the central issues in health care today, was
never directly confronted. Then and now the best method to achieve
both goals is education that convinces individuals to adopt healthy

[e] Background Statement Re: Public Health Educator; 20 February 1951, found in Commonwealth Fund archives, but apparently typed on an HMC typewriter. RAC, CF. Such an approach verges on radical in light of the thinking of that time, when it was rare indeed for
medical professionals to emphasize the wishes and self-defined needs of either individuals,
families or population groups. Professionals who served in an advisory capacity, or as sources of
information, did not see themselves as negotiating with autonomous individuals who planned
for their future health, although Spence, cited elsewhere, came very close.

life styles. If Hunterdon could have performed what Trussell planned, it might have come very close.

THE PUBLIC HEALTH DEPARTMENT

Plans were laid for a referendum to be held in the autumn of 1952 on the subject of a county health department. A select group of local activists was appointed, including political figures, representatives from every association, voluntary agency, farm group, and so on. Trussell obtained the endorsement of the N.J. Medical Society.[32] That summer, the League of Women Voters obtained the necessary signatures on a petition to place the question on the ballot. Trussell was very careful in handling this project. Perhaps sensing how the voters would react, he was careful to defer to the public will, adding that the Medical Center would make every effort to give good service, with or without a health department.

In the proposed department, Trussell was to serve in the dual role of HMC Director and County Health Officer. The projected budget of about $100,000 included support for the 10 or 12 nurses already working for the county. The issue became entangled in an extraordinary mess of legal requirements; for example, the Board of Chosen Freeholders would have to approve the formation of the Health Department in advance, without knowing which, if any, of the municipalities had voted to join it. The necessary referendum on a unified County Health Department was soundly defeated. HMC's Board did not have the will or the resources to proceed on its own. In Trussell's assessment

> There were no precedents anywhere else in the state. We were
> the first to try it out. It was too soon, too much and we were
> defeated by a substantial margin of negative votes . . . It be-
> came politically involved. We had one lawyer who I found to
> be particularly antagonistic about the whole thing, and in
> spite of extremely strong support of the *Hunterdon County*
> *Democrat* and an awful lot of public speaking, it was turned
> down . . . Wescott felt really put down by it.[33]

After the vote, which was the only issue over which Trussell saw Lloyd Wescott become upset, Trussell and Wescott differed over employing a public health nurse, which had been funded by a Commonwealth grant. Wescott opposed the idea because "the vote against the Public Health Department . . . made it imperative that we avoid, in every way, seeming to implement a specific program that the community had voted down."[f] After a meeting of Wescott, Trussell, and Seward Johnson with Commonwealth, the Fund agreed to allow employment of a nurse under their grant for a variety of educational, administrative, professional training and liaison activities, predominantly in the pediatric area.

Eventually a County Public Health Department became a reality. From a survey they conducted in Hunterdon County in 1961, the League of Women Voters concluded there was no countywide coordination of health services, and this was much needed.[34] There was a need for better understanding of public health standards, environmental sanitation including water, sewage and food, dental health, improved school and municipal nursing, and many other aspects of a comprehensive public health program.

Several years later, the N.J. Health Department, then led by Roscoe Kandle, began to enforce longstanding regulations requiring each municipality either to hire an approved Health Officer or contract for equivalent services. Under state pressure, a committee, led by August Knispel, a local farmer, recommended formation of a County Health Department to perform mandated services. Municipalities would be charged a dollar a year, a notion that all thought ludicrous. With this combination of carrot and stick, the Health Department opened in April 1967.[35] At the time the Board of Trustees made one last effort. They authorized Medical Director Henderson to write the Freeholders explaining all the reasons why the proposed County Health Department should be based at, and a part of, the HMC complex.[36] Nothing of the kind happened. Hunterdon County sensitivities were still raw. John H. Scruggs, the Department's first Director, arranged for complaints to be screened by municipal boards of health before being dealt with at the county level: "We hope to show that we are not trying to usurp their powers."[37]

Over time the County Health Department has gradually become a more pervasive influence, as originally envisioned. The current director, able and thoughtful John Beckley, has worked closely with HMC and other agencies. The Health Department, HMC and a

[f] Memorandum from Wescott to Executive Committee, in Minutes, 15 January 1953. Board of Trustees file, HMCA. This is one of only two situations I am aware of where Wescott fully retreated after a rebuff. In everything else he would pause and then try a new tactic.

large proportion of community nonprofit and governmental agencies concerned with health and welfare, have joined to form a Partnership for Health. This group has performed multiple community health assessments and identified special populations in need of new or increased services."[38]

PUBLIC HEALTH NURSING

STARTING A NURSING SERVICE

Hopes for a highly professional nursing service, staffed by nurses at master's level in public health, were abandoned when voters defeated the referendum on a County Health Department in 1952. Following the defeat, the Hunterdon County Public Health Association, stimulated in large part by Bobbie Knocke, wife of orthopedist Fred Knocke, explored public health nursing resources in the county. Fifteen part-time school and municipal nurses, with no special training, and two supervisors provided by the N.J. Department of Health, provided a patchwork of uncoordinated services. Miss Lela Greenwood, HMC's Director of Nursing, mentioned the need for public health nursing to Mrs. Knocke, who had thought of employment at the Medical Center, but was told that policy forbade the hiring of physicians' wives.[g] Miss Greenwood steered her to the local Public Health Association, where Mrs. Knocke became President. Over a period of five years support for home health nursing was nurtured. The Association decided to open a visiting nurse service as a private not-for-profit agency in cooperation with HMC.

THE FAMILY NURSING SERVICE

The Family Nursing Service initially opened for business in a small area of the hospital that also housed the social worker, speech therapist, Public Health Association, Dental Clinic, Public Relations, and the office of Marguerite Moore, who supervised volunteers and fund-raising. Lloyd Wescott (inevitably keeping his finger on the pulse of health care issues in the community) offered the nursing service larger quarters in the old Butler farmhouse (the "Pink

---

[g] This policy apparently did not last very long. Hunt's wife, Lotte, was a nurse on the maternity floor. John Fuhrmann's wife, Jane, was a nurse on the pediatric floor.

House") on the Medical Center grounds, near the highway. One of the candidates suggested by NYU's School of Nursing to head this new agency was Henrietta Siodolowski, herself ready for a change after nine years of work in Hoboken.[h]

The Medical Staff felt quite comfortable in hiring good bedside nurses with R.N. degrees. However, the Public Health Association and the National League for Nurses did not, until it was pointed out that hiring an R.N. would not lower standards, because the master's level nurse in charge would actually help to raise them. There had never been such a credentialed nurse in the county before. A major problem was resentment from the nurses already serving schools and municipalities when the Family Nursing Service proposed to contract services by better trained nurses to both. The new organization, its well-trained leader and consultant understandably threatened existing staff. Rather than seek constructive ways to improve existing services, the nurses asked for, and received, help from the N.J. Educational Association to combat the new agency. Eventually the Department of Education specified the training required for school nurses and the Department of Health did so for municipal nurses. The Department of Health provided funds for the new nursing service for the first three years.

Convincing municipalities to contract for nursing services was not easy. Siodolowski performed this task between home visits and bedside care, because she served as both Director and staff for the first few months. Municipal officials insisted that if they were to purchase services, they should be provided with both patient identification and diagnosis, for they feared being billed for someone living in another municipality. Siodolowski also had to provide coverage when the first staff nurse was hired, because she did not have school nurse certification—no one in the area did—and it was necessary to send her for schooling. As the nursing service grew, programs from the Public Health Association were absorbed, including the Crippled Children's program, work with the Cancer Society, and all school nursing. Income for services increased, but could never keep up with the budget, so a fund-raising event was discussed. Siodolowski, well aware of Bobbie Knocke's interest in

[h] Born in Jersey City, Siodolowski was raised in Hoboken where she attended public school. From an early age she always wanted to be a nurse. She chose a five-year program through the Jersey City School of Nursing, leading to a degree in Health Administration, an R.N. and certification in school nursing. She was awarded a Master's in Public Health Administration from NYU in 1957.

horses and shows suggested a Family Nursing Service Horse Show. Siodolowski pointed out that a show would offer excellent public relations in a relatively affluent community where many young people kept horses or enjoyed riding. The show enjoyed immense popularity for a number of years. Medical staff supported the event by maintaining an emergency tent with a physician available, lured in part by free tickets. The Family Nursing Service had a booth where they gave out brochures and educational material.

The Family Nursing Service maintained a close relationship with HMC and with the County Medical Society. Work with school nurses was facilitated by the full-time nurse at North Hunterdon Regional High School, Evelyn Lawson, who was cooperative and helpful. In contrast, the Public Health Association found that the agency it had sponsored had grown into a behemoth and some of its Board members were not entirely happy with this change. A Visiting Homemaker Service was established as an independent not-for-profit agency, and the two services worked together, but not without some rivalry. Ultimately, the Family Nursing Service was merged with HMC, primarily as a result of changes in Medicare reimbursement regulations, which made it wiser for the two to function as one.

Today a Public Health Nursing and Education Service, directed by Marianne McEvoy, is financed by a mixture of state and federal grants, including funds from the tobacco settlement. The moneys flow through the Hunterdon County Health Department to Hunterdon Healthcare System, which hires and pays the nurses to perform a panoply of public health nursing and educational services in child health and immunizations, nutrition, epidemiology, adult health screening and education and disease control. The Dental Clinic mentioned earlier is directed by this group. They are housed a few yards off campus in county buildings.

School Health

Trussell and HMC's Associate Director of Nursing, Margaret Wiles, looked closely at the local schools and agreed that none offered a modern school health program.[i] Students with learning difficulties

---

[i] Wiles graduated from Hood College and the Johns Hopkins Hospital School of Nursing. She majored in Public Health Nursing at Catholic University and obtained a master's degree at the University of Chicago. She came to Hunterdon from Baltimore where she was Nursing Consultant in Pediatrics with the Maryland State Department of Health. At Hunterdon, she made many contributions to the mental health, obstetrical and nursery programs and to the

were not evaluated, provided with tailored curricula, or offered appropriate services. The County Superintendent of Schools, Eric Groezinger, a farseeing and secure administrator, welcomed the opportunities that an infusion of talent and grant money might provide.

A committee formed in 1951, representing the Medical Society, the schools and school boards and HMC, considered the content of a modern school health program. It outlined steps to improve existing services, hoping to "integrate school health services with the broad community health programs of the Medical Center."[39] The committee's composition typified so many similar groups in this community. In addition to Groezinger and Trussell, it also included Frank Dalrymple from Pittstown, in Franklin Township.[j] Board minutes repeatedly refer to the school health program, which was initially to operate in the Franklin Township school, where the administrator, school board *and* Dalrymple had expressed interest.

On 23 May 1952, HMC's Board agreed that Trussell could serve as county school Medical Inspector, appointed by Groezinger. Trussell was asked to develop policies and standards for school health services, promote their improvement throughout the county, supervise the school nurses, assist the county superintendent and consult with the schools. In 1954, through the influence of Groezinger, Dalrymple, Kenneth Myers (later a member of HMC's Board) and others, representatives of Franklin Township school invited HMC staff to work with them, perhaps as a pilot program for other districts and as a training site for resident physicians.[40] Pediatrician Hunt served as school physician there for several years. When Hunt left, the program was turned over to a family physician; family physicians have continued to serve as school physician. Over time, legislative and regulatory requirements gradually tightened, so that programs for developmentally disabled children improved, and members of HMC's Pediatric Department began to serve as consultants to the schools. When the Child Evaluation Center, dis-

Chronic Illness Survey. Hunt and Trussell regarded her as a particularly valuable member of the nursing staff.

[j] Dalrymple (pronounced locally *D'-rump'l*), owned a grocery store famous for its fresh meats, and was a member of the Board of Chosen Freeholders. He was much respected and admired and had typical country canniness. The day after my family and I moved to this area, my wife went to his store. As he was checking out her order Dalrymple said to her, "You Mrs. Katcher?" She answered, "Yes, but how did you know?" Dalrymple replied, "Figured that's who you ought to be." In those days everyone knew who was moving into the area.

cussed in the section on the Department of Pediatrics, was formed, consulting work was performed by this unit of HMC.

SOCIAL SERVICES

Many social supports—old age assistance, public assistance, aid to the blind and aid to dependent children—were fragmented, competitive and uncoordinated when HMC was being planned. Many of these services were controlled at the municipal rather than county level, which meant geographic as well as functional fragmentation. HMC sponsored other services—Social Service, Multiple Screening (which grew out of the Chronic Illness Survey), rheumatic fever control (sponsored by the local Heart Association and the N.J. Department of Health, and staffed by Pauline Goger), parenting classes, weight control, and school health. The list is much shorter than what had been envisioned in the original planning.

In a letter to the Medical Director in early 1960, Wescott expressed regret that, because of lack of space, HMC had never been able to carry out the Corwin report recommendation that the "Center should offer space to all voluntary community health and welfare agencies in the county." There were really two different reasons. The first was lack of money to build space. The second was anxiety that building the space, and attempting to cajole agencies to move in, would be seen as too aggressive a change in county traditions and would call down wrath upon heads, impairing HMC's ability to perform its mission. Wescott believed that "working in close relation to one another . . . the agencies could make their work both more productive and rewarding."[41] He expressed confidence that a new facility, then in the planning stage, might remedy this lack. That did not come to pass, and to this date nearly all public and private agencies in the county are located in their own structures; relationships with HMC remain on a more formal working level.

WELLNESS CENTER

In the late 1980s the Board took note of a lack of medical services in the northeastern part of the county. A community-based wellness center was the preferred response, and polling was used to verify interest. A car dealership in Whitehouse had left a suitable building;

reconstruction was performed and the center opened in January 1998.[42] The center includes a lap swimming pool, large numbers of exercise machines, on-site babysitting, locker facilities and sauna, and is staffed by trainers, physical therapists, cardiac rehabilitation specialists and counselors. It has been so successful that enrollment had to be closed for lack of space. The center's plans include space for physicians' offices. As of 2002, Hunterdon Pediatric Associates and Hunterdon Cardiovascular Associates have taken space there. The former was the first to move in, only after a conflict with a local family physician who vigorously opposed the project. The YMCA and a separate private partnership have constructed wellness centers not far away. HMC has firm plans to open another such center in the northern part of the county, also in conjunction with physicians' offices and a center for alternative therapies.

DENTAL CLINIC

Twenty years before HMC opened, experts were recommending predominantly hospital-based, urban dental clinics emphasizing preventive dentistry for children and the poor. In 1930 two million people a year were treated in such clinics.[43] An existing dental clinic was incorporated into HMC, one of the few integrated community ambulant care programs. As Trussell described, Hunterdon County was challenged by a sizable number of serious dental problems among children from families of limited means or understanding.[44] Confronted with the challenge of barriers to care, the community responded by organizing a Dental Clinic to provide restorative dentistry for these children. Funds from the N.J. Department of Health, the Hunterdon County Board of Chosen Freeholders, the Red Cross, and donations raised by a citizens' committee were pooled to hire a part-time dentist, a dental assistant, supplies, administrative services and transportation. Initially housing was offered in the county Welfare Department; when it opened, HMC provided space on similar terms of operation. Restorative dentistry for school children was offered until 1999 when the administrator retired. The situation was then rescued by the county Department of Health. Using a line item budget from the Freeholders, 20 local dentists were recruited to offer restorative dentistry and dental hygiene in their private offices for children who were on the Federal school lunch program. This has worked well, but does not include children on Medicaid because of conflicting regulations. Those children are being transported to clinics out of county. Negotiations to include the Medicaid children into the existing program are under way with no success thus far. The county Health Department also offers materials for dental health education to school nurses for classroom use; an unknown number take advantage of this aid.[45] Clearly what all these events chronicle is a series of actions to transfer funds among nonprofit and governmental institutions in order to pay for dental services. The issue is money, not availability of dentists. Of course that is true of dental services in general, not only those for children in need of restorative work.

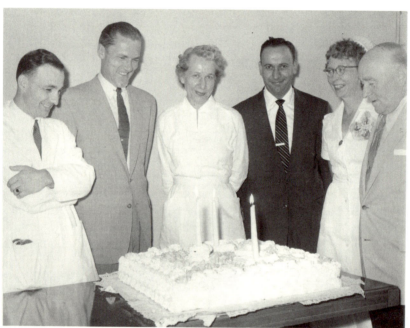

The third birthday celebration at HMC. From left to right, Edmund Pellegrino, Medical Director and internist, Lloyd Wescott, Katherine Booth, HMC dietician, Murray Rubin, administrator for finances, Miss Lela Greenwood, Director of Nursing, and devoted Board member Joseph Moskowitz.

CHAPTER 16

Years of Stress and Change

This chapter deals with events at Hunterdon Medical Center as an institution no longer seen as an experiment—as it was labeled by many during the first few years—but a viable and successful health care organization. The evolution of intrastaff and staff–Board relations is described in roughly chronological order, including attitudes and relationships that eventually led to radical changes in staff structure. I was an observer and often an actor in all the events noted from 1959 on. In particular, I served part time as assistant to the Medical Director from 1969 to 1977, focusing on a proposed HMO, as well as other administrative duties. I have endeavored to chronicle the era as objectively as possible. I apologize if in preparation of any part of this record my effort was not successful.

THE LONG-RANGE PLAN—WHAT KIND OF MEDICAL CENTER?

As early as March 1958, the Board was already considering long-range plans. Now we had a hospital, but just what kind? For example, how would the quasi-academic specialist staff, engaged in professional and public educational activities, as well as a clinical program, develop a center of excellence in a small community hospital?[a] The Board considered many issues, in particular, the limits of growth, the future role of the specialists, and the relationship with the community. At that time Medical Director Ed Pellegrino emphasized to the Board the importance of a broad

---

[a] Quasi-academic refers to the activities of the specialists. Like university academics, the specialists taught and endeavored to deliver exemplary care and consultations. But unlike true academics, they were not involved in research. Cowles Herr, as noted elsewhere, spoke of this as "JV academic."

range of services, quality control by full-time specialists with university appointments, maintaining a modus vivendi between the specialists and family physicians, community participation, and economic feasibility of all programs.

Questions about specialty services, subspecialty services, and what could and should be done in a small community hospital were chewed over for years in a rapidly changing medical climate. For the first time in human history physicians were able to modify the course of illness, cure or ameliorate. The explosive growth of basic and clinical research fueled the growth of subspecialty medicine and powerful new treatment tools. For many patients the best care for serious sickness was to be found in institutions large enough to see sufficient numbers of unusual disorders and to do research both on them and on more common serious problems. An institution the size of HMC clearly could not provide this level of care for all. Board and Medical Staff recognized this problem, and patients were referred elsewhere as indicated.

In 1959 when I came to Hunterdon it seemed clear that the choice was either to remain a small community hospital and grow with the community or to build selective regional consulting services. There was then only one medical school in New Jersey, founded in 1957 at Seton Hall College. The neighboring hospitals, although most were larger than HMC, were not accustomed to deliver regional services. The possibility of expanding services was considered by the Board, Pellegrino, Fred Knocke (orthopedic surgeon and Assistant Medical Director) and Ed Grant, the administrator in 1958, when they were explicitly looking at expanding the market area and the range of services HMC offered.[1] But whether it was the fear of the inability to fund expansion, the community's reaction to using local contributions for structures designed to treat residents of neighboring areas, the response of the staff, or simply innate reluctance to change, HMC elected not to become a regional resource.

With respect to expanding services, Board direction and the interests of the Pediatric Department appeared to differ. Hunt and I had a special interest in child behavior and development, and we began to consult regularly on patients with developmental or behavioral problems, which often required other health services such as psychologists, psychiatrists, and therapists trained to work with children. Developing such a specialty on a regional basis would require HMC's support by way of space, salaries, and so on. However, such a regional resource might not become self-supporting, even though it would offer major benefits to county residents. Extended discussions with administration, then led by Medical Director Henderson, and the Board, led by Wescott, could not convince them to move—the decision was made. Today, regional centers for children with neurological or developmental disabilities exist now within an hour's drive from Hunterdon. Years later, HMC began to add self-supporting subspecialty services, most notably an oncology service collaborating with a tertiary care institution. Other regional services include a cardiac catheterization unit, ambulant mental health facilities, a full-time neonatology service, a sleep center, and extensive patient education facilities.

At the time of the above discussions, there was no recognition on my part or, in my opinion, on the part of the Medical Center, of the notion that sometimes in the world of health care, more may not be better and sometimes may be worse.[2] It is not clear even now, how much recognition of this concept exists. Data and tools were not then available to determine diagnoses with greater precision and plans of care with greater safety. Examples of too much care include the widespread overuse of antibiotics, adoption of new surgical procedures without controlled study and frequent use of drugs as a substitute for life style changes.

Fencing among Staff and Board

Over time, family physician–specialist relations and the relations of each with HMC's Board frequently became antagonistic, and at times hostile. Eventually Wescott and many Board members spoke and behaved as if the specialists were interested primarily in their own welfare, and not at all in the high principles with which the institution was founded. There is little evidence that they recognized the specialists' sense of frustration and anger, which arose from distribution of income, the Board's paternalistic attitudes, lack of effective administrative support services and specialists' perceptions of institutional constraints on how they conducted their affairs. In turn, when it came to the family physicians, many specialists had little idea of the realities of private practice. From the early days some specialists viewed the Board with unmitigated suspicion. Communication on both sides became confrontational. In general, the Board played the controlling parent role, and the specialists played the rebellious adolescent role.

SPECIALISTS AND FAMILY PHYSICIANS

The educational and supportive relationship between family physicians and specialists was one feature of a love–hate affair. Friction appeared early and persisted. Relationships between family physicians and specialists were disturbing and disturbed from the start of the Medical Center. What initially held physicians together was good will, particularly among early members of the closed specialist and the open family practice staffs. In March 1953, even before HMC opened, records of staff meetings outlined with clarity all the problematic areas affecting staff relationships. At first, everyone was carried along on a wave of enchantment with their remarkable new hospital and its revolutionary staff structure.

At the end of 1954, after 18 months of operation, Trussell organized a series of meetings. Fifteen of the most active family physicians and eight of the specialists most concerned with direct patient care were asked to fill in a lengthy questionnaire. Several roundtable discussions were held, each time with four or five specialists and seven or eight family physicians. Summarizing the results, Trussell found that there was general satisfaction of both groups with the system. Criticism was scattered over many areas, with the exception of two issues: the business office and the relationship with Pediatrics. Family physicians and some specialists reported many patient complaints with business office procedures. Pediatrics was a sore point because many parents wanted their children to be offered an annual health evaluation by the pediatrician; however, caring for children was one area where family physicians felt very comfortable and saw little need for consulting advice. Many satisfied comments about Hunterdon were also noted.[3] In a letter to Lester Evans, written in the spring of 1955, as he was transferring responsibilities to Ed Pellegrino, Trussell referred to "frank, and I really mean frank, discussions of how well we have done and what we can do to straighten out any bugs. The fascinating thing has been the friendliness and the frankness . . . There really wasn't anything more to fuss about and that in the future these things could be handled on a day to day basis."⁴ Would that it had been so.

Some of the interactions described below should be considered in the light of Trussell's thoughtful discussion in his book. However, I feel there was more tension, even as he left, than Trussell recorded. In 1958, Trussell's successor, Ed Pellegrino also decided to move on. That October, the Board offered pediatrician Andrew Hunt the position, with Robert Henderson serving as Chief of the Medical Service. One month later Hunt took a position elsewhere, and in late November Henderson agreed to become Medical Director.⁵ Psychiatrist Morris Parmet and obstetrician Herman Rannels left soon after. With these departures and the death of Carl Roessel, whose stabilizing influence cannot be overemphasized, tensions that had always been present came to the surface. Problems described in the March 1953 meetings of the Medical Staff had not been resolved, only camouflaged by the efforts of the pioneering staff members to cooperate to make the system work.

On my arrival it was apparent from many private comments made to me that interpersonal friction had increased beyond what Trussell reported. There were multiple causes. Specialists' pay elsewhere had advanced beyond levels at HMC. Some specialists reacted by avoiding work where possible. Some family physicians took advantage of the system. In some instances specialists believed informal consultations were used to avoid formal, more costly consulting advice. For example, a family physician who purchased an x-ray machine for his office, brought to the radiologist those films which puzzled him for "teaching conferences." On the other hand, some specialists continued to treat patients (perhaps on patient request) rather than return them to the family physician. When there was disagreement over care plans or a family physician did not follow informal advice given in the hallway, specialists felt at risk for malpractice liability. Busy family physicians made inpatient rounds at 6 and 7 a.m. Busy specialists held teaching rounds at 8 or 9 a.m., when the family physician had already left to begin house calls or office schedules. There was little opportunity for face-to-face talk about the patient. Reasoned discussion no longer easily reconciled differences. Intimacy and warmth decreased; in the case of new staff members, they never had a chance to flourish. Gradual shifts in attitude presaged the major disagreements that appeared at the end of the second decade.

SPECIALISTS AND THE BOARD

Those interviewed agree that the specialist staff accepted appointments at Hunterdon fully understanding and agreeing with HMC's principles. No one interviewed indicated to the contrary. The atmosphere was idealistic; the word "Camelot" was used, at times cynically. Many specialists came to work at HMC for salaries significantly less than they were earning in prior positions.[b] What happened was reality testing: specialists who produced the largest amounts of fee-for-service income, typically the surgeons, were exquisitely aware of who contributed how much to the pooled earnings. In addition, after a few years, incomes in academic as well as private practice exceeded those at HMC. The idealism did not last— many of the knights of the round table at the rural New Jersey Camelot became unhappy with their lot. Income and autonomy became a source of friction between the specialist staff and the institution, as well as within the specialist staff. Ophthalmologist Nicholas Daukas left over low income. Otolaryngologist Walter Petryshyn approached the Board's Treasurer in 1958 to discuss income sharing based upon productivity, asserting that peers in private practice were earning much more than he was. Others valued the tradeoff of money for advantages at Hunterdon, such as the ability to practice high quality medicine without compromises, the convenience of office and hospital all in one building, the quasi-academic atmosphere, the professional camaraderie or the rural life style. Another advantage, protection from competition by a closed staff, however, was not commonly recognized. For still others, Hunterdon meant the opportunity to earn a reasonable living without working too hard.

In 1958, when I negotiated joining the specialist staff, it was explicitly stated that pooling earnings from professional activities was a basic and unchanging characteristic of HMC. In April 1959, when I arrived as successor to Andrew Hunt, at the monthly meetings of the specialist staff I heard blunt and intensely felt discontent with the financial system and with staff relationships. The outline of what the system was *intended to be* was clear. It was the *performance* of that plan, and the differences of opinion on the result,

---

[b] On interview, Barad and Katzenbach, and the widows of Roessel and Knocke so stated. In contrast, Woodruff said his initial salary was competitive, but what happened was that soon salaries elsewhere outstripped his, which remained much the same.

that produced ongoing debate and, at times, acrimony. The institution was always abuzz with discussions in hallways, over coffee, in meetings of the specialists and of the Medical Staff. Everyone acknowledged the need for a cooperative spirit on the part of all to make the system work, but as time went on reason no longer so easily reconciled differences. As the pediatrician operating under the existing "rules of the road," there were insufficient consulting and hospitalized patients for me to cover my salary and overhead. Pressure, sometimes overt, but principally covert, came from more than one member of the specialist staff to be more "productive." Pressures also came from parents who wanted their children seen by a specialist pediatrician. If they had donated money to HMC, why could they not see, and pay for, the services of a specialist when they wished to? Even before my arrival Hunt had developed a modest practice among families who had children with interesting or unusual conditions, who were politically or financially well connected, or whom he knew socially. This question was not explicitly dealt with in Trussell's memorandum or the By-Laws as adopted June, 1953, setting forth staff rules and regulations.[6] Specialists were to work in the Diagnostic Center (a six-room suite which encompassed all the outpatient space there was), might maintain special clinics there and were to see consultations on referral. The issue of periodic health examinations was dealt with in a sentence: "The Medical Board did not have time to discuss this problem further." The first Medical Staff minutes likewise clearly raised the question of patients who wished to see specialists directly, but report no conclusion of opinion or action.[7]

Another important source of discontent for specialists was practice management. This was, and remained, haphazard. Offices were makeshift and crowded, support systems uneven. The building that housed the specialist staff quickly became overcrowded, a facility that had been bare bones basic from the start. Within five months after HMC had opened, Trussell reported to the Board that the Diagnostic Center, the wing for ambulant visits, was "approaching maximum utilization."[8] The number of specialists outstripped the limited facilities—six examining rooms and five or six offices. No action was taken for over five years; then a construction trailer was sited in the parking lot and divided into makeshift offices, with limited space and partitions transparent to sound. Finally a large new building was opened in 1966, 13 years after Trussell's warning. Much of the delay was due to fiscal anxiety. HMC was barely afloat financially, and longtime Board members were acutely aware of the first years of daily financial crises—and the loss of nearly $100,000 in the first year. Board and staff had conflicting ideas about where money might be found to pay for more space. From the Professional Service Fund? From Medical Center funds? Why should the community be asked to contribute to capital to provide enhanced facilities from which physicians made their living?

There was the rub. Were specialist physicians employees or independent contractors? Both HMC and the specialists tried to have it both ways. For tax purposes, for fringe benefits and pension, they were employees. For new ventures, new staff, new buildings, they were independent contractors. The intent of the Board, Trussell and the original staff had been a structure to facilitate the delivery of best possible health care—not to benefit either HMC or the doctors. Every document of the time and every person interviewed for this book agree on this point. For comparison, consider a group of specialists in private practice that required larger or improved physical facilities. They would borrow money and build or remodel. The loan would be repaid from earnings. Staff would be added on the same basis. Community contributions would not enter into consideration. That same group, however, would be competing openly for patients and probably would not have as a major activity a supportive and educational relationship with family physicians. So HMC and the specialist group were doing a rather delicate balancing act. This became harder when relationships became adversarial.

Administrators expert in hospital management, even if devoted to the specialists' welfare, were not trained to manage medical practices. Collection procedures were antiquated and ineffective, hampering further the building of a positive balance sheet. Community complaints about bills, insurance and collections were heard on all sides. Procedures to manage patient flow to specialists' offices were inefficient and distastefully managed.[9] There was a mounting need for sophisticated office administration, yet few specialists had experience in this area, and most felt that one of the tradeoffs at Hunterdon was not being required to manage practices. They wanted others to do this for them, but hospital administrators were not then, nor are they now, trained in physician practice management.

Specialist dissatisfaction, therefore, arose not only from salaries but also from working conditions. The perception with regard to income was real. Long-tenured specialists may have also remembered the controversial Board debate with respect to the degree of control that the Board should retain, as employer, over physicians' charges to patients. For example, in February 1955, Louise Leicester maintained that physicians' charges were too high and the Board had the absolute power to set them. "The complexities of this were discussed and the opinion voiced that it was doubtful the doctors would accept this."[10] Whether or not all these concerns of the specialists were valid, they were not addressed by the Board. And in the event, no action was taken.

I was not unhappy over money issues, but was very aware of working conditions. Specialists felt that they had no control—no means to alter the state of affairs. As it turned out later, this was one of the rocks on which an attempt to start an HMO crashed. Had we been a private group, we would have borrowed capital and built a suitable office building, hired a trained practice administrator, and organized an efficient service. Had we been a private group, we would have pursued an aggressive marketing strategy, and fees might have increased. But this was not possible in the institutional framework in which we worked. In the 1960s the specialists did not yet have the will to insist. Board and administration served other constituencies as well: family physicians, the public, particularly those who gave donations, and the overall framework of operations. In my view, one great failing of Wescott and the Board was not recognizing the importance of marketing HMC and its distinguished staff, both specialist and family physician, to the community in Hunterdon, and the region round about. Had this been done early and well, it might have been possible to overcome the financial problems, the tawdry work environment, and at the same time maintain, if not enhance, the quality of care. An entrepreneurial spirit built Hunterdon; an entrepreneurial spirit might have spared it from the troubles of later years. Actually, an entrepreneurial spirit pervades the institution and the staff today.

In early 1961 Wescott prepared, and the Board approved, a document intended to promote good relations.[11] It summarized the give-and-take of Hunterdon's structure, with emphasis on advantages. Long lists of reasons were given why that arrangement offered many advantages to all parties, and the various ways in which the arrangement was constricting were constructively acknowledged. Although the document was meant to resolve problems, unfortunately that did not happen. The reason was that *dissatisfaction did not arise out of conflicts on interpretation of what the system was supposed to be. Dissatisfaction arose out of disagreement with the efficiency, wisdom and advisability of what the system was—and the need for a change.*[12]

At that time I wrote to Wescott suggesting the hospital hire full-time family physicians (i.e., physicians trained in the specialty of family medicine), to be supervised by a Director of Family Medicine. In my view, a full-time family practice staff would create among the community of family physicians a center of quality, a model of excellence and a focus of identity. Family physician–specialist relations would be improved if the former felt on a par with the latter. Wescott quickly vetoed that idea—"This would be a grave mistake." He was fearful that this might cause anxiety among the privately practicing family physicians.[13] Pellegrino equally disagreed with such a radical change. A few years later, when a Family Practice Residency program was founded, and satellite ambulant care centers established, the result was a center of quality, a model of excellence and a focus of identity.

The Board, led by Wescott, chose to focus on money as the reason for discontent. At annual meetings, with specialists, administrators and representatives of the Board of Trustees in attendance, expenses charged against the Professional Service Fund (PSF) (i.e., overhead) were reviewed with a fine-toothed comb by the specialists. Invariably Wescott attended, because satisfaction of the specialist staff was essential—like a builder attempting to seal the cracks in the foundation with wallpaper. Staff members reviewed the annual audit of income and expenses looking to reduce expenses, typically by transferring an identified item to the Medical Center side of the ledger. Wescott would make a pro forma argument, ending by asking Rubin and Grant if there were not some merit in the points being made. Accordingly, the identified item would indeed be adjusted.[c] Eventually, this excursion into creative accounting was of insufficient magnitude to soothe the specialists.

In 1961 specialists complained about a portion of the Medical Director's salary being charged against the PSF. In early May of

[c] For a typical example, see the Board minutes of 22 April 1960, which provided for a 15 percent reduction in the cost of secretarial services provided to specialists as compensation for the fact that the specialists provided a measure of care to the medically indigent.

1961 Wescott's report of a meeting with the specialists ended with his recommendation that none of the salary be charged against the PSF, even though, he asserted, a portion of Trussell's salary had been charged against the specialists.[d] Wescott added, "This was less than a convincing argument, as they had not liked that either." Henderson, who was Medical Director in 1961, did not practice and thus did not contribute to the PSF. This was the feature that most bothered the specialists, in contrast to the period when Pellegrino served both as Director of Internal Medicine and as Medical Director. Wescott's note to the Board reads in part: "I would prefer to have Henderson paid entirely from general funds, and not charged in any amount to PSF. This is obviously an academic argument, as *it is all hospital money in reality*" [emphasis added].[14] Legally, he may be correct, because in order to avoid burdensome double taxation, the specialists gave up their rights to moneys earned from patient care. But in a psychological sense, specialists felt very strongly that the money was theirs, and theirs alone. They saw the legality as a fiction for tax purposes; the reality was they had earned the money and were entitled to it and to a greater say in what was done with it. On its side, the Board saw no reason to give up the control that was part of the heritage of HMC from its beginnings.

In 1953 starting salaries for specialists ranged from $12,500 to $15,000 for a Director of Service ($82,200–$98,600 in 2001 dollars). By 1963 the range was $13,500 to $21,000 ($88,700–$139,000 in 2001 dollars). Salary increments of $1,000 per year ($6,800 in 2001 dollars) for five years were given. These figures applied to all specialists, the pediatrician, psychiatrist and surgeon alike. Junior specialists were losing ground compared to the cost of living; the senior specialists were gaining. By 1963 there was a full program of fringe benefits, including 10 percent of salary for each specialist to a retirement program with TIAA-CREF. In June, 1963, Wescott reported these figures to the Board to refute a groundswell of opinion in the community that the specialists were earning enormous salaries. His conclusion was that "active GPs in the community can earn comparable salaries, and specialists in private practice many

---

[d] Trussell says flatly that this was not so (handwritten emendation to draft of this book), because Commonwealth had funded his salary. He had feelings about this matter, for he regarded the Medical Center as not particularly openhanded.

times earn much more . . . Our salary scale must be considered reasonable. We attract men who are not primarily interested in money."[15]

By 1963, relations had so deteriorated that the specialists refused to accept HMC's presentation of the PSF by an independent auditor. They suspected costs that should have been charged against the hospital were on their side of the ledger, making their income in some mysterious way disappear. As surgeon Felix Salerno, later the spokesperson for the specialists who most objected to the system, said: "We were charged with part of cafeteria costs, which were subsidized, because office employees ate there. Or rent of the medical records space because doctors' charts were stored there. Or part of administrative costs. Or rental of the new office building [built in 1966]."[16] I believe the real issue was lack of control and independence.

Specialists insisted on meeting privately with the auditor. Wescott was not happy about the idea, but resignedly agreed. He pointed out that "if the Full Time Staff ask to meet with the auditors separately before meeting with us, we will probably do the same. Thus we will come together, each defending a preconceived idea of what is fair, rather than together trying to reach a mutually satisfactory settlement."[17] It is difficult to disagree with this statement, and nowhere in the records nor in private conversations in my presence is there any suggestion that Wescott or the administrators were thinking of breaching the principles of the PSF. Nonetheless, as a participant at the time, I can attest to the atmosphere of distrust and suspicion, which no protestation or demonstration could alleviate.

While some of this jousting was rooted in financial matters, it soon became an issue of power. The idealism of the Camelot days having vanished, different parties tested their strength. Wescott seems to have been clear about the primary role of the Board in assuring that medical care of the highest quality was delivered by selecting and meeting objectives for physicians of the finest caliber. He did not grasp that the concerns of the specialists needed to be addressed in some fashion, with respect to money and working conditions. And so the physicians would test the system, with the twin goals of increasing their income and gaining the ability to locate and organize their practices as they would. Inefficient and ineffective support services gave them some justification.

In the midst of this strife, public anxiety and anger over the costs of care came to the surface, sometimes as complaints about a bill or as rumors and word-of-mouth expressions of unhappiness. In 1963 Wescott felt it necessary to ask Board members to be on the lookout for such rumors. Unhappiness also resulted from continuing difficulty in the business office, which had been rescued in 1954 by the work of Murray Rubin backed up by Ed Grant and Bill Lamont (Board Treasurer). When Grant and Rubin left around 1967, the situation then deteriorated to the point that the auditors, a year later, strongly criticized the work of billing and keeping of accounts. That same office also provided billing and fiscal services to the specialist staff.

REVISIONS TO STAFF STRUCTURE

The original Summary Statement of the Objectives, as approved by the Board, gave initial descriptions of the status of the family physician staff (described previously) and the specialists. The latter were to serve as heads of departments, supplement, supervise and guide the work of family physicians, render needed specialist services, supervise the house-staff teaching program and have responsibilities at NYU.[18] The same document also provided for use of the fees earned by specialists as already described, and created a Professional Service Fund. None of this appeared in the first By-Laws of June 1953.[19] Later that year, excerpts from the December revisions of the By-Laws of the Board were incorporated into the Professional Service Plan which specialists signed as a contract of employment.[20]

Because of concern arising from smoldering specialists' feelings, considerable debate on Medical Staff structure occurred within the Board during 1961. In March a statement written by, and pushed along by Wescott, was adopted in principle. Later it was incorporated into the HMC By-Laws to accomplish two goals: to provide a constitution of sorts, a clarification of staff structure, and to send a message to the specialists that the Board had taken a stand.[21] The statement summarized in idealistic language drawn from earlier documents the various ways in which the existing staff structure was beneficial to family physicians and specialists, and, above all, to the community. It differed from the earlier documents by adding language that the heads of each specialist service (or delegated junior members) would participate in the care of each patient to the extent needed to assure high quality of care and were responsible for providing needed specialist services or arranging for a substitute. This placed upon the specialists clear responsibility for quality of inpatient care. As before, outpatient care was not discussed except relative to consultations.

A Needs Committee was formed in 1963 to evaluate requests for additional specialists and to perform ongoing evaluation of needs in all specialist areas in order to establish a rational framework.[22] A consistent and fair structure was needed so that expensive additions to the specialist staff were made in the best interests of patients, community and specialist staff finances, rather than on the basis of which doctors were noisiest. All this contrasted with the family practice staff, for whom merely setting up a practice in Hunterdon County was sufficient to entitle a physician to a staff position, although "to different positions of different grades," and, of course, only after undergoing the usual selection process. On the Needs Committee were specialists, family physicians and Board members. Staff appointments in the specialties required the committee approval of the opening. If approval was granted, a recruiting process followed, and candidates were then screened in a process managed by a Selections Committee. Family physician Ray Fidellow, who served on the Selections Committee during this period, felt the system worked well.[23] The committee screened applicants to ensure they were well qualified, agreed with and would support HMC's principles, and whether they would fit in with the existing group. That was the selection process in theory. In practice, the candidate had often already been chosen by the department; the function of the Selections Committee was to approve a fait accompli.

In other circumstances, the Needs Committee could be problematic. For example, around 1964 the Pediatric Department (that is, me) proposed moving from a one-physician department to two. My caseload had now increased to troublesome proportions and the burden to be on call every night and weekend, particularly to help with the sick patients of family physicians, lay heavily. Administration openly, and some specialist colleagues less visibly, felt that fiscal matters trumped all; whether the department could earn its own way was to them primary. The real stumbling block was a system that could neither change nor grow as then structured. Eventually I made enough racket to win the point, and a second pediatrician arrived in 1966. In 1977, when the organization's structure was changed, the Pediatric Department was quite able to earn its own way and progressively expanded. Meanwhile, in the intervening decade the structure of the Needs Committee changed little, and dissatisfaction gradually increased.

FURTHER STRUGGLE

Staff concerns and disagreements did not subside. By 1965 it was felt necessary to convene a special investigation in the form of a Medical Staff Liaison Committee chaired by family physician Louis Doyle to review the topics that had been chewed over since the first Medical Staff meetings in March of 1953, three months before the institution was open. The committee prepared a list of questions; Medical Director Robert Henderson compiled a corresponding list of responses designed to interpret the principles of staff organization.[24] He finessed the issue of whether the principles should be changed. Who should care for the indigent was one question. The response was that each physician treats indigent patients similarly to paying patients and does not transfer them because they are indigent. Another was whether the specialists should accept patients without a referral. A significant number of residents preferred to see a specialist for regular care. Henderson responded that specialists should take patients without referral only if the patient was insistent or threatening. He did not discuss the issue of whether family physicians should refer patients to out-of-area specialists.

Specialists complained that more seriously sick patients remained on the service of a family physician in hospital, while the specialist really provided the care, and in addition spent time teaching medical students and house staff. The response was that the physicians involved should have a frank open discussion. Referrals were a bone of contention because patients did not get appointments as promptly as needed when the specialist's office staff were unaware of the reasons for the referral; the response was that any physician initiating a referral should make a telephone call to indicate how urgent the problem was. On the part of the specialist, they should respond promptly and courteously. All of the childish behavior referred to, occurring daily in the halls and rooms, was now codified in formal records. Most physicians could not imagine needing to be reminded of the basics of professional relations.

Ten years later yet another special staff committee was convened.[25] It was again felt necessary to place on paper such kindergarten admonitions as the response of the consultant in an emergency situation is expected to be immediate and that it is the responsibility of the referring physician to provide significant history, lab data, etc. Soon thereafter a major change in staff structure, discussed below, produced a more conventional relationship with responsibility thrown to the individual physician rather than a committee.

FIGHT OVER SPECIALISTS' STATUS—CONSENT DECREE

During the second decade of Hunterdon's operation, stresses mounted. Many specialists were seeing more patients without referral and for primary care, viewing this as an appropriate response to community pressure. Citizens of a now more affluent community expected to consult freely with the "specialist" when they thought it necessary. Many family physicians saw this turn of events as an abuse of a well-designed system and deemed it unacceptable that anyone but they should deliver primary care medicine. Not every physician felt this way. Lou Doyle, who had chaired the Medical Staff Liaison Committee in 1965, commented:

> I never believed in the business of compulsory [allocation of care] through the family physicians or the specialists, even when I came in 1958. If someone preferred to see the gynecologist or have her care obstetrically, fine. I didn't object to that. Many family physicians did . . . At a certain family practice meeting, there were individuals in tears about the fact that they would liberalize inhospital specialist access to patients . . . They were absolutely terrified . . . I was very unsympathetic to that nonsense. If they couldn't generate a practice they shouldn't be here anyway.[c]

As will be shown, Wescott and his followers concentrated on upholding the structure of HMC's staff as the most important element over which to struggle. No one, including myself, saw the

---

[c] Doyle L. Interview by author, 30 January 1996. As noted elsewhere, it was Doyle who chaired a liaison committee, who raised questions that continue to be aired to this day about the points noted at the first meeting of the Medical Staff in March, 1953.

importance of the original mission for the Board and Staff, as noted by Corwin so long ago, that HMC existed to further the health of the residents of Hunterdon County.[26] It was to do so by healing and comforting the sick, promoting health in the well and providing access to health care for all. Now, as all along, Wescott could not focus on the central principle; instead he focused on the tools to accomplish that. How this was to be achieved would depend on what tools were available and what attitudes characterized those who would use them. Wescott could have learned from the approach of President Abraham Lincoln during the 1860s. Lincoln made plain to all that his goal was to preserve the nation. He believed northerners and southerners alike were citizens of the United States. He was not conducting a war; he was dealing with illegal acts of citizens. He said, "If we do this, we shall not only have saved the Union, but we shall have so saved it as to make and keep it forever worthy of the saving."[27] He went on to make clear that the central task was to save the Union, by the shortest means possible. One can only speculate what might have happened if Wescott were able to say that his goal was to save a health care system capable of offering comprehensive health care to all the residents of the community. Then, with that in mind, perhaps it might have been possible to consider what to do to alleviate the distress of specialists, family physicians or any other group, without losing sight of the primary goal. Instead, a war was conducted.

The growing unhappiness of the specialists eventually led to a lawsuit terminated by a Consent Decree breaking the closed, geographic and financial full-time specialist staff open.[f] This section will describe in brief how this played out. In response to specialist concerns, the Board, in the early 1960s, took several steps. HMC began a much-needed expansion, particularly of space for doctors' offices and ambulant care, culminated by the opening in 1966 of a new building, with greatly enlarged, handsomely decorated space for the specialists, the emergency room and other HMC departments. Accounting practices, a focus of attention by all, were complicated in 1966, by an incentive pay program for the specialists.[28] At the end of the calendar year a joint committee of specialists, administration and Board reviewed the status of the PSF. Money

---

[f] A closed staff means that a physician may not win appointment solely on merit; there must be a determination through the Needs Committee that a need exists for a new staff member. Geographic full time means office on the hospital campus. Financial full time means salaried.

for distribution to the specialists as incentive pay was identified. Criteria were a mixture of productivity (how much the individual billed for collection), and how much the individual contributed to the teaching program and other HMC activities. A rather complex point system was created for the latter. In principle, it corresponded to programs used by many medical groups. The system at first was welcomed; through the years it aroused more and more dissatisfaction, because the proportion for productivity was too small. A set of Personnel Practices codified the activities of the specialists after approval by the Board. This had not been rigorously done earlier. The prior rules were incorporated into the contracts signed by the physicians as individuals, noted in this chapter in the section on Revisions to Staff Structure.

In February, 1963, Henderson wrote to Lloyd Wescott:

> I am sure the Board is only dimly aware, if at all, of the abdication of some of its rights over the first 7 years of HMC's operation. I know you agree that they must be faced with this problem at the time Personnel Practices are brought up for approval and before they further abrogate their present authority.[29]

Henderson regarded the revised Professional Practices document, which was one component of the Personnel Practices of the specialist staff, as tantamount to setting up an autonomous organization within HMC's structure and opposed the degree of self-regulation implied by this revision. Wescott and Henderson recognized at least some of the concerns of the specialists—salaries, compared to elsewhere, or office management.[g] Records are really unclear to what extent either side was able fully to understand the other's position or freedom to negotiate.

Trussell stated in strong terms his disagreement with the incentive program, calling the plan "the biggest mistake Lloyd [Wescott] ever made."[30] He felt that a pay plan such as that which had been introduced at the University of Iowa Medical School would have worked out better. This included equal salaries, combined with recognition of income production and some agreement on distribution of that income between physician, institution, and between

---

[g] For example, one of many aspects of office management was how bills were sent out. Previously, specialists' bills were sent under a hospital letterhead. Specialists wanted bills under their names, and collections managed in a separate department. They and administration fought—the former concerned with lack of control of a crucial area, the latter with legal aspects of whose money it was.

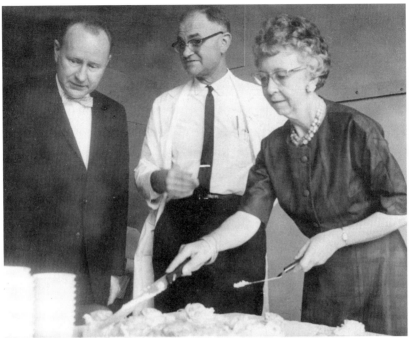

Miss Lela Greenwood leads another cake-cutting with Administrator Ed Grant and Medical Director Fred Knocke.

education and research. From my conversations and correspondence with Trussell, although he did not directly address the issue, I think he might have changed his mind had he been there, at least so far as favoring a program similar to the one at Iowa. In hindsight, had this been done five or more years sooner it might have avoided some of the bitter struggle. But the distribution of money was only one of the problems confronting specialists and Board. Difficulty in support services has already been described. By 1973, the twentieth anniversary of HMC's opening, there was open and serious discontent. Much of it was understandable.

For years a majority of the specialists negotiated with HMC's Board about changing their status. They sought fiscal and managerial autonomy. However, a contemporaneous article by Wescott betrays no sign of the turmoil.[31] During some of this time I served both as Chair of the Pediatric Department and as Assistant Medical Director to Fred Knocke who was appointed Medical Director when Henderson left. In that dual role I led the unsuccessful effort in the early 1970s to open a prepayment insurance program—an

HMO. I regretted the outcome, but have already indicated in Chapter 14 my present doubt that it was workable. It was not possible for me to ally myself with the specialists who wished to change the staff structure. I enjoyed my work status and felt the HMC organization to be a fine one. When it became clear that change was inevitable Glenn Lambert (my colleague in pediatrics, who joined me in 1966) and I decided to remain as geographic and financial full-time employees of HMC.

As the backbone of HMC's Board weakened under the combination of controversy and financial pressures from New Jersey state regulators who controlled hospital income, Wescott endeavored to stiffen it by bringing back Ed Pellegrino to address the Board about his fervent belief that a salaried full-time staff with responsibility for quality of care and education was central to the institution's mission.[32] He criticized the incentive pay plan as destructive, favoring negotiated, but equal salaries. Finally he recommended that specialists who could not agree could enter private practice while the institution hired new full-time chiefs. In an interview 20 years later, Pellegrino spoke of his tenure as Director:

> In the later years, there began to be some dissonance in the staff about the full-time salary idea, and the idea that we were employees. I never fought that. The medical staff wanted more control of finances and practice income than I felt appropriate . . . Bob [Henderson] and I did not agree on fiscal matters. Bob introduced the idea of incentives. I never believed in financial incentives. When I was there, only one person left and he left under interesting circumstances. It was Nick Daukas, the first ophthalmologist . . . He said he was going to leave. He said he had never seen such good medicine in his life. He didn't expect he would ever see as good again. But, he had to "see the color of his money." And I said, "That's fine. God bless you, the world is waiting for you, go."[33]

As surgeon Felix Salerno, who served as spokesperson for a majority of the specialists, recalls, the situation that made confrontation irreversible was the decision of an ophthalmologist, and, separately, an otolaryngologist to practice independently, outside of HMC's campus on a fee-for-service basis. Salerno said the group of specialists really saw no problem with the wish of the two doctors, and might have recommended hiring salaried replacements.[34] What happened at that time was that orthopedist Fred Knocke, the Medical

Director, for personal reasons, resigned and moved away. Triggered by this, under increasing pressure and now almost 70 years of age, Wescott retired as president in 1976. He felt that he was the lightning rod for all the feelings of the specialists, and that the institution would fare better if he were out of the way. Wescott's final annual report to the Board of Trustees aimed to be conciliatory: "Areas of potential disharmony between the staff and institution have increased. There is little question that our unique staff organization impairs, to a degree, the freedom of action of every doctor concerned. It has offsetting advantages . . . But the problems exist . . . [I am] hopeful that the problems can be resolved."[35]

The HMC Board hired Henry Simmons as Medical Director to replace Knocke. Cowles Herr, Vice-Chairman of the Board, was involved in recruiting Simmons. Herr believes Simmons was Wescott's handpicked choice, brought in to save the staff structure.[36] Salerno, who served on the Selection Committee, also recalls Wescott pushing Simmons' nomination. He remembers Simmons as cold and dogmatic. Indeed, as the new President (the office of Medical Director had been retitled, and now encompassed both medical and administrative responsibility) Simmons was determined not to compromise on the status of the full-time specialists. The Board voted against change. Simmons became the catalyst that brought the years of struggle to a head. Negotiations, or even constructive discussion, became impossible. To this day the mention of Simmons' name elicits anger from physicians there at the time. The unhappy specialists resigned.[h] Counsel was hired, a lawsuit initiated and after a delay a consent decree issued, by which the parties agreed to a settlement with approval of the court.[37] Simmons has described his point of view, which seems to recognize none of the key issues underlying the hullabaloo.[38]

I shall not attempt to describe the emotional intensity of those years, the lawsuit, or the feelings about its outcome. Salerno felt that the core of the matter was the ability of specialists to practice outside HMC, geographically and financially. He does not believe that salaries were the major issue, saying, "This was the ideal way of practicing medicine if the physicians could be more independent but yet a part of the system."[39] I believe that three proximate

[h] Salerno F. Letter of resignation on behalf of 32 members of specialist staff. Advertisement in *Hunterdon County Democrat*, 9 June 1977. These were all the staff except for pediatricians, family physicians and some internists. Later a group of family physicians joined the suit as defendant-intervenors on the side of the institution.

causes, not fully articulated, were involved: management and control, money and lack of trust on both sides. In any case, the result was irreconcilable differences. HMC's Board, now led by Willard Young, agreed to every change the specialists were seeking: freedom to leave salaried status and practice independently, freedom to open offices outside of HMC, to obtain privileges at other hospitals, and freedom to compete with each other and with the family physicians. Specialist staff status was now similar to other institutions. The Board compromised out of anxiety over what might happen to the institution if they remained intransigent.[i] Young felt that it was time to put things back together and move ahead. Cowles Herr, Board member and Vice-Chairman during much of this time said:

> I had always been a firm believer in the basic idea that the plan engendered . . . I knew that the problems which the doctors were expressing were to them real problems and if they were real problems to them they had to be real problems to the Board of Trustees who were responsible . . . But there was a great lethargy amongst the Board to do anything to try to solve this problem. Some of the Board members refused to accept the idea that there was a real problem—wanted to adhere to the basic tenets which were laid down.
>
> The strongest voice on the Board [had been] obviously Lloyd Wescott . . . [who was foremost among those] who could not accept the compromise of the full time system . . . It was a difficult proposition for an individual Board member to speak out forcefully against Lloyd Wescott who was the father . . . the rock upon which this institution based its foundation. As it went on even he became cognizant of his own mortality. Eventually he quit. That was a noble gesture if there ever was one. He realized in his own mind he was the lightning rod for the discontent. That is why he quit. Subsequently he never spoke to me of the Medical Center days.[40]

By this time Wescott had been out of office for two years. During his tenure, however, he summed up his feelings in a series of candid letters to Seward Johnson, who strongly supported a full-time closed specialist staff.[41] The frequency and emotional tone of these communications suggest intense effort to maintain Johnson's

[i] All through this time, another expensive expansion was underway. HMC's finances were precarious. Wescott was no longer in charge.

relationship, which was obviously changing. Wescott said now he was not opposed to restructuring the staff to allow specialists to practice as individuals, while maintaining full-time salaried chiefs of service. An incentive system for pay, based upon both earnings and other types of contributions, could not gain agreement on a formula that would content all. As in so many medical groups, dividing the pot left some individuals unhappy. There was no alternative to change; further struggle would be detrimental to health care and destructive to the institution. The existing principles were likely to be unenforceable in court. Should the specialists resign, as they threatened, it would be impossible to deny them privileges in any event. Yet Wescott was at heart ambivalent. In a written Annual Report to the Board in 1976, he attempted to rally the troops: "To abandon the staff structure which has existed from the first would be regrettable."[42] In one letter to Johnson his point of view was:

> The relationship between the Board and the staff and actually within the full-time staff itself took on the character of an angry marriage from which neither couple could escape by divorce, or separation, who could not move out of the same bedroom or even out of the same double bed.
>
> The demands of some of the more irresponsible money-hungry men have been really quite astonishing. How can doctors who last year were paid $60, $70, and even $90,000 a year challenge costs charged against them for using plastic liners in wastebaskets . . . One even insisted that he was entitled to have his wife come in and clean his office.[43]

A few years later, he added in an interview, "to some of the doctors, being employed by a hospital was an anathema in the sight of God."[44] Wescott wrote a summing up in 1980 to Donald Davis, Simmons's successor:

> I feel very strongly about the future of HMC. There is no question in my mind it is at the cross roads. It can have a new lease on life or it can slowly degenerate into a third rate institution. The person who can determine that is you.
>
> Camelot is dead. At its best it was unique and quite wonderful but this is a different world . . . It is futile to think that further compromise with the past would be useful or that some modified version of the "status quo ante" would satisfy anyone.

Henry Simmons came in convinced that Camelot could be reconstructed and he could do it even if it meant replacing most of the staff. That of course blew the place apart.

The present situation is intolerable from an administrative, medical, and moral point of view. Chaos reigns . . . Doctors, hospitals, outpatient services—exist to serve people. This is particularly true at HMC to which so many thousands of people have given so many millions of dollars. It can be made to work for them again.[45]

A Separate Building for the Specialist Staff

The consent decree in 1977 did not help allay suspicion between family physicians, the specialist staff and administration. Following the consent decree, most specialists wanted to practice independently on the Medical Center grounds. A medical office building was suggested. Led by three physicians who had been deeply involved in the lawsuit against the Board, the specialist staff began negotiations to construct a physicians' office building on the hospital grounds.[46] Despite general agreement that the project was highly desirable, the specialists and Board required seven years of negotiations, at times quite acrimonious, a mixture of progress and confrontation, before coming to terms. On interview, Donald Davis said of fall 1978: "The relationships between the Board and Medical Staff . . . were probably about as bad as they could be . . . There was absolute distrust on both sides."[47]

Although impasse seemed to exist several times, the two groups persisted in returning to the table. The key issues were whether, if the building was constructed and owned by a partnership formed for this purpose, HMC would compete for rentals by offering space being evacuated in the existing structure (they agreed not to); whether a long-term ground lease would be offered (it was, for 99 years); whether HMC would agree to be a partner in the venture (it did); and whether majority control of the partnership would remain with the physicians (it did).

The members of the Pediatric Department had not been allied with the specialists who brought the lawsuit and entered into the consent decree. But when it became clear that a medical office building was likely to be built, the Department joined the partnership, and I became President of that venture. There were several reasons behind this step. First, it was convenient for patients, and it was clear that most specialists wanted to see the building erected and to have offices there. Second, Pediatrics felt it would be injudicious to be located separately from the other specialists, particularly in light of any residual feelings based on not having joined the lawsuit years before. Third, eventually perhaps a fully integrated medical group would evolve, and if the pediatricians were there, we might be able to further the process. Finally, I felt I could facilitate construction of the offices. It was indeed trying. A great deal of time was spent stroking various specialists who would throw a tantrum if something occurred with which they disagreed. Fortunately, a construction firm specializing in medical office buildings (The Erdman Company) had been engaged; the representatives of this organization displayed exemplary patience and ingenious professionalism, all of which played no small role in the ultimate success of the venture. Donald Davis said that construction of this building was the most important achievement of his term as HMC's President: "I thought it was extremely important to maintain as much of the geographical full-time nature of the Medical Center as possible."[48] The building was constructed by the specialists and hospital cooperatively, on campus, and connected to the patient care wings.

FURTHER CHANGES

In the 1990s when many physicians felt that formation of an Independent Practice Organization was a good idea, negotiations dragged on for years, without resolution. Several surgeons opened off-campus offices; others, including several leaders of the specialists' group, did not. Of those who did, almost all either reopened offices on HMC campus or nearby, in some instances maintaining multiple offices. Several opened a freestanding, same-day surgical center a mile from HMC; Midjersey Health Corporation, a for-profit subsidiary of the HMC complex, eventually joined the venture. Almost all surgeons left salaried status, recognizing that although they might compete with family physicians, they also were dependent upon them for referrals. Following a bit of seesawing, what evolved appears to be a more coherent staff, with a more conventional structure and unwritten code of behaviors.

During the many years of struggle, the quality of health care at

Hunterdon did not fade. The residency program has continued and strengthened. As of this writing, there are 64 family physicians on the staff, compared to 122 specialists. Even when institutional animosity was at its most intense, every physician I knew, without exception, gave primary attention to the needs of the patient. Perhaps the most striking instance was when Wescott needed surgery. He asked Felix Salerno, spokesperson for the specialist group, to operate. Today, staff physicians are more concerned with the demands on them from the variety of payment plans than with any other aspect of their work at Hunterdon Medical Center.

DEPARTMENT OF PEDIATRICS

The author's experience in pediatrics may be illustrative. From arrival in 1959, until 1966, I practiced alone. Limited coverage was available from a pediatrician who lived some 20 miles away. In 1966, a second pediatrician was added after lengthy and at times contentious negotiations with HMC's administration and specialist staff colleagues who were aware that the Pediatric Department either did not or could barely earn sufficient funds to "break even." Two of us then maintained a consulting practice alongside of an increasing primary care group of patients. Many in the affluent community that Hunterdon County had become insisted on a specialist seeing their children.

We had not been participants in the lawsuit when the consent decree was entered, but we soon recognized that under the new structure we must choose either to maintain our practice as it was or enter active primary care pediatrics. We chose the latter. It had long since become clear that subspecialty pediatric skills at tertiary care hospitals made it injudicious, as was true 20 years previously, for a generalist to provide most nonsurgical care for children with serious problems. Failure to expand—to bring in pediatricians with new abilities—would mean consulting services of decreasing worth. The demands of modern newborn care required backup from younger, more recently trained pediatricians. We saw no reason to change from full-time geographic and salaried practice.

Accordingly the Department expanded progressively, to reach a total of 12 pediatricians and 3 nurse practitioners by 2001, including physicians trained or experienced in medical genetics, infectious diseases, intensive care, sports medicine, adolescent medicine, nutritional disorders, and development and behavior. Three offices in other parts of the county were opened, and a child development program and a lactation consulting program were created. Pediatrics and Robert Wood Johnson Medical School (formerly Rutgers Medical School) discontinued an affiliation for teaching medical students by mutual agreement in 1995. Pediatrics was the last department to give up primary student rotations. Students from the medical school are still seen for teaching physical diagnosis.

In 1991 Robert Wise succeeded Donald Davis as President. He asked me to comment on information he had received that Pediatrics was not interested in inpatient care, but referred sick children or those needing surgical care elsewhere. I responded, for the Department, in writing, that the Department referred out few patients except for those truly in need of intensive care or tertiary care subspecialists.[49] Pediatric staff members were sitting up all night with many children who might be referred and handling more newborn problems than many other pediatricians, all with excellent results. In addition I pointed out that it was the surgeons who had in some instances discontinued certain types of infrequently performed surgery because they were concerned about quality of care and malpractice risk.

By 1989 it was clear that HMC administrative staff was unable to keep up with the administrative requirements of an expanding practice and the demands of the changing health care environment. Accordingly, the Department of Pediatrics engaged a full-time administrator, and in 1991 entered private practice. I retired and left practice in 1994. By 1998, the environment had changed. Now there were needs for large amounts of capital to provide technologically sophisticated office systems. After a review of many options—merger with another pediatric group, buyouts from various entities—the Department agreed to be bought out by HMC, and is now again on a salaried basis, but with the distinction that it provides its own administrative management. HMC has embarked on a program of purchasing practices; there are now 50 salaried physicians, both specialists and family physicians, and a pediatrician now directs this complex.

CHAPTER 17

Hunterdon Medical Center up to the Present

EVOLUTION OF RELATIONSHIP WITH COMMONWEALTH

By 1954–1955, as Trussell laid plans to leave, a series of letters between HMC and Commonwealth indicated that Commonwealth was making a serious attempt to wean the Medical Center from dependence on grant money. With chirps of pleasure HMC would report that the Specialist Staff was financially more than breaking even or that the operating deficit of the hospital was less than expected. Trussell attempted to increase Commonwealth's support of his salary but without success.[a] One example that typifies the direction of the relationship is a letter from Pellegrino, as Medical Director, to Evans requesting transfer of $300 from some $4,000 remaining in the funds supporting the mental health program—the purpose: providing air conditioning for Morris Parmet's office. Evans replied, tongue in cheek: "It will be impossible for us to approve this request, but I have no doubt that with things going so well at the hospital you will be able to provide from other sources."[1]

During these years the proportion of letters from Hunterdon to Commonwealth written by Trussell or his successor, Pellegrino, decreased as the proportion from Wescott increased. There is a contrast between them: the former always informative, direct and meaty, the latter more oblique, often more politic and, regrettably, with less substance.

In 1958, Commonwealth's interest was rekindled when Hunterdon proposed a series of trips to other comparable ventures in commu-

[a] Despite all that he had done, his salary, which was never munificent, was increased only by small increments. In 1954–1955 he received many offers of prestigious positions, one of which he finally took.

nity medicine. Pellegrino wrote: "[The sites] have been chosen with some malice aforethought as . . . examples of good plans . . . others as examples of the future possibilities of medical care, and others as, perhaps, *a deterrent to those who might have a tendency to revert to the more usual way of practice*" [emphasis added].[2] In his reply, Evans expressed his hopes that they would explore group practice and staff–board relationships. It is clear that leadership at both institutions was aware of staff ferment at the Medical Center.

Before these trips could be undertaken, Pellegrino was replaced by Henderson, and some years elapsed before the funds Commonwealth provided could be utilized. In late 1959 Henderson noted in a memorandum on his visit to Commonwealth, that President Malcolm Aldrich "looked at us as lost cousins."[3] Subsequently Henderson wrote long position papers describing Hunterdon's accomplishments in hopes of obtaining additional support. Henderson's efforts were for naught. Commonwealth said it was now concentrating its efforts on education of medical students and would no longer be able to be of significant help.

In 1967 Commonwealth awarded HMC $11,100 in support of Henderson's plan to write a follow-up on Trussell's monograph, a project never accomplished. In 1972 Reginald Fitz, a Commonwealth staff member, and Wescott exchanged letters indicating that the Commonwealth grant had been spent and nothing had, or was likely to, come of it. Meanwhile Wescott attempted without success to obtain funds from Commonwealth for the prepayment insurance program and a health survey in connection with the family practice satellites.

When Henry Simmons became HMC's President, he did obtain in 1977 a grant for over $100,000 for long-range plans, including a study of HMC's functioning. At that time, turmoil over the specialist staff relations was at its height. One outcome of that struggle was a Board vote to "close the office which would handle these new developments."[4] The terms of the grant were never fulfilled.

There have been no further communications on record.

FISCAL EVENTS

HMC's early financial situation was typically precarious, a tight-wire act, seesawing from near disaster to adequate and back again. Wescott said "we were dead broke in 1954." More detail will be provided in the profiles of Murray Rubin, the fiscal officer for many years, and Ed Grant, the first administrator. When these men left in the late 1960s, HMC was barely afloat. New Jersey's attempt to regulate hospital rate-setting proved to be extremely difficult for HMC. During the 1970s when there was open warfare between groups of the staff and the Board, the institution continued to function despite preoccupation with strife. Administration did its best to keep the hospital functioning; more significantly, all the other employees and volunteers—orderlies, nurses, clerks, laundry workers, maintenance, all the people who made HMC function,[b] and I mean all of them, despite their dismay about what was going on around them—continued to carry out their work of exemplary patient care with courtesy and thoughtfulness, as if nothing had happened. My hat is off to all of them for their contributions. The unhappy professional staff at no time compromised patient care and kindness.

By 1978, when Donald Davis arrived as President, years of losses had left HMC in no position to undertake the urgently indicated renovation of its 25-year-old plant, planned just after World War II. During Davis's tenure, HMC began to move towards improved operational profitability. Losses were stemmed and money saved so that capital improvements could be carried out with no more indebtedness than the institution could carry in the new managed care environment.

That shift to profitability continued during the presidency of Robert Wise, and HMC has enjoyed a number of financially productive years. Decisions will soon be required to determine how to stay on a fiscally healthy path. Individual staff practices have not all enjoyed improved financial circumstances; many have found income lowered by the combination of capitation pay systems, discounted fee for service, and increased overhead arising from the need to add auxiliary staff and information services to deal effectively with health care companies and, with soaring malpractice premiums.

The 2001 report of the Hunterdon Healthcare System (the current name of the controlling corporation) shows total operating expenses of $115,508,000 and total revenue received or to be received of $119,346,000. Inpatient income was 49 percent of the

[b] See the profile of nurse Jeannette Ash.

total; outpatient income was 46.4 percent of the total. There were 7,678 admissions with an average length of stay of 4.8 days. There were 5,555 same day surgical procedures. Ambulant care visits were 102,314, of which just over a third were to the Behavioral Health Department.

PLANNING FOR HEALTH CARE SERVICES

In the beginning, Hunterdon aimed at unified use of community, physician and HMC resources to maintain and improve overall community health. Trussell represented a public health approach, even though the effort to create a county health department failed. Trussell's successor, Ed Pellegrino, as much as anyone, represented an individual health approach. Were they to be working at HMC today, Trussell would ask what allocation of scarce resources would do most for the present and future health of the largest number of persons. Pellegrino, while not unmindful of these needs (just as Trussell would not be unmindful of the needs of the individual), might argue the importance of scrutinizing one patient at a time, with a moral obligation to recommend what was best for that patient, regardless of material resources required. For a period of time in the 1980s there was some uncertainty about the mission of HMC. A mission statement, adopted in 1980, said: "First, and foremost, the Hunterdon Medical Center is an *acute care hospital* [emphasis added]." Wescott's response to this was typical: "If that is really so now, I consider it disgraceful and a betrayal of the thousands of people who gave millions of dollars to support it."[5] Subsequently there has been no doubt. Hunterdon is a health care system dedicated to the health of the community.

In the first decade or so after HMC opened, change was the product of less organized, more haphazard efforts. Sometimes recognition of major need sparked change. Trussell early on reported that specialist staff practice facilities were inadequate. In less than 10 years the inadequacy turned into a major crisis and a significant source of specialists' dissatisfaction. Accordingly, in 1966 after five years of planning and fundraising, a huge new addition, larger than the original inpatient wing, was opened, cleverly suspended over the tiny original ambulatory care wing on huge trusses shaped like an inverted letter *U*. The addition cost $4.5 million, compared to the $2.7 million cost of the entire original structure.

The next major additions resulted from a combination of need and circumstance. The Mental Health Department was greatly enlarged and received its own dedicated building due to the efforts of Lloyd Wescott. He had learned of federal grants for comprehensive community health centers, and with his unique approach pushed and prodded until one was created at Hunterdon. The new structure's cost was $1.05 million. It is named the Louise B. Leicester Pavilion in honor of her ongoing interest in mental health. A continuing care facility connected to the main complex was built to replace the original small convalescent center unit. In 1970, the Large Foundation, a local foundation originally dedicated to care for the elderly and whose Board included key Medical Center individuals, determined that a continuing care facility would fulfill that purpose. The facility, one floor, cost $2.4 million and is named the George K. Large Pavilion.

By the mid-1970s it was clear that the original inpatient wing was no longer adequate: the operating room was minuscule, the emergency room was too small, and an intensive care unit, which occupied the space of the earlier continuing care unit, was now constricted. A two-stage building program in the 1990s, added first the Emergency Department, a large new surgical suite, and a large adult intensive care unit plus additions to several other departments. On top of this, a complete new inpatient wing was constructed. The original unit was vacated and today is used for a variety of functions. Total cost was $21 million.

The most recent building program includes three phases. Phase 1, the Hunterdon Regional Cancer Center, which includes a radiation therapy unit, was completed two years ago. The cancer center is the product of an affiliation contracted in 1991 with Fox Chase Cancer Center, a major institution in northeastern Philadelphia. The backup available from this institution, combined with the skills of HMC's staff, have enhanced both services and utilization. There is now a cardiac catherization laboratory. The controversy over whether Hunterdon would be a general hospital-health service for the community or a regional resource has been settled. The medical and diagnostic imaging center, including a women's imaging center, has been renovated. A new Emergency Department will be constructed, replacing the present one, and the Intensive Care Unit will be reconstructed.

CURRENT SERVICES AND FUTURE PLANS

Since 1995 HMC has been engaged and allied with the Hunterdon County Health Department and representatives of community agencies and the public in planning for services based on the health status and health concerns of the county population. Two surveys of residents' health behaviors and one of high school youth risk behaviors have been performed. The alliance has selected ten health priority areas to concentrate upon, including heart disease and stroke, cancers, mental health, respiratory infections and injuries in residents over age 65, substance abuse, and several others. The goal of this venture is to encourage healthier life-styles in county residents, and to enable them to avoid preventable illness.

Despite original hopes for countywide integration, an array of community agencies functions independently of HMC. Local and national philanthropic organizations and county and state funding support agencies dealing with almost any social or medical problem one can think of. These local units are protective of their autonomy; HMC has not sought structural affiliations. To the extent that integration is achieved, it is the product of good administrative and interpersonal relations rather than a structural relationship. Even if a closer association with HMC were desired, housing on its campus would be almost impossible.

HMC's structure has become far more complex. A corporation, Hunterdon Healthcare System, is now the parent of four entities:

➤ Hunterdon Medical Center, a member corporation.

➤ The Hunterdon Medical Center Foundation is the fund-raising arm to promote investment by the Hunterdon community in quality health care services via charitable giving. In 2001 the Foundation raised over $3.6 million.

➤ The Midjersey Health Corporation is a for-profit entity. Its goals are to develop programs and services that expand, diversify, protect and/or improve the system's health care market, promote improved relationships with physicians and other providers, and finally provide a financial return. Projects include a nearby day surgery center owned in partnership with several physicians, a second health campus in the northern part of the county in Clinton, including space for comple-

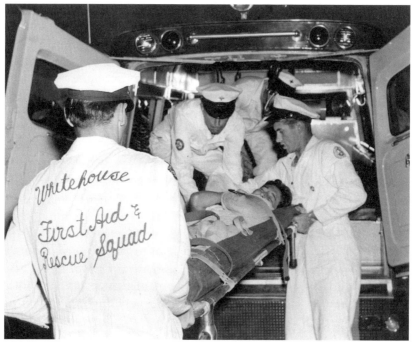

Among the many autonomous community agencies that collaborate closely with HMC is the county-wide network of rescue squads, supported by three mobile resuscitation and intensive care units.

mentary and alternative medicine, expanded behavioral health, pediatric and other medical and physical medicine services, part ownership of the on-campus physicians' office building, and shared ownership with radiologists of two MRI units.

● A three-year-old corporation, Hunterdon Regional Community Health, operates programs all heavily dependent upon fund raising. The focus is on home health care. At this time, the most widely known is Hospice care for patients in the final phase of terminal illness. Hunterdon Community Care provides home infusion therapy and durable medical equipment, and the Visiting Health and Supportive Services is the current name of the Visiting Homemaker service that began nearly four decades ago. In addition to home health aides, services have been expanded to include companion and volunteer visitors and respite care. However, recent reductions in government payments have resulted in cutbacks of care.[6]

These programs are an adjunct to the certified home health care agency operated by HMC, which also offers home health aides as well as visiting nurses, physical and occupational therapists.

Several years ago HMC began to rethink the issue of salaried full-time physicians. Family physicians at the health centers had always been employees of HMC. The institution moved cautiously at first, because its purchase of a family practice in a nearby community aroused a storm of protest from staff, who felt they had not been consulted. Communications were improved; now 47 physicians, including 2 internists, 1 obstetrician–gynecologist, 5 psychiatrists, 11 pediatricians, and 28 family physicians and 4 nurse practitioners, are employees. As Dr. Harry Woske, the senior cardiologist, has pointed out, although a majority of all physicians practice independently, in one way the status of specialists and family physicians has reversed: more of the latter are now employees of HMC. Specifically, 38 percent of family physicians and 11 percent of specialists are employees. They are grouped under the rubric Hunterdon Health Care Practices, an administrative entity of the Hunterdon Healthcare System led by Vice President George Roksvaag, a pediatrician. The Department of Pediatrics returned to employee status as a unit to obtain access to capital for expansion. HMC currently has no strategic plan to target practices for purchase, nor does the institution wish to compete with physicians practicing independently.

The Medical Center helps newly trained physicians to enter practice in parts of the county most in need of family physicians by offering employment arrangements. In today's medical environment, many new physicians have difficulty starting a new practice because of the delay, averaging six months, in obtaining managed care contracts. While some will accept employment and when ready buy back their practice, most who finish training do not wish to practice independently.

The financing of all this has required a commitment from the Board. Nationwide, each employed physician in the average hospital produces from $80,000 to $120,000 less than overhead costs. A principal reason is lowered productivity. HMC has dealt with this by implementing productivity driven compensation. Physicians receive training in the business side of medicine, billing practices, coding, etc. in order to develop revenue to cover expenses. A central billing office for employed physicians is in action. Plans to use the Internet are being studied. Those practices working on such a system are in the black. The overall totals for all physicians remain in deficit. The practices are growing: six new physicians in 2001.

Hunterdon Health Care Partners is an Integrated Delivery System. Hunterdon Practice Association is the IPA that contracts with insurance companies. Over 130 physician members of the HMC staff are members, as well as the Hunterdon Healthcare System. Membership is contingent upon delegating contracting power to the Director. The Association has been successful at obtaining reasonably priced contracts. All institutional affiliates, such as a day surgery center and an MRI center, are involved. Clinical management systems have been implemented, with use of guidelines for preventive health care first for children, patient satisfaction surveys, chart audits and immunization surveys. Immunization rate is 91 percent with a goal of 95 percent for year 2000.

Resource utilization remains conservative. A survey conducted in 1995 and again in 1997 by the non-profit affiliate of the New Jersey Hospital Association showed that Hunterdon County has the lowest rates in the state for inpatient treatment of disorders that usually respond to ambulatory care (Ambulatory Care Sensitive or ACS).[7] It is true that ACS hospitalization rates usually correlate inversely with income level, and Hunterdon County is one of the most affluent in New Jersey. The key intermediary circumstance is access to primary care, where Hunterdon is also a leader. The finding suggests that Hunterdon physicians remain conservative in use of expensive inpatient facilities. Finally, a formal structure for care for the medically indigent has been adopted.

HMC has focused its attention on overall community health, and plans are made with that primary goal in mind. These efforts include a women's health center, in existence for over a decade; several mobile intensive care teams serving the entire county and portions of adjacent counties; child evaluation and early intervention programs and genetic consulting services for children with neurodevelopmental problems have been in existence for two decades and are integrated with hospital and ambulant care functions. A full-time, board-certified developmental pediatrician and a pediatrician board-certified in genetics supervise these activities.

The founders' hopes to offer special programs in geriatrics have been fulfilled. A physician with board qualifications in family medicine and geriatrics has offered geriatric services at Phillips–Barber Family Health Center in Lambertville for a number of years. In 1999 a physician with board qualifications in internal medicine and geriatrics assumed a full-time position at HMC. He is also Medical Director at several nearby nursing homes. Assessment services, care plans and educational programs on healthy aging are also offered, and outreach is emphasized.

The Mental Health Department changed its name to the Behavioral Health Department and greatly expanded outpatient services. Offices have been opened in two neighboring counties and in a part of HMC's complex separated from the inpatient and day hospital services. The department is reaching out to the community in a fashion reminiscent of the origins of mental health services at Hunterdon.

Planning has become a much more formal process. Research, although often mentioned in the early days, has not been pursued with either vigor or consistency. In 1976 at the time of Henry Simmons's arrival as president, $150,000 was obtained from Commonwealth Fund for outcome of care evaluation. I have found no evidence that anything came of this. Teaching of family practice residents remains a very important part of HMC's program; however, teaching of medical students in other specialties has been largely abandoned.

With some initial reservations, HMC's Board approved a Healthy Hunterdon Wellness program. An enormous array of programs is available, including access to the medical library and HMC's web site, a variety of exercise and training programs for adults, children and even the newborn, instruction in CPR, life style management, and specific teaching about self-care for many disorders including diabetes, asthma, cancer and obesity. Mailings to the community encourage joining; enrollment is without charge although there may be a modest fee for specific programs. A health and wellness center, including a large fitness center, in the eastern portion of the county has a waiting list for joining. A second wellness center and other buildings for offices are in the planning stage.

As is true of other hospitals, the Hunterdon system finds itself with more and more programs operating at a deficit. It will become more difficult to sustain the mission of the health of the community as changes in Medicare payments and other federal and state actions constrict options. One way in which the Hunterdon health apparatus might be able to support its community approach is to document on a regular basis the outcomes of care. Both individual physician practices as well as the institution as a whole need to show the results of resources allocated for each division.

CHAPTER 18

Conclusions

This chapter is designed to comment on what has been accomplished, what objectives were not reached, what might yet be aimed for, what risks are visible. Of course these thoughts are my own, culled from six years of work on this book.

THE MEDICAL CENTER AS A MANAGED CARE ORGANIZATION

HMC and its staff organization as originally conceived can be compared with the organization and function of a managed care plan. I have used a modified version of the conceptual framework of Devries and associates to organize my comparison.[1]

- Terminology: The term family doctor was in use in 1953, long before anyone had invented managed care. In contrast to "primary care physician," or "general manager," the original nonspecialist physicians were referred to as "local practitioners," "general practitioners," or "family physicians." What we now call "health care" was then called "preventive medicine." Most important of all, the person who came to see the doctor was the patient, and not the consumer. The professional person whom the patient saw was the doctor, not the provider.

- Goal: The Hunterdon system was explicitly designed with the welfare of each patient *and* the overall health of the community in mind. Every element of the system served to maintain and improve the health of the population served. Financial stability was not overlooked, but patient welfare was considered first. The Chronic Illness Survey and a screening program helped identify at-risk individuals. Managed care plans are fiscal structures organized around mechanisms to allocate finite funds; HMC was primarily concerned with the health of the patient who pays the premium.

● Focus on Quality and Ambulatory Care: Hunterdon, as managed care organizations, strengthened the primary care physicians' bonds with patients by the care manager or gatekeeper concept (a concept not used in 1953). Without capitation or other incentives, HMC strove to focus on quality by reducing expensive inpatient and ambulant care. Implicitly, rather than explicitly, the staff adopted the suggestion made in 1950 by Lester Evans with his characteristic prescience: "The whole problem both of general staff-senior staff relationships, of consultation, and of payment for specialized service could be approached more constructively if it were oriented to ambulant care as the basic service rather than to bed care."[2]

● Open Primary-care Staff: Unlike managed care organizations, all primary care physicians were admitted to staff, because it was believed that a physician of marginal skills would do a better job on the staff, and involved, rather than working in isolation. In 1953 there was no grave threat from malpractice lawsuits. The Joint Commission for Accrediting Hospitals was then a tiger cub. State regulatory bodies in effect did not exist. Today regulatory mechanisms and the pressure of legal liability deny to staff organizations and hospital boards the freedom to implement such an open staff policy. Instead, physicians whose work is of questionable quality are subject to censure by state licensure authorities, placed under probationary or supervisory status, and, overall, dealt with in a disciplinary and punitive rather than an educational framework.

● Closed Specialist Staff: Hunterdon created a closed specialist staff as a consulting group. Like managed care plans today, consulting opinions were offered on the request of the primary care physician. Initiation of a request for consultation depends on either the physician recognizing that such need exists or the patient being upset enough to demand it. Many plans specify mechanisms for partial payment of out-of-plan opinions. Those who can afford the cost will see whom they will. Hunterdon planned no out-of-plan consultations. The specialist staff agreed they would not accept patients without a referral, an agreement that was breached even before the hospital opened. For this there is no either/or solution. All solutions will be imperfect. The test of any solution is whether it provides a reasonable fit that does justice to all parties, in particular, the patient first.

❧ Staff Self-education: Hunterdon designated the specialist staff not only as a consulting resource, but also as an educational influence offering continuous improvement to the practice skills of the family doctor, via clinical experience and didactic encounters. Specialist staff members in turn were influenced by the university–regional affiliation. Managed care plans lack this feature. They make no provision for education, and the financial structure discourages utilization of time or effort for other than patient care.

❧ Outcome Evaluation: Managed care plans (but not Hunterdon initially) overtly require evaluation of outcomes, use of algorithms indicating productive and economical patterns of care, and provide complex information systems to examine and document these activities.

❧ Restrictions on Resource Utilization: Hunterdon, in contrast to managed care plans, created no structural mechanism for approval of actions of the primary physician. Ordering a complicated test, a hospital admission, or other procedure was the responsibility of the primary care physician. Fiscal considerations were only infrequently explicitly recognized. Hunterdon achieved its impressive conservative levels of resource utilization by mutual education at all levels from specialists to nurses, including family physicians, house staff and medical students. Individuals in each group are able to query and stimulate the others. Today managed care plans do not approve procedures that exceed cost limitations.[a]

❧ Payment Mechanism: Despite four trials, HMC was not able to create a prepayment program. Today, a consortium of physicians and HMC negotiates with managed care companies as an integrated delivery system.

❧ Finally the enormously complex problem of reconciling the

[a] In reaction to this particular problem, the N.J. Department of Health and Senior Services promulgated regulations in February, 1997, to require HMOs to provide "medically necessary" services, to deny authorizations only after consideration by a physician in a like specialty who must, if requested, speak to the personal physician and to provide an internal complaint system for providers, parallel to that for consumers.

care of the individual, with the care of the community population, given that there is a finite amount of health care resources available, was not solved by Hunterdon, and has not been solved anywhere in the United States. At Hunterdon, it was the clinician vis-à-vis the public health physician (i.e., the medical staff and Ray Trussell). The issue has been joined in the health literature. Lamm has noted that health care professionals (but really the public at large) "assume that society could pay for everything they need for their patients." He goes on to say that "government [read "society"] is not about what we 'need'; rather it is about what we can afford."[3]

What was Achieved?

Rarely has such a comprehensive effort to resolve major problems in health care services for an entire community been accomplished. Hunterdon Medical Center was a project of broad historical significance for issues in the policy and practice of health. A major goal was to develop methods to incorporate an extensive array of advanced solutions to health care challenges. This history describes the intertwining and reciprocal influence of distinguished national experts and determined local groups. Their work influenced at the local level issues that played out and still are playing at the national level. Despite certain flaws, HMC was an extraordinary achievement. No element of the health care system at Hunterdon was novel. No technologic breakthrough was included; the structure integrated original concepts from many sources, skillfully combined.

PROJECT GOAL

Board, Administration and Staff recognized HMC's mission as the best attainable health of Hunterdon County residents.

REMOVING BARRIERS TO ACCESS

A trusted health adviser—the primary care physician—provided the first point of care and introduction to other health and social services as needed to each resident of Hunterdon County. This adviser was conceived as a gatekeeper, with staff privileges, before the term was invented. As a source of health and sickness care accessible to every resident the family physician offered a "medical home" connected to specialized care as indicated. Where family physicians varied was in the extent to which they endeavored to promote health, compared to preventing or treating illness. This book has shown that family physicians continue to provide a large proportion of primary health care. The remainder is offered by pediatricians and gynecologists; general internists are uncommon.

Financial barriers were in part overcome by agreement between HMC and staff that all residents would be treated comparably in the same facility, in the same manner, regardless of ability to pay. At Hunterdon there was no inpatient ward for the indigent, no public clinic for the poor. All inpatients were admitted to the same semi-private rooms, and seen by the same physicians in the same offices. Medicare and Medicaid did not then exist. Today they are widely accepted. Family physicians and specialists, then and now, practiced conservative care with emphasis on prevention. The resident training program supports this attitude. Well-documented low utilization of expensive inpatient care resulted. Willingness to treat in ambulant facilities was readily accepted by the community. Surveys in 1972, 1977, 1995 and 1997 suggest significantly lower health care costs for Hunterdon County residents than other areas of New Jersey or the nation.

Structural barriers were attacked by efforts to integrate health and social care entities rather than suffer further fragmentation. This was partially successful, more by personal relationships than structural bonds.

Attitudinal barriers were lowered because this was a hospital of, by and for the community. Residents felt this was "our hospital." HMC Board, staff and employees shared a spirit of idealism and a sense of togetherness. The institution arose from actions of enlightened, energetic and idealistic community leaders supported by and responsive to the overwhelming majority of residents. In this fashion, a sense of responsibility was formed, today much diluted by an influx of families not involved in the earlier events.

Barriers of understanding were lowered by programs of education for the public and for individuals; these programs have become more organized, more comprehensive and more related to measured local needs. A focus on disease was superseded by recognition of the needs of the individual considered in the light of his or her niche in a family and social setting.

Emotional barriers were breached by a mental health department dedicated to outreach and interaction with community leaders and significant organizations. After an interregnum concentrated on closed inpatient care for serious disorders, an outward-facing program of behavioral health is in place.

Geographic barriers were lowered by encouraging primary care practices throughout the county and by moving segments of HMC ambulant care to peripheral locations.

Ethnic, linguistic and cultural barriers were not explicitly discussed nor attacked, perhaps because of the homogeneous character of the population.

ATTAINING A HIGH QUALITY OF CARE

Setting High Standards. Local leaders decided not to construct "just another hospital." They insisted on a health care institution of highest attainable quality. Health care experts were consulted frequently to ascertain functional and structural features most likely to enhance quality. At each decision point in implementation, quality of care was considered primary.

Combined Medical Staff. The staff consisted of family physicians, with staff appointment, available to every resident, fortified by geographic (i.e., maintaining offices only at HMC), full-time salaried specialists teaching the latest health care advances. Family physicians and specialists shared appointments equally to the Medical Board, which set professional policies. Each specialist had a faculty appointment and attended regularly at an affiliated university medical school. Specialists saw patients on a noncompetitive referral basis, recommended needed tertiary care services and hosted the educational program including residents and medical students. This structure is no longer in place, but staff remain devoted to quality of care.

Integration of Health and Social Services. As planned, one institution was to serve as a central focus and communication node for health and social services—an acute care hospital, an ambulant health center, and a source of specialized programs designed to integrate public and private agencies with an array of health, diagnostic and preventive services. In the event, integration of agencies has taken place to some extent functionally, but to a much smaller extent structurally. School health services are not now involved.

Geriatric and Mental Health Services. These services were organized on a population basis, with planned outreach to key individuals and groups in the community. The latter developed early; the former more recently.

The One Class System. The system has been sustained for inpatient and outpatient care.

A Comprehensive Approach to Inpatient Child Care. This approach incorporates behavioral and physical health, including rooming-in for the newborn infant and mother, relaxation techniques and family participation in obstetrical care, and round-the-clock visiting for parents with their sick children. To this has been added comprehensive ambulant services for all children, particularly those with developmental disabilities, and neonatal and lactation consulting services.

Ambulant Care. Ambulant care was identified as the core activity of health care. Hunterdon was built to make the hospital a vital factor in the lives of people who were not in the hospital. To meet this goal, the original plan included a Diagnostic Center providing ambulant studies and consultation with specialists. Planned home care was explicitly developed at a later date. Other approaches included a Survey of Chronic Illness, a multiple screening program, a variety of public educational programs, a cancer center, wellness centers, a Hospice and other home care services.

Medical Education. Medical education included a house staff program, now offering three years of training in preparation for board certification in family medicine. Medical student rotations were active for the first 15 years, then thinned, except for elective rotations on family medicine. Specialists offered education for family physicians and each other. Every patient in the hospital or Diagnostic Center was a teaching patient. The community accepted this concept. Affiliation with a medical school was ended by mutual agreement.

Preventive Health Services. Such services were initially a central part of the program. More recently a full-fledged, community-wide wellness program reaches out to all.

PLANNING

Planning was performed by the local group in collaboration with invited consultants. This process was initiated before the decision to build a Medical Center was made. This resulted in a complex process with continually changing attitudes on the part of consultants and local leaders. The Commonwealth Fund facilitated this process by providing several knowledgeable and inspirational leaders. These men and women did more for the project than the direct financial support that was offered. The latter served as much for emotional support as for bricks and mortar.

No one individual can be credited with leading this venture from start to successful conclusion. A number made contributions that were necessary, but not sufficient. Those included, in chronological order, Rose Angell, Louise Leicester, Clifford Snyder, Lloyd Wescott, Lester Evans, Ray Trussell, Clarence de la Chapelle, Lela Greenwood, Andrew Hunt, Morris Parmet, Edmund Pellegrino, Murray Rubin and Edward Grant.

Overall, *the planning process* was ad hoc, as individual contributors came and went. There was no design, in the sense that the word might be used to characterize the approach of an architect. Instead, the Medical Center group seized upon one problem after another, agreed upon a solution in the light of past experience, and moved on to the next that loomed up. Today planning is performed in collaboration with a community-based Partnership for Health. It is hoped this will result in more novel ventures and willingness to innovate

EVALUATION

Innovation in systems of health care delivery is no more likely to be an improvement on the existing order than are new drugs, diets or operations to be an improvement on existing therapy. Just as new treatments must be compared, in rigorously designed and conducted trials, against the natural history of disease, placebos and existing therapies, innovative health care systems must also be compared against existing patterns of care. For a new therapy the question is the patient's total well-being compared to alternative treatment. For a health care system, what is the well-being of the population compared to some other system? If I were to identify one failure of the Hunterdon project, it is that formal, ongoing, carefully constructed methods of outcomes research were not designed as an integral part of the whole.

There has been no formal comprehensive evaluation of this project other than the book that Trussell wrote and the staff dialogue that he conducted. Trussell's comments remain pertinent:

> If despite intense efforts . . . the community still fails to provide adequately for the health of its individual citizens, a strong argument exists for outside intervention in local health affairs . . . Will the project serve merely to reduce the local problems to the point where they no longer attract serious attention . . . Or, will it go the whole way, through continued community action and professional cooperation, in providing a practical range of health services?[4]

Lessons for Innovation in Health Care

NEW CONCEPTS ARE NOT ALWAYS NECESSARY

It is not necessary to conceive new, sweeping ideas in order to innovate. At Hunterdon, decades-old concepts were combined in one organization.

Hunterdon demonstrated and taught a lesson not well understood to this day—ventures aiming to produce change must arise from the beliefs, values and perceived needs of community residents. Those residents must see such ventures as participatory and capable of being influenced. This is true for health care and for political change.

Innovation may depend as much on the politics of individuals as on the rationality of ideas. For example, Rose Angell, Louise Leicester and Ann Stevenson came before a county Board of Agriculture that possessed political power and political will at just the right time. Louise Leicester convinced the staff at Commonwealth of the value of this project.

Chance influences events as the House that Jack Built: As in the nursery rhyme—because Louise Leicester utilized James Alexander Miller as her physician, who knew personnel at Commonwealth and who had worked for years with E. H. Lewinsky-Corwin, who for decades had been at the center of changes in health care, who was delighted with an opportunity to design the health organization of his dreams, and who also knew Clarence de la Chapelle in the regional hospital program at New York University . . .

STARTING WITH A CLEAN SLATE—HELPFUL, BUT NOT NECESSARY

Creative advance is easier when an organization is opened new, from foundation upwards. Creation through renewal may occur when administrative, professional and public groups are willing to aim for high levels of quality. Crisis may be an opportunity for improvement, as well as a chance for failure. Innovation appeared blocked at Hunterdon in the 1970s, during an era of turmoil when individuals and groups failed to recognize each other's needs. HMC reconfigured itself on this occasion, starting with efforts to resolve a need for improved ambulant care space, and culminating in 1999 with the opening of an admirable regional cancer care center. Being an established institution need not be a barrier to change or improvement.

The myth of all-knowing experts was shattered in creation of policy and in the development of Hunterdon Medical Center. Consultants were used frequently, but those who were working on the scene made decisions.

Fiscal or political barriers may be overcome in different ways. The contrast between Bassett and Hunterdon illustrates that a high quality community health care system dominant in a service area may arise either from massive, community-wide public involvement or from small professional groups bolstered by generous single-source funding.

Quality of care is based upon the practitioner who interacts one-on-one with patients, but who relates for service, education and standards with local health systems integrated with secondary and tertiary services. Regardless of the configuration of entities, public and private, which manage payment for health care, their organization should be designed to emphasize quality, encourage wellness but be able to treat illness. Both the practitioner and the health system should be devoted to collaborative efforts that enable families to promote their own health as well as to make thoughtful decisions about illness. This is as true today as when the new HMC exemplified what was known about how to achieve this goal.

WHY WAS THE MEDICAL CENTER STRUCTURE NOT REPLICATED?

Long-term planning—over five years before opening. The period of gestation, most of which occurred before the specialist staff came on the scene, allowed principles of approach, definition of goals, and selection of solutions to take place with fewer constraints. In almost all existing hospitals there is already a staff in place. It is more difficult for such a group, no matter how motivated, to accept the loss of autonomy implied by a full-time salaried and geographically located position.

Pressure to Change. In Hunterdon County, because there was no hospital, a major movement to construct one appeared. To this was added the desire to create a center of excellence. Pressure to proceed would not be as acute when the community perceives itself already served by a hospital.

Timing. The postwar years were a period when a spirit of optimism was more pervasive, and novel ideas that had been floating about for some time now drifted up into sight.

The Quality of Local Leadership in Hunterdon County. This leadership involved both a long-settled group of more conservative attitudes and a newer group of more adventurous individuals who also desired integration with the "old-timers."

Participation of the entire community, encouragement by leaders to involve all, and foresight emphasizing fund-raising in smaller amounts from many over efforts to seek out a few major donors.

Parochial Attitudes. National leaders in health care often did not recognize or believe what happened in Hunterdon County.

Community Wealth. What was not a barrier at Hunterdon was being a relatively cash-poor rural community. Although Hunterdon is now one of the wealthiest counties in the United States, that was not true in the 1940s and 1950s. Although some of the leaders were wealthy, their financial contribution was relatively small. Many other leaders, such as Rose Angell, Clifford Snyder, Waldo McNutt, Ray Trussell and the first professional staff on hand prior to opening were not well-to-do. The community involvement was due to almost total participation of families—over 80 percent—not the size of individual gifts.

WHAT HAS BEEN BROUGHT TO THE HEALTH OF THE COMMUNITY?

HMC was founded as a community hospital, by, of and for the people who lived in Hunterdon County, who supported it with passion, money and hard work, confided their trust to the staff and rejoiced in its success. And to this day it is, even in these competitive times, the *Hunterdon* Medical Center. The staff from top to bottom provides high quality, personal and thoughtful care.

Outreach and education are a product of expanded service to the community. Programs seek those in need of help, to educate those who wish to maintain and prolong their state of health, and to influence each resident in the direction of a healthier life.

Family medicine has remained primary. A family practice residency program, enjoying an eminent reputation, thrives, filling all openings every year with graduates of prestigious U.S. medical schools.

Although the closed full-time staff exists no longer, the specialist staff, of uncommon ability, upholds a tradition of conservative practice and low utilization, willing to obtain consulting advice or to refer for care whenever it serves the best interests of the patient.

Hunterdon is fiscally sound and continues to innovate in the organization of economical and efficient methods to offer health care. It is administratively and professionally devoted to close cooperation with public and private community agencies in any appropriate field.

WHAT MIGHT BE CONSIDERED FOR THE FUTURE?

Evaluation. Ongoing evaluation of results should be a function of every department or division of the entire HMC complex, including the level of the multiple interlocking boards. For this purpose, the planning process of the Partnership for Health could be expanded and adapted, using existing data for ongoing reassessment of community health.

Research. This may have been a major lack, understandable in the light of what was accomplished, but regrettable. As new units are opened a research component should be an integral part of the program, incorporated into initial plans. The cancer center has shown the way by affiliation with a major research center. In late 2001 two new smaller services have opened: neonatology by the Pediatric Department and pediatric orthopedics by the Orthopedic Department. Staff of these services have an excellent opportunity to devise clinical projects of academic value. Other HMC components should be so encouraged. HMC should plan creation of an endowment fund to provide seed money for such projects.

Education. Consideration should be given to incorporating leading theory and practice into HMC's already extensive efforts in patient education, behavior change and provision of information of health significance.

Structure. Many volunteers serve on the rather complex set of interlocking boards that oversees the many components of the Medical Center complex; a number serve on several boards in the group. This might be simplified, not only to reduce volunteer stress, but also to reduce administrative costs. Each of the above services has its own billing, grants management and scheduling services. Consideration might also be given to comparable changes in other hierarchical areas—examination of both trees and forests.

What is special about Hunterdon Medical Center is not a novel discovery or new way to deliver care, but rather that the best known was brought together and integrated into a package; the persons involved were motivated by a desire for excellence; the halo of glory which surrounded the institution and its staff was energized by a spirit of idealism not commonly seen at the close of the 20th century. To quote Winston Churchill, *"This was their finest hour."*

PART III

The People Who Created the Ideal

CHAPTER 19

The People

Early Members of HMC's Board and

Other Important Contributors

P rofiles of seminal figures in the creation of Hunterdon Medical Center, such as Rose Angell, Louise Leicester, Ann Stevenson, Clifford Snyder, Lloyd Wescott, E. H. Lewinsky-Corwin, Lester Evans, and Ray Trussell, were part of the main narrative. However, there are many others who made contributions, great and small. The profiles that follow are of individuals who were involved in the early years (i.e., before my arrival). Their tales are presented for many reasons: to reveal the enormous breadth and variety of human enterprise; out of my admiration for these persons; and as testimony to their achievements. The profiles were developed from interviews with relatives and friends or from archival records. Unfortunately, in many cases the record is scant or incomplete. This part of the book consists of profiles, with chapters organized by role—early Board members, specialist staff, family physicians, house staff, administrative and nursing staff—with individuals listed alphabetically within chapters, except for Chapter 20, where the profiles of key specialists—Andy Hunt, Morris Parmet, and Ed Pellegrino—are presented first, with other specialists following in alphabetical order.

SAMUEL LOUIS BODINE

Bodine is an old county name. Samuel Bodine, a power in Republican politics, earned his livelihood from a lumber company founded by his father in Flemington. Born 22 January 1899, Bodine was educated in the Flemington public schools and at Lafayette College, class of 1920. He served as mayor of Flemington and as county freeholder. He played leapfrog with Wesley Lance in the state Senate, elected in 1943, 1945, and 1948. In the Senate Bodine won respect from his farmer constituents by reporting regularly on political developments to the Board of Agriculture. County Agricultural Agent Bill McIntyre regarded him as a "good member of the Board [of Agriculture and] a strong supporter of . . . [its] activities."[1] Bodine was one of the eight original incorporators of the HMC. He continued to serve on its Board until 1955. His opinions there, marked by fairness and thoughtful open attitudes, won him high respect. His community influence was also quite useful to HMC. In later years he was very active in Republican party politics, serving as a mediator to settle destructive conflicts. He served five years as state Republican Chairperson. He died unexpectedly at 59, in September, 1958.

George I. Bushfield

George Bushfield was a member of HMC's Board from 1949 to 1969. Born at home on 13 January 1900, he grew up in Hunterdon County, attending a one-room schoolhouse in Stanton, Flemington High School and then graduated from Columbia College in 1922. For the next 30 years he was in advertising in New York, attaining great renown and many national awards for creativity; he then retired to his family home to work as a freelance consultant. Bushfield was extraordinarily helpful to the Board in fund-raising and in measuring community responses. Voluminous correspondence between him and Wescott testifies to his ready availability, how highly his opinions were respected and his ability to influence others. He served the Board as Vice President, a member of the Executive Committee, and Chair of the Public Relations Committee. In the community he was active in many areas, establishing zoning and planning boards, working on environmental issues, promoting better education, and indeed almost any cause he felt would better the people of Hunterdon County. I remember him and his wife, Elizabeth, as two immensely charming and handsome people. He died in June, 1969.

CHARLES HENRY CANE

Charles H. Cane was born 6 July 1900, raised in Lambertville in southern Hunterdon, and educated at Rider College, near Trenton.[a] He started his career as State Extension Poultry Specialist and Agriculture Agent in Cumberland County. In 1927 he became a poultryman in Rosemont in southwestern Hunterdon County, where he developed an efficient, model showplace egg hatchery, producing up to 500,000 chicks a year and shipping to farmers all over the northeast. This was made possible by the insight of a poultry raiser from nearby Stockton, who had, in 1892, realized that since newborn chicks lived on the yolk sac for several days after birth and did not need food, they could be shipped by mail without injury.

Cane had a hand in another significant development for local farmers. He, Ed Gauntt, Hunterdon's first County Agricultural Agent, and Jim Weisel, another member of the HMC Board, developed the first auction market for eggs in Flemington in 1930. The auction enabled farmers to obtain better prices for their eggs. At its start, the split between the conservative farmer and the optimistic entrepreneurial farmer was never more clear, but its early success soon converted everyone. Cane served on the Executive Committee of the Board of Agriculture for over 30 years. As a Director of the Phillips Memorial Fund, he was instrumental in establishing the Phillips–Barber Family Health Center in Lambertville.

ALMENA DEAN CRANE

Almena Crane was a thoughtful, sincere and sweet woman who tirelessly worked for the best interests of the community and of HMC. She was a sterling example of the virtues of Hunterdon's traditional farm families: hard working, efficient and effective, recognizing the needs of others and willing to share, but aware of the importance of obtaining the most value for a dollar. Crane was born in 1907, in Nichols, New York. She graduated from the Cornell

[a] In those days Rider was a very popular college for young people interested in agriculture, particularly in poultry husbandry. An uncle of mine, raised in the county, graduated from Rider, where he met his future wife, and managed a hatchery in southern New Jersey his entire active life.

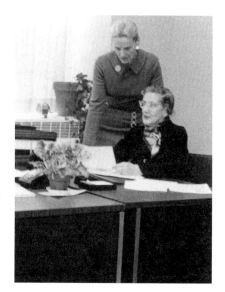

Almena Crane, on the right, discussing hospital affairs with Eleanor Claus, Director of Nursing and acting HMC Director. Mrs. Crane, who managed the family farm for 30 years after her husband's death, was an HMC Board member and worked actively helping with hospital affairs.

University School of Home Economics. She married Robert Crane and moved to Franklin Township, Hunterdon County, where they raised poultry and grain. In 1942 he died in a manner peculiar to farmers—his tractor turned over. She took over the farm and managed it for 30 years, until she retired and moved to Flemington.

Crane went on to be active in the community:

> I'd lived in the county several years before I became active in women's groups . . . I observed a bit of controversy over the role women should play . . . I was asked to become a member of the women's committee [which] became known as the Associated Women of the Hunterdon County Board of Agriculture . . . We became a very strong group.[2]

She was a member of the Board of Agriculture's committee, appointed in 1946 to examine the need for a hospital. She became a member of HMC's Board in April 1954. She was active in farm affairs, in many organizations, and after retirement painted until her eyesight failed—and then wrote poetry. She was typical of many farm women who were active in affairs. She died 21 October 1993.

REV. EDWARD C. DUNBAR

Rev. Dunbar was a short, roly-poly, sweet-tempered, witty and very sharp clergyman. Little escaped his eye. His awareness of human frailty did not diminish his concern for each person he met.

Following graduation from Colby College, he attended Newton Baptist Seminary in Newton, Mass. In World War I he served in the infantry and was discharged as a first lieutenant. He was ordained in 1922 and served in Massachusetts, Connecticut and finally at the Flemington Baptist Church.

When the drive to start HMC began, he was a member of the Board of Agriculture, where he represented the County Council of Churches. He knew at once that it was a project of major importance. After the hospital opened, he supported its chaplaincy program. He was a member of the Board for 28 years, much of the time as Secretary. Similarly to Joe Moskowitz, Almena Crane, and many other HMC Board members, Rev. Dunbar was an active and vigorous contributor to innumerable community organizations and programs, as well as a person who engendered affection in others. He was active helping migrant farm workers' children get an education. He was a long-time member of the Welfare Board. Dunbar always enjoyed meeting and speaking with people and learning about new ideas and was said to have been a favorite of many outside his congregation to perform wedding ceremonies. He reached out to include everyone he met regardless of background.[3] Rev. Dunbar retired in 1965 and died 6 August 1983 at the age of 89.

RAYMOND J. GERMAIN, M.D.

Ray Germain played a dual role as an HMC Board member and a family physician. He was the first, and for decades the only, physician to serve on the Board. Germain was an original Board member, one of eight incorporators of the Medical Center. He played a key role in swinging the Hunterdon County Medical Society to unanimous acceptance and support for the hospital plan and was extraordinarily helpful in cementing relationships between the Board and family physicians. He had a record of civic activity. In 1941 he helped create a doctor's bill insurance program, sponsored by the N.J. Medical Society, for families of limited income. He encouraged county residents to join, but the program never really got off the ground. In 1942 he was named Head of Emergency Medical Services for the Civil Defense program.

Despite Germain's contributions to HMC, the Board of Trustees voted in 1951 that no physician could serve on the Board; Germain resigned on 7 December 1951. Many Board members told

me in personal conversations that physicians serving on the Board
had an inherent conflict of interest because they regarded the hospital as a workshop, to be modified to suit their interests. Board
members felt a responsibility to serve the best interests of community health. Why presumably selfish interests of physicians would
govern behavior more than those of Board members was never
explained. I am not convinced that this was why Germain was
shown the door. The real reason may be found in a presentation
given by Lloyd Wescott to the American Hospital Association.[4]
He strongly advised against physicians as board members. In the
event, physicians were barred from Board membership until the
Consent Decree of 1977 took effect.

Germain founded a nursing home in Hunterdon County, which
he sold about 1970. He and his wife separated, and he left the
area. I was unable to locate other information about him.

GEORGE HANKS

George Hanks was President of Taylor–Wharton Iron and Steel
Company of High Bridge, during the first half of the 20th century
the largest employer (over 600 employees) in the county. Taylor–
Wharton was the oldest continuously operating iron and steel pro-
ducer in the United States, dating back to 1851, and located on the
site of Union Furnace, where iron was made during the Revolutionary War. Attorney Wesley Lance recalls Hanks as

> a no-nonsense man; a graduate of Princeton University, the
> class of 1915, I believe. My first contact with George Hanks
> was through baseball since I organized the Tri-County Base-
> ball League around 1937. George Hanks was also connected
> with the First National Bank of High Bridge. I imagine he
> was chosen because he was a large employer. Taylor–Wharton
> . . . often lost money or barely broke even.[5]

The obituary in the *Hunterdon County Democrat* records that while
Hanks was still at Princeton the then president of Taylor–Wharton
offered him a job because his college record as a center fielder
suggested he could help the company team. His service on HMC's
Board did not last; he worked on the board of Somerset Hospital,
a competitor in a neighboring county, for many years. Hanks died
12 October 1975 at the age of 85.

J. SEWARD JOHNSON

Seward Johnson was one of the most remarkable of those who created HMC. Many thought that his money had done the job, but records and comments from the time indicate that while he did give generously, his gifts were far from dominant. He contributed far more by lending his name as a backer so that others would follow; by bringing in ideas based on his own strong concerns about health; and by serving as a stimulus to others and as a conscience to all. Just as the critical contribution of Commonwealth Fund was its consulting help, so the critical contribution of Seward Johnson was his presence.

BACKGROUND AND CAREER

John Seward Johnson (1895–1983) was the son of Robert Wood Johnson, one of the founders of Johnson & Johnson, the pharmaceutical company. Seward Johnson was raised in New Brunswick, and later in New York. He was tutored at home, perhaps because he is said to have suffered from a learning disability that led to difficulty both with reading and writing.[b] His father died while he and his older brother, Robert Wood Johnson Jr., were adolescents; the Johnson brothers inherited great wealth in the form of Johnson & Johnson stock. The elder brother, a person of formidable qualities, managed the company. Seward's son, J. Seward Johnson Jr., attests to this: "In 1910 when he was 14 or 15 years old, my father developed appendicitis and was in need of surgery. His brother . . . was two years older. Father had died, and mother was away. My uncle arranged to have an operating room rigged up at home with full antiseptic technique."[6]

Seward Johnson, who inherited equally, was occasionally but not deeply engaged in management. However, after his older brother died, he took a much greater interest in the company. In addition to raising prize-winning registered Holstein cattle, his interests included competitive sailing (he won a number of international competitions) and oceanography. During World War I he requested

[b] Goldsmith B. *Johnson v. Johnson*. New York: Knopf, 1987: 7–10. I have reviewed hundreds of his letters; unless he hired someone to clean up spelling and language, I found no evidence of any expressive problem. To the contrary, he wrote clearly, concisely, and to the point.

sea duty, commanded a subchaser, and earned commendations and a promotion to lieutenant.

INTEREST IN FARMING

After World War I Johnson farmed and bred cattle in Oldwick, Hunterdon County. He lived the life of a gentleman farmer, de-voted to milk production and breeding his cattle. His farm was something of a showplace, according to Bill McIntyre.[7] Farmers met there to see the glass-lined silos and the coal mining machines used to unload silos from the bottom. During World War II Johnson attempted to make farming more efficient by producing more with less staff. He started a commercial dairy in Morristown, because he felt that he could bypass the "middlemen and unions [that] drove up prices."[8] He and Lloyd Wescott were involved in the development of artificial breeding of cattle. Johnson provided signifi-cant financial help to the N.J. Agricultural Experiment Station at Rutgers University.

INTEREST IN HMC

Almost surely Johnson was brought in by Wescott.[c] They shared an interest in farming and a life style. Seward's son pointed out that his father would not have been interested in "just another community hospital, such as Princeton Hospital, for example," but was intrigued by the tie with NYU Medical School. Wesley Lance, an attorney and legislator from Clinton and an early mem-ber of the Board, described Seward as a

> very quiet, very selfless, unassuming man. He would be the
> last man at the table you would probably pick out to be
> [wealthy]. But he was dedicated to the hospital, the prin-
> ciples on which it was founded, and whatever was good for
> the community. What he did was to be available to come to
> the rescue when needed, providing financial stability, more in
> the nature of potential, than of actual funds. He would match,
> or promise to match donations.[9]

Wescott regarded Johnson as a last resort when things seemed

[c] Seward's uncle, Carter Nicholas, Jr., was also for a time on the HMC Board.

black. When criticism was made of the size of his gifts, relative to his means, Wescott wrote:

> He, like many other rich men, dreads being played for a patsy. If he feels something is the responsibility of the community at large, and that they can manage it, he will not pick up the check . . . He gave $25,000 . . . when few other people in the County would even listen . . . When the chips were down and no one—but no one—would give us enough credit, he guaranteed a loan of $300,000 and put up J&J stock to cover. When we were dead broke in '54 he put up $65,000 to keep us from closing down entirely.[10]

Wescott listed a total of $590,000 that Johnson had donated; the timing of these gifts had an enormous effect on donations from others.[11]

Johnson provided more than money. His response to Trussell in 1950 is illustrative. Trussell had polled Board members on HMC's future direction. Johnson wrote out his reply by hand. It is worth quoting:

> We should first acquire a site that has all our immediate requirements plus capacity for at least 200 percent expansion. We should then plan buildings that will house all the basic ideas that have made our hospital planning interesting to people in the hospital world and to the people of our county . . . As a first consideration the hospital must contain facilities to service the general practitioner . . . Equally important will be the facilities for the administration and clinics of public health work. In the building of our hospital *no matter how limited our funds may prove to be we must not depart one fraction from the ideals that have brought us to this point* [emphasis added].[12]

Seward Johnson was always interested in personal hygiene, physical condition and diet. His son recalls that he was concerned with fundamental things—pure air, water. "At one time grapefruit were very important. He used to send me supplies of grapefruit when I was at school."[13] In 1961 he became intrigued by the notion of public health education at HMC (see Chapter 17). He wrote to the Medical Director that "the only path which will result in complete public health services without tax support or heavy endowment will be the education of the people from the cradle to the grave, to understand the advantages of health services to them."[14]

He saw health education covering a spectrum from physical fitness and nutrition through parks and conservation to Christianity. He proposed a Department of Public Health Education for HMC (see Chapter 15); the idea did not advance at that time. More recently, HMC has created a large, effective Health Education Department.

Seward Johnson was interested in many other areas of health care. He corresponded regularly with Trussell, Pellegrino, Henderson and Wescott. For example, in 1959, he indicated he would consider funding research by the staff in conjunction with NYU: "Our staff would be more welcome . . . if they brought with them funds."[15] For some reason, his offer was never made known to staff. Two years later, he wrote: "At the HMC we go to great lengths to study the background of the doctors who come to work with us, but it has never come to my attention that we ever make what might be called an 'audit' of the quality of their work after they once join us."[16] At other times he initiated correspondence about home care programs, physical fitness for the public, progressive patient care, a community college, and schools of nursing. Unfortunately, none of these ruminations were discussed with the staff, because at least some of them might have led to productive research to enhance HMC's reputation and solidify what Cowles Herr called the status of Hunterdon as "a JV academic center." After 1970 or 1971, the files reveal Johnson's diminishing interest in HMC. Wescott complained of difficulties meeting with him, and Johnson refused a number of requests for assistance.

Johnson was a man of slightly less than average size, serious in demeanor, neatly built. I can recall being interviewed by him as a candidate for staff appointment at HMC. He wore what I called an "ancient mariner" white beard, shaven around the mouth and front of the chin. He was described by some as reserved or shy, but kind and gentle. On the other hand, Walter Petryshyn, the otolaryngologist, said that they socialized with the Johnsons. "He liked to dance . . . he loved to do the polka with Mrs. Petryshyn who taught him [the dance.] He was a party person."[17] Indeed, a book chronicling the Johnson family, as well as a bitterly contested fight over the disposition of his estate, describes him as quite charming and a roué.[18]

WESLEY L. LANCE, ESQ.

EARLY CAREER

Wesley Lance was born in Lebanon Township on 21 November 1908 and grew up in Glen Gardner, Hunterdon County. He graduated from Lafayette College in 1928, where he was on the baseball team. He taught school for a time before graduating from Harvard Law School in 1935. He returned to New Jersey to practice law and formed the Tri-County Baseball League, which had teams from Hunterdon, Warren and Northampton (Pennsylvania) counties. The League's President, Col. Arthur F. Foran, a power in local politics, offered him an opportunity to run for the Assembly as a Republican in 1937.[d] Lance, at this time a Democrat, felt that with the cushion of some inherited income, he could afford to run. He was successful, was re-elected in 1938, 1939 and 1940, and went to the state Senate in 1941 and 1942, and after World War II, in 1953 and 1957. He was President of the Senate in 1959. Lance provides some detail on his political career:

> [Foran] was honest enough to tell me that in those days Republicans didn't win the Assembly very often. But he said it won't hurt your law practice as a young lawyer. I ran, and much to my surprise, and a lot of other peoples' surprise, I won as an Assemblyman, and then later, I was a State Senator. Then I resigned to go in the Navy, came back and was the County Judge for five years and then went to the Senate the second time. I was Chairman of the Joint Appropriations Committee, President of the State Senate, Majority Leader of the State Senate and Acting Governor which was purely ceremonial . . . I served in two constitutional conventions, '47 and '66, and also I was . . . a Presidential Elector . . . for Nixon and Agnew. I apologize for Agnew but I always thought Nixon was a good man in foreign policy. So, that's my political background of which I'm proud although it never made me much money, I'll say that.[19]

[d] The Foran family owned a foundry in Flemington, established in 1893, the source of family wealth. Col. Foran had three sons: Walter E. "Moose" Foran became Hunterdon County's senior N.J. legislator, with long service first in the Assembly, then in the Senate; Richard became a cowboy movie star known as Dick Foran; and Arthur has been very active in many voluntary organizations in the county.

SERVICE ON HMC BOARD

Lance was invited by Lloyd Wescott and Louise Leicester (whom he represented from time to time) to join the Board. "I think that flattery was part of it, to tell you the truth." At the time, 1950, Lance was in his early 40s and had been interested in organizations. He desired community service and was not unaware of the favorable effect upon his reputation. The unique aspects of the institution were not a major motivation, although he did understand that Hunterdon was a national model. But "on the technical aspects I was helpless, because my whole life in politics and government had been more or less on economic lines, taxation and revenues rather than the social welfare lines and I was entirely out of my field of expertise." The timing, he felt, was right also, because he was then a county judge, and his appointment to the Board would not make the other attorneys jealous. His most important reasons for joining were that he felt the idea of a hospital was a very good one, plus his immense admiration for Lloyd Wescott and his contributions.

Although not on the original Board, and thus not an incorporator, Lance served on the Board before HMC opened. He did much pro bono legal work for HMC (a tradition carried on to the present by other attorneys), including land acquisition and legal matters related to construction. The entire construction process, he felt, was blessed in that none of the many pitfalls that can dog such ventures occurred—no bankrupt contractors, unpaid suppliers, subcontractors, laborers, no untoward delays, and so on. He left the Board in 1954 because he was re-elected to the N.J. State Senate and had insufficient time to devote to both.

Lance tells of one of his more memorable interactions with Board members and others in a position to be of help.

> [HMC] obtained from people written pledges or IOUs: I promise to pay you $500 or . . . whatever it was [and] needed to raise money on these IOUs. Obviously this type of collateral is not like Moody's Investor Service where you're rated as triple A. People in their enthusiasm may pledge $1,000 but whether they pay it or not is another thing. I was asked to make an appointment with . . . the National State Bank of Newark . . . I called Paul Stillman, whom I knew through politics, and

said I want to bring down a couple of Hunterdon County
farmers. So we go down to Paul Stillman's office in Newark
with Lloyd Wescott and Seward Johnson. Paul peeked out,
looked at the three of us sitting there and then he beckoned
me in. He said, "Did you say a couple of Hunterdon County
farmers?" I said, "Yes." He was referring to the beard of Lloyd
Wescott and the beard of Seward Johnson . . . I have often
wondered why Seward Johnson, who could have bought us
all out 1,600 or 1,700 times, relied on me to set up the temporary financing where we borrowed money from National
State Bank in Newark using the pledges as collateral.

Wescott's comments and Ray Trussell's story of the same event, in
which Johnson co-signed the loan, make clear that Johnson wanted
the community to manage on its own as much as possible.

Lance was always interested in politics. Although a Republican,
he worked closely with Lloyd Wescott, who was a prominent Democrat. As a member of the N.J. Senate, he twice led the Senate in
confirming Wescott to high governmental appointments under
Democratic Governor Robert Meyner. Lance recalls often being
asked why Wescott did not run against him for the Senate. "It
would have been an interesting battle and I think Lloyd would
have probably won. But I think Lloyd . . . probably thought that I
was doing a satisfactory job in the state legislature." Wescott's pledge
to his wife not to engage in politics was apparently kept to the
confines of the Wescott family.

WILLIAM J. LAUDERDALE

Although he never served on the HMC Board, Bill Lauderdale was
involved in many aspects of progressive agriculture in the county.
He was appointed to the Committee to Study the Possibility of a
Hospital, but apparently does not appear on the final report. Lauderdale was a Director of the Lambertville National Bank and a
"lifelong and outspoken Republican."[20] According to his obituary,
among the biggest thrills of his life was meeting President Calvin
Coolidge and later President Herbert Hoover to explain to them
the problems of the farmer.

WALDO REYNOLD MCNUTT

Waldo McNutt became interested in a hospital when on the Executive Committee of the Board of Agriculture. He helped arrange for Rose Angell, Louise Leicester and Ann Stevenson to appear before the Board. He followed through by becoming a member of the study committee, an incorporator and founding Board member. McNutt was deeply involved in planning and fund-raising activities. He remained on the Board until the day after HMC opened.

According to Don Shuman, a real estate broker with whom McNutt worked briefly, McNutt was a cherub-faced man with a round face and a rosy complexion, outgoing and pleasant, gregarious. He lived in the Frenchtown area.[21] McNutt came to Hunterdon as a poultryman, and an organizer and representative of the Farmer's Union. He had a reputation for "liberal" views—a local euphemism for socialist or communist. County Agricultural Agent Bill McIntyre described him as helpful to the [farmers'] cooperative, a good active member of the Executive Committee of the Board of Agriculture whose views were thought provoking for the strong conservatives.[22] McNutt graduated from Wabash College in Topeka, Kansas, with an LL.B. When he came to Hunterdon he said he wanted to enter hospital administration. Accordingly, in 1951 he matriculated at Columbia University School of Public Health, (where one day Ray Trussell would be Dean), graduating in 1954 with an M.P.H. Meanwhile he served an administrative residency at Cumberland Clinic, Cumberland, Kentucky, an affiliate of the United Mine Workers group of hospitals. When he resigned from HMC's Board, he was already employed by that group.[23] Unfortunately I was unable to locate further information about him.

JOSEPH E. MOSKOWITZ

Joseph Moskowitz came to Ringoes in southern Hunterdon County in 1940 to take over a farm of 213 acres for dairy and poultry farming. He was born in Brooklyn, N.Y., in 1891, one of nine children. He spent his career manufacturing leather goods until he decided, for reasons I cannot determine, to become a farmer. Once in this area, he was a hard worker and also looked beyond the borders of his land. He was a founder of the Delaware Valley Farmers

Cooperative, one of two in the county that on a group basis helped farmers market their produce and engaged in collective purchasing.ᵉ Moskowitz was also active in Republican politics and in religious affairs as President of the Flemington Jewish Community Center. Bill McIntyre said, "He understood the need rural folks have for medical care."²⁴ Probably Moskowitz's affiliations led to his being asked to join HMC's Board in 1949. His own character and devotion led him to come in four and five days a week to attend Board meetings and serve as Secretary. He died on 3 April 1959. Although I never knew him, I was touched by the extent to which his loss affected those who had worked with him. The Board felt strongly enough that a grove of beautiful trees behind the hospital, with picnic benches installed in the shade, was named for him, the only named feature on the hospital campus for many years.

KENNETH B. MYERS

Kenneth Myers was born on a farm at Allen's Corner, not far from Quakertown. "If you come down from Quakertown toward Croton, you would turn to your right and it would be the second place on your left."²⁵ Birth was "reluctant" because he was a ten-pound baby. His great-grandfather purchased the farm in 1850, but it was a working farm before that: "There was about 100 acres, dairy, poultry, turkeys and the usual general farm practice." The stone farmhouse had no electricity or central heating.ᶠ It was cold and damp in the winter and warm and damp in the summer. At the end of the lane was a small schoolhouse built on land donated by his grandfather to the local school board. Myers attended this one-room school until eighth grade, and then went on to Flemington High School. His first year there, they were bused to school in a feed truck.

ᵉ Eventually this co-op was absorbed by the larger one founded by Richard Schomp, which ultimately became Agway. In a typical change of the times, Moskowitz's silo and building were converted into an upscale manufacturers' outlet, where makers of clothing, jewelry, and household items sold their seconds and discontinued lines.

ᶠ My father and his family lived in a farmhouse like that in Raritan Township, less than two miles from where HMC is now. My father talked about breaking the ice in the water jar in the bedroom to wash his face, or lighting candles and lanterns. I can remember as a young man saying to myself, "Yeah, Pop, sure, Pop." But after moving here, one day I took our children to see the ruins of the old house. We found no pipes, no plumbing, no electric wires and no heating plant.

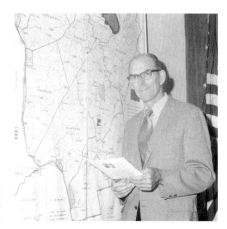

Ken Myers in a typical
pose at a meeting of one of the
governing bodies of the community.

Little Wilson Deets had a feed business in Pittstown and they
had a canvas-covered truck. They would take the canvas off
and use it as a feed truck after they delivered the school kids
to the Flemington High School . . . It was cold and the snow
would blow in and it was about a three-quarter mile walk
from our farm to the crossroads up on the hard road. The
second year, we had a closed-in bus and that was a better
trip.

Myers left the farm when he graduated from high school. He
had been lonely long enough, never really cared for the farm, and
longed to be where there were people. During his second semester
of college in Philadelphia he was called home by Dr. Leaver because his father was seriously ill. The doctor met him at the door,
told him his father had died and his last words:

"Tell Kenneth to take care of his mother" . . . I didn't have
any choice with that kind of admonition from Dr. Leaver so I
gave up my schooling and returned home. I operated the farm
for a couple of years. I didn't like it. I went to work for a
fellow named Chester Niece who had a lumberyard in
Frenchtown.

Myers came to the attention of Senators Bodine and Schenck
and when the Republicans were successful the following year and
controlled the Board of Freeholders, Myers was appointed clerk,
one of the few patronage jobs.

My job was full time and I was excited about getting into the

> political picture. I was quite happy as clerk to the Board of Freeholders for three or four years. Then World War II was coming along and I knew that this was a political appointment every three years and that the complexion of the Board changed. I knew, just as I had replaced somebody, somebody would replace me. I thought I really ought to have something a little better. By this time I had been married with one child. So I took an exam to work with the Internal Revenue Department and except for the three years . . . in the service, I worked there. After that I came back to be County Treasurer.

Other than help with fund-raising, Myers did not have early connections with HMC, although he knew almost everyone involved on the Board or influential in county affairs. In 1973, in the midst of the financial crises and staff turmoil, Lloyd Wescott invited him to join the board and Myers became Treasurer, reorganizing Board finances, instituting regular Finance Committee meetings and seeing that cash reserves were suitably invested.

Myers remained very active in the community until his death in July 1995. In person, Myers was a lanky, lean man, with a wide mouth, long jaw and friendly face. He was easy to talk with—when you could get a word in. Like many other local activists, he tended to look for positive qualities in people, but when he could not find them, he managed to be critical in a way that would not cause offense. He was a hard worker, always on the go. He seemed to spend a great deal of time in conversations, but these were with his enormous social network, which provided him with the resources he needed to get things done. As was true of a number of other local political figures, he always had time to stop, listen and attend to someone's needs. And, like Lloyd Wescott, the man he admired so much, he always had time to help by identifying a pathway to someone with a possible solution. His livelihood, which was never great, came primarily from accounting and bookkeeping services.

REEVE SCHLEY, JR.

Reeve Schley, a powerful figure, large, with a blocky head, wide jaw, firm features, and a pipe always in his mouth, appeared to be the person of wealth and position that he was. Although he described himself as a farmer, he was from a family of wealth and social position. He married well and moved in distinguished circles his entire life. His father, Reeve Sr., St. Paul's School, Yale and LL.B. Columbia, was a Vice President at Chase Bank, President of the Somerset Trust Company and active in Republican politics. More important to the history of HMC, Reeve Sr. was for many years on the New Jersey State Board of Control, which managed a large proportion of the state's penal, social and medical institutions. He eventually became President of the Board of Control and was succeeded by Lloyd Wescott.[26]

Reeve Jr. was born 7 September 1908 in Monmouth County and was educated at St. Paul's School and at Yale, where he graduated in 1931. From there, he moved on to Columbia University Law School and received his degree in 1934. His wife, Elizabeth, was sister to the wife of Webster Todd, long-time head of the New Jersey Republican Party.[g] Schley brought to the HMC Board, in addition to his experience and network of connections, a relationship to banking; the younger Schley succeeded his father as President of the Somerset Trust Company. He coordinated a consortium of 10 local banks to obtain a badly needed loan, saving HMC when fund-raising was about to founder.

Another side of him emerged at a party, one of innumerable affairs for HMC Board and Staff given by Lloyd Wescott. Also present was a friend of Schley's from Australia, who after a few drinks, talked of Schley's record in World War II. From him we learned that Schley had volunteered in 1942 and became a lieutenant in the horse cavalry. Apparently dissatisfied, he volunteered for the O.S.S. and parachuted on several occasions into Occupied France in 1944 and Italy in 1945 to work with the French resistance and the Italian partisans. For this he received from the United States the Bronze Star twice and from France the Croix de Guerre.[27] He died 18 October 1993.

---

[g] The Todds' daughter, Christine Todd Whitman, eventually became governor of New Jersey and serves as the head of the Environmental Protection Agency in the administration of President George W. Bush.

RICHARD S. SCHOMP

Dick Schomp was born in 1888, in Pluckemin in neighboring Somerset County, raised in Flemington, and graduated from Reading Academy in 1906.[h] He attended the State Agricultural College, the precursor of Cook College, Rutgers University, and was one of the group who managed the affairs of the Board of Agriculture in Hunterdon County for more than three decades. He was the perennial secretary, a leader in the efforts to modernize agriculture. Schomp was a farmer and also managed the GLF (later Agway) feed store. He was instrumental in enlarging it to a cooperative farm store. He pioneered in the artificial breeding of cattle. Schomp was active in many farm organizations, including the Grange, the State Board of Agriculture, and the Board of Hunterdon Central High School, the first regional school in the county. His daughter, Ann Sauerland, grew up on the farm. She helped in the dairy with registered Holstein cattle, feeding the chickens, collecting the eggs and throwing hay bales around in the barn. It was work, but she looks back, with some nostalgia, "not a bad life."[28]

Schomp's opinion was always respected, and he had a thoughtful demeanor. If he was upset, he never let it show. His daughter does not remember his ever losing his temper. He, along with Almena Crane, Herbert Van Pelt and Bill Lauderdale offered balance to firebrands like Leicester and McNutt. He served on the HMC Board from 1954–1961. Sauerland believes that in that post–World War II period, the community attracted a group of forward-thinking farm families unique in this community. A certain type of person was attracted who was open to new ideas, up to date in current thinking, and good at listening to what others thought. All these qualities were characteristic of Richard Schomp, as well as Snyder and Lauderdale. Schomp died 15 June 1961 at age 73.

HERBERT D. STEM

Herb Stem was active in local Democratic politics. He was born in Milford in 1894 and died 1 April 1978 at the age of 83. He was President of the First National Bank of Milford, as well as of a

---

[h] Reading Academy was the name of the Flemington High School; a member of the Reading family, an old one in the county, had donated the building. It still stands and is used as a middle school.

savings and loan association, and was active in the insurance business. He served on the HMC Board from 1949–1959.

HERBERT E. VAN PELT

Herbert Van Pelt descended from a family settled in the area before the Revolution. He was born in 1882 and began his career "crying" as an auctioneer in 1917. Van Pelt was the auctioneer at the Flemington Egg Auction, which established his connections with the county Board of Agriculture. Van Pelt's appointment to the Study Committee of the Board of Agriculture may have been because of his delightful personality—people often attended his auctions just to laugh at his jokes and antics. He did not serve on the HMC Board, but organized and managed several successful fundraising auctions at the Flemington Fair to benefit HMC. He always had more work than he could handle, and his auctions typically brought top dollar. In addition to everything else, he was the president of two banks and an insurance company, a director of the Flemington Fair, and a trustee of neighboring Somerset Hospital. He died on 15 March 1968.

MARGARET (MRS. CHARLES) WAGG

Margaret Wagg was known for her civic-mindedness throughout south Hunterdon where she lived. She and her husband Charles, a dentist, owned a farm and residence on High School Hill above the city of Lambertville. Dr. Wagg practiced in Trenton. She had administrative and organizational skills that often led her to a leadership role.[29] She served on the HMC Board and its Executive Committee from 1949–1959.

JAMES WEISEL

James Weisel, along with Clifford Snyder, Charles Cane, William Lauderdale, Richard Schomp and others, was a major figure in the organizations and politics of agriculture in Hunterdon County. He earned this distinction by hard work and professional skills as a farmer, by willingness to work for the community, and by a blend of careful and realistic conservatism with an open mind towards innovation, and by his contributions to ventures that benefited farmers. It is not hard to understand why he was asked to serve on the HMC Board. His influence within the farm community was immense; he had a record of accomplishment; his personality was winning. I remember him as an unassuming man who seemed concerned only with how the Board might best support the functions of the hospital. Weisel was an incorporator and served on the Board from 1948–1970.

Born in Brooklyn, New York, 11 May 1898, Weisel was raised on a farm in Newfoundland, Sussex County, New Jersey. He graduated from Rutgers in 1920 in poultry husbandry. Subsequently he was a breeder and then general manager for Kerr Hatcheries near Frenchtown, a major shipper of chicks. At one time they maintained 15 plants and incubated up to 1,000,000 eggs at a time. He was one of three innovators who developed the Flemington cooperative egg auction in the depths of the Depression, a story outlined earlier. Eventually he set up his own hatchery in Rosemont. In addition to his local work he eventually became a member of the New Jersey State Board of Agriculture and its president in 1942. He was active in Republican Party politics, serving at one time on the state Republican committee. He died 3 August 1984 at the age of 86.

CHAPTER 20

The People

The Specialist Staff

Ofne of the reasons why HMC enjoyed unusual and productive staff and community relationships was that Ray Trussell, supported by a grant from Commonwealth, brought in three key members of the specialist staff—Andrew Hunt, Morris Parmet and Edmund Pellegrino—before the hospital opened. I have interviewed Hunt, Pellegrino, Parmet's widow and other physicians or their relatives, selected on the basis of having worked at HMC before I started. These interviews have reinforced my admiration, respect and affection for this extraordinary group. Note the common threads in their stories of why they came to Hunterdon and what they liked about it—the chance to open a new department and "do it my way," the camaraderie of peers who were deemed to work at a high level of quality, the chance to teach and to practice in the best manner, and, finally, the community's life style. Chapter 20 begins with the profiles of these three first, with other specialists following in alphabetical order.

ANDREW DICKSON HUNT, M.D.

Andy Hunt grew up in Haverford on the Main Line suburbs of Philadelphia. After graduating from Haverford College he attended Cornell Medical School. There one of his classmates was C. Everett Koop, who became chief pediatric surgeon at Children's Hospital of Philadelphia and later Surgeon Ggneral of the United States.

After a rotating internship and a year of pediatrics at the Hospital of the University of Pennsylvania, Hunt's training was interrupted by World War II and military service with the 98th General Hospital in England, Germany and France. He returned to Children's

Hospital in 1945, finished as Chief Resident in 1947, and then remained on staff as Director of the Clinics. Research activities included extensive work on antibiotic blood levels, for which he was elected to the Society for Pediatric Research, biochemical investigations including the first demonstration of a genetic aberration resulting in unusual dependency on pyridoxine (vitamin B$_6$), and, finally, an abiding interest in behavioral pediatrics. Mentors included Joseph Stokes, Chairman of the Department of Pediatrics, McNair Scott, and for behavioral pediatrics, John Rose. Hunt described the change from bench researcher with a focus on antibiotics to behavioral medicine:

> [I] became for a few years an authority on antibiotic treatment in pediatrics in the United States. But I became sort of disillusioned with the process in which we would give these babies in the nursery a dose of antibiotics and then go out and take their blood and do blood levels with nothing like informed consent or anything of that sort. It was just done. Gradually, I decided that there was something about this with which I was unhappy and indeed with the whole paradigm of that kind of research. I began working with a fair amount of intensity with Dr. John Rose.[1]

Hunt learned of the new hospital in Flemington from Rose. "[Rose] heard about an operation which was going to be big in mental health in Hunterdon County, New Jersey. They were talking about a hospital, full-time specialists." After interviews with Trussell, Wescott and Leicester, he decided to accept the position. Trussell recalls Hunt's response as not quite so deliberate: "I told him what this was all about and he just asked for the job."[2] Morris Parmet, a child psychiatrist and colleague, had already accepted a position at Hunterdon. The salary was more than twice what Hunt was earning at Children's Hospital. It was a chance for him to have his own pediatric service, to have "this consulting relationship with family physicians which I thought quite challenging and interesting and because the opportunity to live here was very attractive." Hunt knew the community because he had attended Solebury School in nearby Pennsylvania, and he and his wife thought it would be a good place for their children. He had just met Lester Evans of Commonwealth, with whom he felt he would have a good relationship. Finally, he was advised by Ray Trussell who suggested that by coming to HMC, Hunt could retain the option of a practice or an academic career: "This could either be something you want to spend the rest of your life at or it could be the beginning of an academic career because the relationship with New York University had been established and because of the . . . Chronic Illness Survey."[3] Hunt feels the decision was wise—Hunterdon helped his confidence, and he profited from the relationship with psychiatry and with social work.

Soon after arriving in 1952, Hunt developed relationships with the family physicians, set up a consulting service in pediatrics, fostered close working relations with behavioral and mental health professionals, and laid plans for innovations in comprehensive care.

> I had learned about the importance of visiting hours and that the hospital is a very good place . . . for studying and understanding parent–child relationships [with open visiting by parents. This] had generally been overlooked amid the enthusiasm for the value of parent absenteeism as promoter of peace, quiet and submission to disagreeable if not painful nurse and physician ministrations.

Hunt went on to say that "the time was right, and that Hunterdon would be a place where free parent visiting as policy could be effected without administrative opposition. This would, furthermore, fit in well with the project's proposed emphasis on mental health."

Hunt exemplified the teacher described by Edwards A. Park in his 1951 address on the opening of the Hospital for Sick Children in Toronto:

> But there is a second kind of teaching which perhaps is the finest of all; I refer to unconscious teaching . . . The men who gave me the most and to whom I feel the most grateful were not those who made the transfer of facts easiest but those who stimulated me to be like them . . . for clearness and accuracy of thinking, for the liberality and generosity of their minds, for the elevation of their standards and ideals, or for the breadth of their outlook, and, perhaps, also for their unconsciousness of themselves.[4]

In this same address Park also spoke of other qualities that informed Hunt's work. One was the importance of being ready at all times to break the rules and regulations in order to provide care tailored to the individual. Another was the importance of a comprehensive approach to the work of the pediatrician, in particular, the importance of attending to behavior as well as organic health, to the goodness of fit between the child and the environment, and to the long-term outlook, decades in the future, of the child and family.

Andy Hunt is a tall, lean, genial, talkative and charming man with whom all say it was a pleasure to work. He is down-to-earth, yet combines scholarly and academic pediatric care with full awareness of child behavior and family dynamics. He brought about change in attitudes without hostility or resentment. He is flexible, able to compromise differing points of view in a positive way.

Aaron Rausen, who was the first clinical clerk on medicine and pediatrics in the summer of 1953, describes Hunt's skills as a diagnostician.

> An infant in acute congestive heart failure from paroxysmal tachycardia [was brought to the emergency room] . . . He may have been one of the first patients admitted to Pediatrics. [Hunt] made the diagnosis. I was absolutely amazed at how clever he was. The child was put on digitalis and had a break in the heart rate within a few hours and the very large liver subsided and the child's 240 or 280 pulse rate went down and then the Wolff–Parkinson–White EKG showed up after the tachycardia subsided . . . a very, very thoughtful pediatrician.[5]

In his work at HMC Hunt combined outstanding skills in "sick kids" pediatrics with a sensitive approach to parents, recognizing that children, like all patients, do not exist in isolation, but are embedded in a context—a family, a community, a culture. Residents labeled patients with such features as "a Hunt-type case."[a] Although his work was to be consulting, he told me he maintained a small primary care practice of families who had become particularly attached to him.

Edmund Pellegrino recalls Hunt as dedicated to pediatrics and children. He influenced staff thinking on developmental features of children with his great clinical skills—and with his sense of humor. He was willing to serve as a consultant, help others, give information without taking all the credit for it.[6] Each of these men went on to found a new medical school and interestingly each school emphasized the interests of the founder: Hunt in

---

[a] Then, and to this day, residents will stereotype a patient with such labels.

environment and behavior; Pellegrino in scientific compassionate patient care.

Hunt was relentlessly curious and able to sum up complex situations in simple words. He developed a well-functioning multidisciplinary group to evaluate and plan for children with complex problems. I can attest to the legacy of experience and expertise that he left. When I arrived at HMC, I found Hunt's group offering comprehensive, sophisticated and thoughtful diagnostic analyses, and care plans for patients with complex medical problems, psychosocial difficulties, dysfunctional families or chronic illness.

When change was afoot at Hunterdon, Hunt, who had several offers of other jobs, chose one at Stanford to develop a new curriculum in which behavioral science would be considered as a basic science. He felt it was time to return to his academic roots with attendant intellectual stimulation and a modest increase in salary rather than accept HMC's offer to replace Pellegrino. It was never possible fully to implement the curriculum at Stanford, but there Hunt developed an interest in medical education. Five years later Hunt went to Michigan State University as Dean of a new medical school. Among other accomplishments, he installed behavioral sciences as a basic science and organized and directed a Center for Ethics and Humanities in Medicine.

MORRIS PARMET, M.D.

Morris Parmet grew up in Allentown, Pennsylvania, about an hour's drive from HMC.[7] His father, a general practitioner, was immensely popular: he would sit by a woman in labor and hold her hand, and be part of that family for a whole day. Parmet worked his way through college running an athletic program at the Jewish Community Center in Allentown. He really wanted to be a camp counselor or coach, but went into medicine because his father and uncles were doctors, and that was what one did. Perhaps this explains how some felt about Parmet: Jeannette Ash, a nurse who worked with him, said: "He was a lot of fun . . . A real person. Not like a psychiatrist."[8]

Following his father and both uncles, Parmet attended Jefferson Medical School in Philadelphia. In his first year he met Belle, a student at the University of Pennsylvania. They married on her graduation day in 1938. He finished medical school in 1939 and interned at Sacred Heart Hospital in Allentown, which his father had helped to found. Those were years of limited funds: Mrs. Parmet recalls that she sent him money for cigarettes! Parmet entered general practice with his father and remained there until World War II. As his widow recalls, "the war of course changed our lives. It took us out of Allentown and we never went back. We had originally thought that we were going to return there and that Morris would be kind of a general practitioner in psychiatry." During his military postings, he met Karl Menninger, a nationally known psychiatrist, who told him: "You know you are a natural, why don't you leave medicine and go into psychiatry?"

After practicing medicine from 1946–1948, Parmet began a residency in psychiatry at the Veterans Hospital in Coatesville, Pennsylvania. While there, he "developed in Allentown a general medical facility for the International Ladies Garment Workers Union." From Coatesville he began training at the Philadelphia Child Guidance Clinic in child psychiatry, supervised by two distinguished figures— Frederick Allen and John Rose.[b] Allen told Parmet about the opening at Hunterdon. In mid-June of 1952, Allen met with the Board and Trussell. Trussell's report to the Board indicates his belief that Parmet should not be allowed to get away. Joseph Moskowitz, Board Secretary, wrote: "[Allen] stated that [Parmet] had all the necessary qualifications for this appointment . . . If we did not take him, Dr. Parmet would eventually be capable of replacing Dr. Allen when his term expires with the Philadelphia Clinic."[9]

Belle Parmet relates: "Our first reaction was what on earth could be interesting in Flemington," because all they knew about it was as the site of the trial of Bruno Hauptmann for the kidnapping and murder of the infant son of aviation hero Charles Lindbergh. Both thought it would be too rural, a "hick town." After meeting Board and Staff, they discovered Hunterdonites were now free of hay behind the ears.

[b] Allen was one of the early great figures in child psychiatry. He founded the Philadelphia Child Guidance Clinic, affiliated it with Children's Hospital of Philadelphia, and was very active in the movement to encourage study and treatment of mentally and behaviorally disturbed children by teams of professionals from the disciplines of psychiatric social work, psychology and medicine. John Rose, who succeeded Allen, was a distinguished researcher on the impact of maternal behavior on infants and initiated an innovative program to train pediatricians in behavioral aspects of pediatrics, in which I participated in 1957 and 1958.

We fell in love with the idea . . . Talk of HMC stirs me deeply
and I thank the fates which brought us to Flemington in 1952
to live and work with a group of wonderfully idealistic but
also practical and competent people who made a difference in
so many lives . . . Everybody had stars in their eyes. When we
heard that Andy [Hunt] was coming to Hunterdon Medical
Center as a pediatrician to work intimately with Morris, that
sort of dotted the 'i' for us and of course we came. That was
the most wonderful personal and professional experience I
think of our lives.[10]

Hunt and Parmet knew each other well. Hunt had a deep interest in behavioral aspects of medicine; he and Parmet shared
interests and beliefs about children, their disorders, and their relationship to their micro- and macro-environments. Parmet, appointed
in June 1952, along with Hunt, worked out of the Medical Center
office on Main Street, Flemington, for almost a year before the
hospital opened. Parmet met with PTAs, the Granges, the Freeholders, and other groups to try to explain why in the world if
everyone had fresh air, pasteurized milk and good country living,
they would need a mental health program. His reception was mixed.
Some thought it would be a very expensive program; others were
skeptical of the need.

Parmet's work included several innovative concepts. He and
Andy Hunt worked closely together on the innovative pediatric
programs of rooming-in and parent visiting. They also added to
the usual ambulatory child guidance structure the option of one
to three days of inpatient study and treatment to clarify mental
health and somatic dysfunction in child and/or family and to negotiate an acceptable route for therapy.[11] The mental health team
pioneered an informal community behavioral health program. Director of Internal Medicine Pellegrino collaborated with Parmet
on the relationship of physical and behavioral dysfunction[12] and
on a program to admit psychiatric patients to the general medical
floor. These programs are described in Chapter 13.

In private life Parmet saw daily, in a variety of social settings,
patients whom he had treated professionally. He told me that a
major reason why he chose to leave Hunterdon was over issues of
anonymity; he was unable to go out without encountering patients.[13] Mrs. Parmet speaks of this:

> Morris began to treat staff members, families of staff members, personal friends, in direct contrast to what is supposed to be true in psychiatry and medicine generally—that you don't get involved personally and socially with your clientele. That was impossible in this small rural area because he was the only psychiatrist for miles around. [At] a fund-raiser given by the artists of the community . . . they worried about where we should sit so that we would not encounter patients. Every table included someone whom Morris had seen and whom we knew socially. He was able to treat personal friends, family friends, and colleagues and to keep the personal and the professional separate.

So it appears that his strong belief that patients with psychiatric problems could see the mental health specialist openly, similarly to patients with other sorts of medical problems, may have, at times, backfired. At least, he and his wife did not always see it the same way.

The Parmets fostered community support by encouraging formation of a Mental Health Association. Belle Parmet, with her M.S.W. from Bryn Mawr, Louise Leicester from HMC's Board, Sara Boutelle[c] and Louise de Rochemont who were community volunteers, and psychiatrist Mary Mercer, married to Ray Trussell, all participated. They held monthly meetings with speakers from Philadelphia and New York. At the annual Flemington Agricultural Fair, just a few hundred yards from the Medical Center, they took a booth, dressed as clowns and presented slide shows and parties for children born at HMC. One result was to attract the interest of many prominent county residents, gradually bringing about a very real change in attitudes towards mental health in the community.[d]

Doing the work that Parmet wished in the way he preferred limited his financial productivity, and there was increased peer pressure to be more "productive." By 1959 Commonwealth support had long since been terminated, and the mental health program could not earn from fees sufficient funds to continue as it

[c] Sara Boutelle's husband, William Boutelle, a psychiatrist, did not practice locally and had turned down the position that Parmet took.

[d] Essie Johnson, second wife of J. Seward Johnson, Lib Schley, wife of Reeve Schley, writer J. C. Furnas and Pat Klopfer, HMC Board member and wife of a co-founder of Random House publishers, among others, were all very active with the association.

was. Finally, Hunt left in 1959. Parmet and Hunt had a particularly close relationship, both professionally and personally, and Parmet did not see how his valued co-worker could be replaced. Parmet was offered a prized position to head a model developmental children's treatment program at the N.J. Neuropsychiatric Institute in Skillman, which would serve as a prototype treatment program for the state. Belle Parmet was a social worker at Carrier Clinic, and the commute from Flemington was not easy, particularly in winter. Since they also wanted better public schools, they moved to Princeton, where he later entered private practice.

EDMUND D. PELLEGRINO, M.D.

Pellegrino is a third-generation Italian-American from a middle-class family, with what he describes as "standard family values . . . a very happy childhood."[14] His parents were not formally educated, but very bright. He became an avid reader, a person of the book, at an early age. He describes reading the *Encyclopedia Britannica* endlessly, as a great joy of his young life. He became interested in science and biology and attended a Jesuit high school with no electives and a rigorous curriculum including both Greek and Latin, as well as mathematics, history, modern languages and science. After graduating from St. John's College in Brooklyn with a major in physical chemistry, he entered NYU Medical School in order to do clinical biochemistry. In his third year he became fascinated with clinical medicine and clinical research. He married in 1944, the year that he graduated from medical school. The Pellegrinos had seven children.

A residency in Internal Medicine at Bellevue was followed by service in the Air Force and a fellowship in renal physiology, interrupted by illness. He speaks of the impact on his life:

> It was a bit of a shock. I had cavitary [tuberculosis]. I had a hemoptysis without warning. Looking back at the whole experience, it made me a better person and a better doctor. This is not romantic. It is the truth . . . As a very bright, ambitious, fast-moving, young person, I wasn't as essential as I thought I was. To my great surprise, Bellevue Hospital and the laboratory went on without me. From my room, I could look out my window and see the courtyard I used to cross every day with the specimens from Bellevue Hospital. I could see my replacement carrying the same specimen bottles fol-

lowing the same route. A wonderful thing for one's humility.
It was also an unexcelled opportunity to read voraciously. I
have done that all my life anyway. I had the time also to take
a look at myself and to learn about myself and my family, to
reflect on what the important things were. I do not look back
at my tuberculosis with regret. I don't think even at that time
I was grieved. The only concern was what would I be able to
do in the future for my family.

After a two-and-a-half-year cure, Pellegrino became supervising
physician at the Homer Folks Tuberculosis Hospital in Oneonta,
New York.[15]

Trussell told me, "Pellegrino, who had just gotten out of the
hospital having had the rest cure for tuberculosis, was looking for
something to do and de la Chapelle sent him out to see me. We
made a deal on the spot."[16] This was another example of Clarence
de la Chapelle helping Hunterdon and one of his former students.
Pellegrino says, "I really had no suspicion that people like Clarence
had that kind of regard for me." Pellegrino, who was 31 at the
time, drove to Hunterdon for an interview with Trussell, Wescott
and Seward Johnson.

> My first contact with Lloyd Wescott and Seward Johnson is
> worth the telling even though it has no great historical signi-
> ficance. They asked me to meet at the Union Hotel. Even
> though I was recovering from a siege of bed rest, I moved
> fast, as I always do, and I ran quickly up the steps to get into
> the lobby. Out of the corner of my eye, as I whizzed past, I
> saw two men on the porch in rocking chairs, in overalls. Both
> had beards. What flashed through my mind was "They must
> be farmers." I dashed in and said to the man behind the desk,
> "I am here to meet Mr. Johnson and Mr. Wescott." He said,
> "Well you just went past them . . . They're out on the porch."
> Well, there they were, two of the movers and shakers, looking
> like they were discussing cows, not a new hospital.

This was not an unusual presentation for either Wescott or
Johnson. Both delighted in a degree of reverse snobbery on such
occasions. Both were shrewd at using reactions to such novelty on
the part of those they met as clues to character. Both were devoted
to agriculture, particularly cattle, and both had been personally
and prominently involved in new developments in animal
husbandry. Delight in the farming façade was not confined to members of HMC's Board. In my early years I learned not to assume

occupation from appearance. A parent who turned up in farm clothes and had an odor from a cattle barn was probably an airline pilot. The man who was clean and well dressed was a farmer.

Pellegrino was made an offer in July, 1952, to begin work January 1, 1953. He said, "I was overwhelmed. The prospect of making $15,000 a year was just unbelievable in those days" (over $99,000 in 2001 dollars, a respectable starting salary).

Pellegrino had many reasons for coming to Hunterdon. He loved being able to open a new unstructured position where he could be chief. "I like to run things . . . I liked the clean canvas. In my subsequent career, I've had the chance at the clean canvas time and time again . . . If I liked the idea, that would be enough. The details could be worked out." Hunterdon's advantages included clinical practice, teaching, research and supervision. The NYU faculty appointment meant his connection there need not be lost. A rural area offered life-style advantages compared to the city or the suburbs. All his hopes and past experiences came together in this position. "It was almost providential," Pellegrino says. At NYU friends and colleagues gave dire warnings. His academic career would be at risk; he would drop out of sight; his chances for further advancement, except, worst of all cases, in private practice, would be lost. But Pellegrino was excited, knew what he wanted, and was unmoved by the prophets of doom.

Pellegrino began work in offices over a store in downtown Flemington in January, 1953, six months before HMC opened. He saw patients in consultation, provided continuing medical education, and helped plan the medical service with Miss Lela Greenwood, chief of nurses. He felt it was important to get acquainted with the local practitioners. Pellegrino went out to visit each in the office: "I was not absolutely certain that I would be able to handle all the interpersonal relationships. I wanted to know them . . . I went to their offices on their terms to ask them their advice."

As one of the three outstanding clinicians who opened the specialist staff before HMC itself, Pellegrino brought his own special contribution to Hunterdon. This was his brilliance, distinguished clinical skills, and ability to relate effectively in consultation with other physicians in order to help them make the most of themselves. He is an immensely hard worker. As of my interviews with him (December, 1996) he still attends early Mass, is in the office every day at 6:30 a.m. to study and write, and then begins his administrative and clinical day. David Sanders, a resident in Pediatrics in 1953, said: "He remembered everything he ever read, ever, and could bring it up on demand."[17] Many recall him with great warmth. Jeannette Ash, who worked with him, regards him as "compassionate" and remembers with affection how when her husband had surgery, Pellegrino came directly from the operating room to report the results.[18]

Trussell saw Pellegrino as

> an extraordinary contributor to the success of [HMC] because he not only worked well with the local practitioners, he was capable of limiting them if he had to . . . He would call the doctor who made the referral and then he would send a letter. By the end of the first year, I think 15 percent of his consults were from out-of-county. His fame was spreading because he was not stealing patients; he was doing a good job.

Trussell thought he had an added dimension: "He was really a very fortunate choice. He had a spiritual quality. Jesuits trained him and that of course has followed through to his present work now. He is a medical ethics leader of real stature."[19]

One of Pellegrino's most rewarding experiences was working with the family physicians. He said he does not remember a stressful moment arising from these relationships in six years at Hunterdon. He began by confirming that as chief, he was responsible for the quality of care of all patients in the hospital on the Medical Service, whether they were on his personal service or on that of a family physician. He made rounds twice a day on every patient. Right from the beginning, he had to fight off taking patients on his service and fight off consultations to avoid being overwhelmed. In 1957, Pellegrino summarized his approach:

> For postgraduate medical education to be most effective, it should be continuous and in relation to individual patients . . . At HMC every effort is made to preserve the role of the family doctor as the attending physician . . . No major change in management is made by the house staff or the specialist without the prior knowledge and consent of the family physician . . . The specialist is always available, and some of the most fruitful teaching occurs on the telephone, in the hallway, or over a cup of coffee.[20]

Although Pellegrino believed his theoretical and physiological knowledge was much greater than that of the family physicians, he wanted to help without being condescending. It was vital not to put the practitioner down. He felt indirect, Socratic questioning would lead colleagues to the most appropriate diagnosis and management. In one instance, a family physician was treating a patient in hospital for pneumonia; Pellegrino thought the patient had tuberculosis.

> I could have just told [him] his patient had tuberculosis. Instead, I said: "We did a sputum on this patient, would you like to look at it with me?" We looked at it and he said: "What stain is that?" I said: "It's an acid-fast stain." He kept looking at the microscope. "Could those be acid-fast bacilli?" I said: "You're right. That's what they are. The patient has tuberculosis."

He also adds, wryly:

> When [the family physicians] had a patient with meningitis, the house staff and I would do all the hard work. They would get the credit and that's okay, that is perfectly okay. I say that most sincerely. I was trained at Bellevue. Treating meningitis was not a "big deal," but for them it was a big thing.

Pellegrino's anecdote illuminates clearly the conflict at the heart of Hunterdon with respect to the family physician and the specialist. Obtaining the sputum test without the order of the family physician was already a put-down. What dialogue could create a differential diagnosis leading to a sputum for acid-fast bacilli? One might need a half hour or more, on rounds or a conference, time that neither the internist nor the family physician could readily spare. Peter Rizzolo, who served first as a resident in family medicine, and then on the staff, said: "Even after the encounter was over you weren't sure what you were supposed to learn. It was very convoluted to get information from Ed Pellegrino, but it was very stimulating because he would question everything. 'How do you know that?' 'What makes you think that?'"[21]

Family physician John Lincoln was very positive:

> At one point one of the doctors demonstrated very clearly that he did not know how to deal with gout. Some . . . were saying that a clinician with that kind of gap in his knowledge really should not be on the hospital staff. Pellegrino . . . took the opposite tack. That is, if the doctor is that deficient, he

needs to be on the hospital staff so he'll bring his patients into the hospital so he can be taught how to handle these things. It served to help people rather than to punish them.[e]

Another family physician Leonard Rosenfeld, explained what ease of consultation meant to him. Before the hospital opened, a local farmer showed symptoms suggestive of a myocardial infarction. Rosenfeld called for a consultation. Pellegrino drove out to the farmhouse, an EKG machine in the back of his car, and performed a history, examination and EKG, concluding the problem was not cardiac and not serious. The patient was successfully treated at home.[22]

Murray Rubin, who became chief financial officer in 1954, respected Pellegrino:

> When he hired you to do a job, he let you alone to do it. He didn't interfere but periodically asked for accountability. When you gave him the information, he didn't question it but relied on your integrity and honesty to be straightforward. He didn't dwell, linger or second-guess . . . Ed didn't like the financial part of it. He wanted me to take care of it.[23]

Surgeon Buck Katzenbach said Pellegrino was a great doctor.

> We would have an emergency and somebody would be in the little original emergency room and needed a tracheostomy, and before Carl [Roessel, the other surgeon] or I could get there, Ed had it either half done or done. He knew what to do and did it and it didn't matter if it was surgical or what, he did it . . . Ed also had a temper.[24]

Dave Greenbaum, another internist, stated that despite his poise, Pellegrino was not used to handling confrontation. He would be "freaked out to some degree" by colleagues such as Loo Looloian, a family physician who would challenge his statements and ask "why?"[25] According to John Lincoln, Bob Henderson, another internist and later Medical Director, was one of the few "who could tell Ed Pellegrino, 'Ed, you're full of it' and nobody would get angry."[26]

---

[e] Lincoln JA. Interview by author, 19 July, 1996. Contrast Pellegrino's approach with that of today when a member of a hospital staff is found to be deficient. Structured educational measures, in a punitive atmosphere, are the order of the day, always with the underlying threat of expulsion from the staff if the erring physician is not compliant. This is not to suggest that physician-engendered errors should be tolerated, but rather to emphasize that the atmosphere was, in those days, a far more constructive and supportive one.

Pellegrino himself says "Patience was not, and is not, my crowning virtue." Once, when the pathologist, Ed Olmstead did not appear promptly for an autopsy, Pellegrino, began it himself, precipitating a verbal battle when Olmstead finally arrived at the morgue. When Pellegrino became Medical Director, he said that Hunt and Parmet

> never let me get away with anything . . . They were always honest with me and brought me down to earth sometimes when I was flying too high. I always appreciated that . . . Andy was a person I could depend on for good judgment and so was Morris Parmet. Morris tended to be negative about things while Andy was more positive.

The Pellegrino family lived further from the Medical Center than some of the other specialists, in the northern part of the county. Their home was on the side of a rather steep hill. On one occasion, in a terrible blizzard, a bulldozer was necessary to open the drive. I have always heard that when Ed Grant, the administrator, came in with a four-wheel-drive army truck, Pellegrino could not wait to get going.

Pellegrino felt that

> one should not stay too long in one position. One shouldn't spend the bulk of his life in a single endeavor . . . in one administrative post. You don't grow that way. If you can't make a major impact in seven to ten years, you're not going to make it. For the good of yourself and everybody else, you ought to move on to something else.

But, he said, it was important to leave a bit of yourself behind: "This is my test whether the things I've done have genuine validity." In 1958 Pellegrino accepted the position of Chairman of Medicine at a new medical school at the University of Kentucky; he helped start a new hospital modeled after Hunterdon. In 1969 he left Kentucky for the State University of New York at Stony Brook as Director of a six-school Medical Center. There he drew on his experience at HMC to emphasize training in family medicine and the humanities. From there, he went to the University of Tennessee as Chancellor, Yale to coordinate its health complex, and to Catholic University as President. He is currently Director of the Center for Clinical Bioethics at Georgetown University Medical Center.

ALBERT ACCETTOLA, M.D.

Accettola, the son of a building contractor, was groomed to enter the family business. He loved working with his father, but influenced by his older brother who had always served as a mentor, he entered Boston University School of Medicine, chose orthopedics, and obtained surgical training at Bellevue Hospital in New York City and in Wisconsin. He married his wife, Rose, at the end of the third year of medical school. Two of their three children are physicians. She died in 1994, and he lives on at the farm they loved near the Medical Center.

Accettola had already established a busy orthopedic practice on Staten Island, New York, and was also an assistant clinical professor of orthopedics at Bellevue when he first heard of HMC. The Chairman of the Department of Orthopedic Surgery suggested that he come to HMC

> to help set up an orthopedic department. I did something that no assistant professor should do. I refused. He let it go and he prevailed on me . . . to reconsider . . . Again, I refused. At that point the Dean of the Medical School [Clarence de la Chapelle] spoke to me . . . and he felt strongly that it would be wise to go.[27]

Accettola's recollections of his interview with Trussell are unique. He asserts that Trussell told him that he expected, in bringing young and well-trained specialists to the community, that, after a year or so, they would work in the community on their own. Neither Trussell nor any other specialist or family practice staff member interviewed recalls any such possibility articulated either in conversation or in writing. Accettola was not in sympathy with the idea of a closed specialist staff and also felt that the pay offered for him to come for one day a week of $50 plus 5 cents a mile for travel, was "ridiculous." In 2001 dollars, $50 would correspond to $330. However, he was so impressed with the quality of the staff and plans for the new hospital that he agreed to come on a trial basis two days per week. Accettola helped plan the orthopedic aspects of the operating suite. He is still chagrined about his first operation there. He was placing a nail in a fractured hip guided by x-rays, which seemed to take too long to develop. "What is going on here?" he inquired. The very competent technician replied:

"Doctor, the operating room is on the third floor and I have to run down to the second floor and the other end of the building to develop the films." Accettola had forgotten to specify including a darkroom in the operating suite. His days were very busy. He enjoyed every minute of it. The nurses were marvelous, had a sense of humor, and the patients were pleasant, courteous and grateful. This was so different from his New York practice.

Had it been possible to obtain hospital privileges as an independently practicing orthopedist, Accettola would have moved his office to Hunterdon County. He would not allow himself to be at the mercy of administration and Board as a full-time employee. He also never felt at ease with the family physicians, who usually wanted him to be the doctor of record and officially in charge. Suppose he were away? In any case, if it was appropriate for the patient to return to the family physician, it was also economical, and built good patient relations.

Accettola continued to consult at Hunterdon until his retirement about 1980. The farm had been a summer home; then it became the family's permanent home. Both he and his wife felt this was a very kindly place to live. In New York, if Mrs. Accettola went into a grocery where she was known, she would be charged double for corn. In Hunterdon County, if she bought a supply for canning, she might be given 25 percent more than she paid for. But it had been hard to manage all the workload at Bellevue, on Staten Island and at Hunterdon. Accettola said of this: "I didn't raise my family. My wife raised three beautiful children . . . She did a marvelous job . . . and I wasn't there. And that's what it did. It's a very unfortunate thing and I just wasn't there to enjoy those children."

GERALD BARAD, M.D.

Barad was raised in Manhattan Beach, New York, in a close family of three generations living side by side. Always interested in biology, he kept a basement laboratory for specimens and took classes at the Brooklyn Botanical Garden. He entered the College of Agriculture at Cornell, but, persuaded by his father, transferred to a premedical curriculum. During his third year he joined the army, serving at Walter Reed Army Hospital and in a laboratory in India. After discharge, Barad married, finished college and graduated in 1952 from Cornell Medical School. His postgraduate training was at Lenox Hill Hospital and NYU–Bellevue.

In 1954, in his first year of ob-gyn training at NYU–Bellevue, Barad met Herman Rannels, Chief of Obstetrics at Hunterdon. Rannels worked at NYU one day a week in gynecological pathology, and the two developed joint interests. Barad thought Hunterdon sounded like a place where he could live and work happily. Initially Rannels was reluctant to take an associate, because there might not be enough work for two. In 1957, when Barad was completing his residency, Rannels asked if he would provide coverage that summer for a six-week vacation. The Barad family, with three children, lived near Flemington in a cabin with no kitchen.

After the summer, Rannels offered a part-time position. Barad accepted. The position sounded interesting, the work enjoyable. He could make maximum use of his training and innovate in the practice of obstetrics and gynecology. In this idealistic atmosphere, physicians, nurses and even the general public cared deeply about the quality of medical care. Barad was impressed by the ability to walk down the hall and ask someone for help in any area of medicine outside his own specialty and get it at no cost: "You just did it."[28] Hunterdon's location was close to family in the New York area, but not too close. He liked the rural area. Barad was still interested in agriculture and breeding plants and hoped to find land to indulge this hobby. In addition, Alexander Mitchell, Carl Roessel and Fred Knocke were specialists he had known and respected at Lenox Hill Hospital.

Barad worked part time for a year; in 1958 he was offered a full-time position at $10,000 per year ($66,100 in 2001 dollars). When he worked part time, the hourly or daily pay was greater than full time. He thinks this was a reason why HMC made the offer. For Barad, a way of life was initially more important than money. The financial differential was compensated by working with a great group of people. Friends and associates in New York laughed at him, saying he could double his income there without difficulty. Later, Barad was to change his mind and join vigorous efforts by the specialists to change Hunterdon's system:

> I had the responsibility for being the head of a family and I
> didn't look far enough ahead at that time. I said to myself,

this is the way I wanted to practice . . . This is the way I want
to live . . . A few years later I began to realize that I had some
problems . . . I harbor . . . an area of distrust which may have
colored some of my reactions toward fiscal affairs in the Medical
Center for many years.

The relationship between Rannels and Barad became and remained

a guarded one . . . Herman and I did things very differently.
Herman's obstetrics was 85 percent under anesthesia with routine
forceps deliveries. I think the few people that didn't get [an-
esthesia] delivered too fast for the anesthesiologist to get there
. . . [As a surgeon he may not have been as gentle with] tissue
as I had been trained to be . . . He didn't always respect my
independence as a surgeon . . . He would come to my post-
ops and [order things differently] than I would have . . . and
at one time I simply said to him, "Herman, if I am to continue doing surgery here, you are going to have to give me
the opportunity to do my follow-up care and leave my patients alone" and he did. We had our confrontation and it
was over.

Although Rannels was a person who elicited strong reactions from
colleagues, some wives of family physicians praised his clinical competence. In addition, in 1954 Rannels commenced a program of
prenatal education, including psycho-prophylaxis in childbirth, which
does not really fit with the idea that 85 percent of his deliveries
were under anesthesia. I am unable to explain the difference.

Barad preferred to allow nature to take its course unless he
suspected an untoward complication. His judgment was heavily
influenced by experience at New York Hospital with the Barads'
first child. They enjoyed classes in natural childbirth and obtained
rooming-in for the new infant. Soon Barad became involved with
the American Society for Psychoprophylaxis in Childbirth:

One of the things which impressed me as being inappropriate
was not to give patients what they wanted . . . Women came
to me and they said, "If I don't want to be asleep why do I
have to be?" My reaction was, "Why do you have to be? Of
course you don't." A husband said to me, "I'd like to be with
my wife when she has her baby." I said, "Well, it's against the
existing policies, but let's see if we can't change them." . . .

That would have been within six months of the time that I
got to be Department Chair [in 1959 or 1960].

Barad took advantage of rapidly changing attitudes about normal labor and childbirth to adopt many techniques of natural childbirth. All this was occurring just at the time that Virginia Apgar was studying the condition of babies at birth, and Stanley James, a perinatologist working with her at Columbia–Presbyterian Medical Center, was doing pioneering studies of blood gases and oxygen metabolism in newborns. Their work led to dramatic changes in pediatric and obstetric attitudes about labor and delivery. Barad would collaborate with couples to conduct labor and delivery as they wanted, as long as it did not conflict with the best interests of baby and mother. When Barad took over, the percentage of deliveries under general anesthesia fell from the majority of deliveries to less than 5 percent. He also influenced family physicians to give up heavy doses of various narcotics, sedatives and other medications. Fathers were allowed in the delivery room in May, 1960. At the time, only one other hospital in New Jersey had comparable policies.

Barad and I worked well together on natural childbirth. He always was devoted to the best interests of his patient and the baby she was to deliver. He would come repeatedly to the nursery to see how babies were progressing. I went to New York to see what Apgar and James were up to. It turned out they were working on a clinic service where almost all the mothers were single, unsupported, very fearful, without appropriate childbirth education, and as a result were terrified throughout labor and delivery. This led to heavy use of sedation and anesthesia, which in turn provided large numbers of infants suitable for their studies. They taught me the importance of prompt intervention and resuscitation when an infant showed signs of depression at birth and, conversely, how to handle an infant who was not depressed. Barad and I often had the satisfaction of seeing a just-born infant, making alert eye contact, and put at once to the mother's breast with the father's help.

Barad is a strong personality who never hesitated to take over a patient from the family physician when he felt he should. He describes coming in more than once to deliver a baby for a family physician who did not monitor labor closely enough. Once, a family physician admitted a woman with an ectopic (i.e., outside the uterus) pregnancy, which calls for emergency surgery. The physician proposed to observe instead of requesting emergency surgery. When others on staff heard of this, they debated whether this physician should remain on the staff. Barad was strongly in favor of retaining him, he said, "at least this way we can pick up after his mistakes." Although Barad was careful to monitor quality of care in supportive fashion, not all the family physicians agreed with him. Family physician Peter Rizzolo, who had a trying time when he began family practice in 1959, taking over from another physician with almost no warning, said that Barad "had a very negative attitude about primary care and family doctors."[29] When he and Barad came to know each other well, Rizzolo found that Barad had more confidence in his work, and Rizzolo felt more at ease with him. Rizzolo made a point of mentioning the supportive teaching which he received from the obstetrical staff, both Barad and Rannels. Barad was years ahead of his time in his use of methods of maternal relaxation, alternative methods of delivery and involvement of fathers.

There were struggles with family doctors who were not accustomed to, and did not want, supervision. Many women were shifting from family physicians to obstetricians. Accrediting organizations specified minimum numbers of deliveries if family physicians were to retain their privileges. Those numbers were large enough to make for considerable stress in a busy family practice. Bambara, Lincoln, Doyle, Rizzolo and others have spoken of this difficult time of transition. The attitude of the obstetrician was an important part of the dynamic, since supervision and support can conflict. Several family physicians told me they felt "under the gun" with maternity patients and gave up obstetrical practice earlier than they might otherwise have done.

Barad left full-time practice in 1987. For many years he has had an interest in cacti, is active in the Cactus and Succulent Association of America and has served as board member and president of the association. He has maintained his own greenhouse since moving to Hunterdon County, travels extensively to regions where cacti and succulents grow and has developed hybridizing and artificial pollinating techniques.

MICHAEL COLELLA, M.D.

Mike Colella died 2 June 1996. The account that follows comes from his wife, Elizabeth, and my personal experiences with him. Mike was the seventh of ten children of parents who had emigrated from Italy. He grew up in Rome, New York, attended public school, Syracuse University and graduated from Hahnemann Medical College in 1939. After marriage to Elizabeth and a two-year internship at Wilson Memorial Hospital in Johnson City, New York, he joined the military in World War II, serving for 42 months with the Army in Africa and Italy, where he was repeatedly under fire in a battalion aid station.

After discharge from the Army in 1946, Colella took a refresher course and entered general practice in Utica, New York. Local practitioners, delighted to have someone who would take night calls for them, welcomed him. The result was that he was deluged or "dumped on," as one would say today, with night work. He developed an interest in anesthesia, and a local anesthesiologist asked him to sit in on cases to gain experience. Mrs. Colella said: "One day he came home and said he had decided that he wanted to go into anesthesiology and he should not wait too much longer—we had two kids and he wasn't getting any younger."[30] Colella took his first year of training at Boston City Hospital and the second at Bellevue.

While Colella was still a resident at Bellevue, the department chairperson informed him of the opening at HMC and encouraged him to apply in the spring of 1953. He interviewed and was hired on 22 May 1953. Board records indicate there had been difficulty in finding a suitable candidate. Consideration was given to nurse anesthetists as a stopgap.

Mrs. Colella says he came because "we had three children and he needed a job." He also liked getting in on the ground floor at the new hospital. He knew none of the other specialists, but he liked Hunterdon for its life style. At the time, Elizabeth Colella was at her family home in Utica, New York, close to term in her third pregnancy and was due for a Caesarean section. She wanted to be cared for by the obstetrician with whom she was familiar. As a result, Colella looked over the situation, and started at Hunterdon without her. She was delivered on 12 August 1953; he came home for the delivery.

Colella loved Hunterdon and was always glad he had chosen anesthesiology. Soon two nurse anesthetists, Eileen Cornish and Cecilia Fetterman, shared the work. The women applied together, having come from Geisinger Hospital in Pennsylvania, together with Clara Anthony, Nursing Supervisor on Maternity, and Jean Moleski, who became Nursing Supervisor on the surgical floor.

Mike was a man of average height, stocky build, wide generous mouth, and a pleasant, low-key demeanor. He avoided fuss, deplored any kind of upset, and relied on his skills and common sense. The result was a near continuous string of surgical patients whose anesthesia was free of complications. At Medical Center staff meetings each month, each staff committee would report on quality of care. Each month the representative of the operating room committee would review statistics, and then, in what became a standing joke, say something like: "Number of anesthetic complications was . . . [pause while staff all laughed] . . . none!"

Mike was so friendly, positive and reassuring. Many a time I watched him with a child about to undergo a procedure. I had the feeling that he used, as his principal anesthetic agents, charm and magic. He would whisper to the child, sometimes sing, and the child would relax and calm. He would always say that the patient's freedom from fear and worry had more to do with uneventful anesthesia and absence from complications than anything that he did. Today an enormous literature accumulates on behavioral techniques for reducing pain, but years ago Mike knew this in his bones. For infants, such as those being operated on for pyloric stenosis, he would use open drop ether, which he administered with a delicate hand. Until surgeons discontinued this surgical procedure at Hunterdon, in the 1970s, there was never a complication of any kind, either from anesthesia or surgery. Part of the reason was meticulous pre- and postoperative care, but much of it was the quality of anesthesiological and surgical skills.

A story illustrates how Mike went about his work. Many years ago a toddler with breathing trouble was sent to me for care. I found inspiratory distress characteristic of croup, but no real evidence of a cause—no fever, no sign of respiratory infection, allergy or aspiration. Something seemed atypical, so I asked for a film. Soon Steve Dewing, the radiologist, joined me at the tot's bedside with wet x-ray films, still dripping from the wash, to show me the results. Not only was the chest clear and the epiglottis not enlarged, but also there was an odd white shape at the entry to the trachea, the main air passage. He had already taken additional films showing something flat and round, with a long thin protuberance from its center extending straight down the trachea.

Otolaryngologist Walter Petryshyn was away at the time, so I called Mike Colella to see what he could do. Mike was in the operating room about to begin a procedure, but he came over at once. He arrived carrying his laryngoscope and a curved Kelly clamp. We took the child to the pediatric treatment room, wrapped him in towels and put him on his back. I knelt on the floor to hold his head, while a nurse restrained his body. Mike pulled up a chair by the treatment table on the pediatric floor. He inserted the laryngoscope, said that he saw a piece of metal, reached in with his Kelly, grasped it, and pulled out what turned out to be a gear from a child's truck or car, with axle attached. The gear was lying athwart the entrance to the trachea, the axle extending down into it. The child's respiratory distress was relieved at once. As soon as we could see the child looking so much better, Mike wiped off his instruments, quietly asked if it was okay to return to his patient, and off he went. No fuss. No muss. No bother or excitement. So to speak—" Ho hum, what else is new?" That was Mike Colella.

The Colellas found a home in Frenchtown and remained there until they left the area. They enjoyed small-town life; the children went to local schools, and they would have remained except for Mike's illness. In 1975, while preparing to administer anesthesia, Mike Colella suffered a heart attack and cardiac arrest. Two surgeons in the room for a procedure, Buck Katzenbach and Felix Salerno, gave resuscitation together. Colella regained cardiac rhythm and was talking by the time they moved him to the recovery room. With this, it was time for him to quit, and they moved to Florida.

STEPHEN B. DEWING, M.D.

Steve Dewing died on 7 February 1996, at the age of 75, after a long illness. His widow, Elisabeth, his second wife, provided biographical information. Dewing was born in 1920 in Princeton, New Jersey, and lived in a number of communities in the United States and abroad as his father was an academic who taught Latin and

Greek. Steve attended private schools, Princeton University, and the College of Physicians and Surgeons, Columbia University, graduating in 1945. After nine months of internship, he entered the military, serving in North Carolina.

As he was finishing his residency, Dewing explored openings in northern New Jersey, preferring to remain near family and in a less urban environment. Mrs. Dewing goes on to say:

> Obviously, HMC met these criteria. Steve's parents were both still living in Princeton, and in failing health, and he wished to be near them. Also, he himself always preferred a rural environment. He settled in a big old house in Ringoes. I am sure the concept of HMC was also attractive to him. Steve was not a "competitor" and was more interested in the treatment of people than in the financial part of practice.[31]

Dewing was appointed to the HMC staff in October 1952. He valued the NYU connection and the opportunity to go there once a week. At that time, radiologists in New Jersey practiced primarily from private offices, and few spent much time in a hospital. A radiologist typically came to the hospital for an hour or two in the morning, spent the day in the office, and returned briefly late in the afternoon to read the films that had accumulated during the day. The radiologist interacted with referring physicians on the telephone, if at all, and rarely saw patients, except for procedures such as fluoroscopy.

Dewing was too interested in his patients and colleagues to work in the traditional pattern. The people side of medicine was too important. After leaving Hunterdon in 1964 for personal reasons (a failing marriage), he worked in an academic medical center, but found it not to his liking. He returned to community practice in Maine for the remainder of his career. He told his wife that he "liked to have patients referred by a doctor and not a department."

Dewing always wanted to know why an imaging request was made. If he did not receive enough information, he called the referring physician. When something unusual appeared, he promptly notified the physician in charge. I remember him walking over to the pediatric floor, carrying a dripping film fresh from the developer, to show me and explain what he had learned and to confer on the child. His style was that of consultant, a tradition continued in the department to this day. Frederick Woodruff, who later joined him as the second radiologist, said: "We got along very well. We didn't have any problems. We really could work together. We could schedule. We could [share] time . . . and we could handle the same patient without the patient, I think, feeling that there was a difference."[32]

Dewing developed techniques for using minimal doses of radiation to treat benign skin conditions and wrote a textbook on the subject. Today this would not be done, because of the risk of stimulating cancerous growths, but for a time it was an accepted form of treatment.

PAULINE ROHM GOGER, M.D.

Goger was born in 1913 and raised in Connellsville, a small town in western Pennsylvania. Her father died when she was very young. After earning an A.B. in zoology from Oberlin and an M.A. from Wellesley, she obtained a doctorate in genetics at the University of Pennsylvania in 1942. Subsequently she taught at Wellesley and Simmons, met and married her husband Milton, and moved to New Jersey, where she taught at Rutgers until she started medical school at NYU. She graduated in 1950, second in her class. She was Phi Beta Kappa and Alpha Omega Alpha. Her postgraduate training was all at Bellevue in Internal Medicine and Rheumatology.[33]

One morning while shaving, her husband heard on the radio about a new hospital in Flemington, to be affiliated with NYU Medical School. Goger was completing her residency at Bellevue, and had already declined an offer from the National Institutes of Health, because the Gogers were established in northern New Jersey where he had a business. Through her chief of service at Bellevue she arranged an appointment with Ray Trussell, at a time when the hospital building was not yet open, probably in the spring of 1953. She was already acquainted with Pellegrino.

Goger keenly felt the need to work in an environment where her special interests and unique training could be utilized. If she could not do research, she wanted a practice with an academic connection. Hunterdon fitted her wishes exactly. Initially Goger, along with Henderson, was engaged to perform examinations for the Chronic Illness Survey, Commonwealth providing $6,000 per

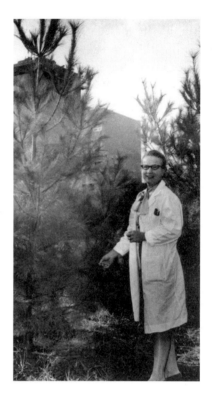

Pauline Goger, first and for many years the
only woman on the Medical Center Staff,
encouraging landscaping on the grounds in
front of the original patient care building.

year for each. She also obtained a grant from the State of New
Jersey to set up a clinic for patients with rheumatic heart disease,
where visiting physicians from NYU came regularly to consult. Tragi-
cally, Milton Goger died of a heart attack not long after they moved
to this area.

Pauline Goger spoke her mind with blunt vigor and honesty.
She could get into "feuds" over minor issues, such as a famous one
with a neighbor over the precise location of a fence between their
properties. Fred Woodruff said that she was the internist he would
call if a patient came down from internal medicine with a radio-
logical imaging request of which he could make no sense. Goger
was sensitive to the needs of older patients with many complications, ensuring that they were handled using a minimum of tests
and treatments and a maximum of useful expertise. She was pep-
pery, down-to-earth, quick to take stock of a situation, and effective
in common-sense management. All it took was a telephone call

and brief explanation to enlist her to take appropriate actions to care for patients. She helped out wherever needed and gave her best to all tasks. John Bambara, a family practitioner, described her as "a lady, well trained, affable, likable, easy to get along with . . . She was accepted as one of the 'boys' by the family doctors."[34]

Jack Elinson recalls a discussion with Goger related to the Chronic Illness Survey about an elderly woman, who was obese, diabetic, had glaucoma and atherosclerotic vascular disease. She did not follow an appropriate diet. Goger argued persuasively that at the woman's age and from her perspective, it might be more harmful to insist on vigorous efforts to change her life style than to let her be, recognizing that her life span might be less. Within the past five years the *Journal of the American Medical Association* has commenced a series of clinical case discussions that focus on incorporating the patient into planning care, in the manner that Goger encouraged.

Goger told me that soon after the hospital opened Trussell asked her to make a house call. Goger agreed:

> It was a lovely September afternoon . . . There was this recluse [who lived near me and] had apparently fallen and broken her hip . . . She kept the door locked and she lived on the old broken down davenport and the house went to wrack and ruin . . . We broke the door down and took her to the hospital. She allowed me to take her because I was a woman.

As the wheel turns in Hunterdon County, the old farmhouse was later sold to our family in 1961. We have lived in it ever since.

Goger contends that gender discrimination was quite evident throughout her years at HMC. She was the only woman on staff for ten years until the second female physician was appointed—an ophthalmologist, Kenette Sohmer. During the first two decades of HMC, the Hunterdon County Medical Society conducted separate simultaneous meetings for physicians and wives—the auxiliary. Many years ago in an interview Goger said that she had been the only woman on the medical staff, and she had never known prejudice until she came to this area.[35] However, in our interview Goger mentioned gender and age discrimination in training. At the time of her entry to medical school, Yale and Harvard did not take women as medical students; Johns Hopkins, where women made up 10 percent of the class, rejected her application, saying that at 29 years she was too old. Her chief of service and mentor at Bellevue,

Dr. Tillet, warned her that in practice, competing with men, she would be given a rough time. She was told by some staff members at HMC that women did not belong in medicine. Others refused to recognize the quality of her work or would conceal information about her accomplishments.

Several interviewees supported Goger's recollections. Jane Fuhrmann, widow of family physician John Fuhrmann, and Catherine Rosswaag, Trussell's secretary, both noted that gender discrimination was pervasive and obvious.[36] Kate Tantum, a laboratory technician, states that Pauline Goger was "probably every gal's heroine . . . because she was a leader, a woman who said 'here I stand' . . . Sexism was blatant, we didn't call it that at the time . . . I don't think it was verbalized . . . There is something that goes on that you sense as a female."[37] Jeannette Ash, one of the first nurses at HMC, said that is the way things were at that time. Nurses who questioned a physician felt such an attitude. Ash also feels the male physicians did not think of Goger as their peer in ability. Ash considers Goger as "the tops."[38]

Financial officer Rubin and I both agree that we saw Goger teased, but we both believe that this took place in an atmosphere of respect for her and her abilities. Never in my presence was anything said that could be considered sexual, hostile or in poor taste. I did not ever hear comments that undermined her personal or professional status. Several physicians on staff at the time were informally surveyed about gender discrimination. All but one denied that gender discrimination occurred. It is reasonable to think that bias, not consciously recognized, was present.

In 1958, when it was time to replace Pellegrino as Medical Director, Hunt was offered the job but declined. Goger and Henderson had equal seniority in the Department of Medicine, but the latter was offered the position, passing over her. Asked about this, Pellegrino stated:

> Bob got the nod over Pauline for the following reasons. First I had known him longer. Second, we had both been on the Bellevue Chest Service . . . Third, we had both had pulmonary tuberculosis . . . Those who had had the disease felt a special bond with their confreres . . . Fourth, Bob and I shared an interest in pulmonary disease . . . I think it was simply knowing one person a little better than the other and also maybe the maleness was in there.[39]

Andrew Hunt said of discrimination: "This might well have been true, although I was unaware of such an issue. I guess we males were all a bit sexist in those days."[40] Contemporaneous correspondence shows nothing further about a promotion for Goger.[f]

When Goger retired from practice, she founded an employee health service at HMC and managed this service until she retired from clinical medicine in 1988. During her tenure she developed an employee preventive health and immunization program, offering checkups and immunizations for those who did not go to a private physician. Eventually she became physically impaired, but continued to live alone in her home with the help of devoted neighbors who cared for her until her final, fatal illness in the autumn of 1996.

DAVID S. GREENBAUM, M.D.

David Greenbaum was brought up in New York City. His father was a lawyer and his mother an artist and sculptor. Greenbaum was educated at the Walden School and Deerfield Academy. He graduated from Williams College and then attended Western Reserve Medical School in the Army after he finished basic training. Greenbaum met his wife Ruth in 1946; they married in 1947, the year he graduated. Following a rotating internship of two years at Lenox Hill Hospital, Greenbaum entered a medical residency at Goldwater Memorial Hospital, both in New York City. At this time he was found to have pulmonary tuberculosis, for which he was treated in hospital for a year and a half. He went to Bellevue in 1951 as a Resident in Chest Medicine, rising to Chief Resident, supervising 30 resident physicians in the care of approximately 500 patients. He then took a fellowship in gastroenterology.

Greenbaum was acquainted with Henderson and Pellegrino: all three had trained at Bellevue and also had pulmonary tuberculosis. Greenbaum also knew radiologist Fred Woodruff from working together at the Bronx VA Hospital. Greenbaum interviewed at Hunterdon in late 1956 or early 1957. He was impressed with the quality of the physicians, and he liked the close-knit group. The principles of HMC were progressive, exciting, appealing and unique.

---

[f] Wescott L. Personal correspondence in October 1958 indicated that Hunt was to be offered the position of Director at the same salary Pellegrino had been receiving. A month later, it is noted that Henderson had accepted the position.

He was pleased by "encouragement for scholarly activities and to visit on a regular basis the centers in New York and Philadelphia."[41] He also found the landscape and rural character of the community very attractive. Money played little part in the decision, because he came from a well-to-do family.

His first year was financed by Seward Johnson for research into producing high-titer-specific antibody milk from dairy cattle by injections of an antigen into the teat. Greenbaum was also part-time in gastroenterology; he became a regular staff member in 1959.

Greenbaum is a quiet soul, of medium size, an academic turn of mind and speech, and a dry wit. He pursued his duties seriously, carefully and thoroughly. Endoscopies were performed in a small room that had been set aside for this and other procedures. Greenbaum was always happy to accommodate referring or other interested physicians, as well as students and residents by allowing them to share in, and learn from, the procedures.

There was a close working relationship with radiology and Fred Woodruff. Woodruff often came to endoscopic examinations, and Greenbaum often attended gastrointestinal fluoroscopic examinations. In addition, pathologist Ed Olmstead was a medical confidant with whom Greenbaum discussed interesting patients. He also found surgeon Carl Roessel very good to work with. They had known each other at Lenox Hill Hospital. Based on shared experience at Hunterdon, they wrote a paper on intestinal tract bleeding.[42] Greenbaum found that his patients displayed a wider variation of problems than he had expected, and the academic opportunities were satisfying: "I was well received [at the urban teaching centers] and I think made contributions, friends and colleagues. I also wrote some papers and was involved with other scholarly things."

Greenbaum felt that his interest in academic medicine was not shared by a number of other specialists. Ultimately this led him to leave Hunterdon in 1969 to pursue his academic interests. He went to the College of Human Medicine at Michigan State University, which Andrew Hunt headed, where he developed new concepts for teaching medical students. He also studied gastrointestinal physiology. In 1995 he became emeritus, but still teaches and sees patients.

C. Buckman Katzenbach, m.d.

Buck Katzenbach was born in Trenton on 31 March 1912, attended Haverford School near Philadelphia, and graduated from Princeton University in 1934 and from the College of Physicians and Surgeons, Columbia University, in 1938. To help finance medical school, Katzenbach waited on tables in exchange for meals. Going into debt at that time was not an option. He met the future Mrs. Katzenbach, the Assistant Night Director at Columbia–Presbyterian Hospital, and they married in 1939. She was immediately discharged since a nurse in an executive position could not be married.

Katzenbach and Carl Roessel barely knew each other at Princeton, but became friends in medical school. After a three-year rotating internship at St. John's Hospital, Brooklyn, Katzenbach began a surgical residency at Cumberland Hospital, also in Brooklyn. After completing barely a year, he entered the military, serving briefly in the United States, before being sent to Australia as commander of a portable surgical unit (the precursor of the MASH unit of the Korean War) accompanying the troops in a series of landings in New Guinea. "I never hit the beach earlier than 15 minutes after the first troops. But then I was young and healthy."[43] Katzenbach remained in service till 1947. He completed training with a residency at Pennsylvania Hospital in Philadelphia.

He began practice as a surgeon in Trenton, New Jersey, while remaining in the National Guard. In June 1948, while bivouacked at the Flemington Fair Grounds, as Battalion Surgeon with the 696th Battalion of the 112th Field Artillery, National Guard, Katzenbach saw a sign in a field across the road: "The Future Home of the Hunterdon Medical Center," but thought no more of this venture until July 1953, when he received a telephone call from a former classmate and long-time acquaintance, Carl Roessel, then Director of Surgery at HMC. Roessel was looking for help at Hunterdon, where he was the only general surgeon. Katzenbach agreed to provide weekend coverage, because he enjoyed "the semi-academic atmosphere as a way of doing things." At first he worked on a fee-for-service basis. "I remember I did an appendix but never got paid for it. That was the service." He was asked to cover for one day a week, then two, for $60 ($394 in 2001 dollars) per day. Because HMC had no full-time orthopedist or urologist, "we did the fractures and everything else . . . We did such things as were necessary." Katzenbach became a full-time member of the staff in 1956, a decision he pondered carefully. His practice in Trenton was going well; he was earning over $30,000 ($197,000 in 2001 dollars) a year. The full-time position at HMC, as second in department, would pay less than half that sum.

Katzenbach was a conservative surgeon who operated only when he was sure that it was the better option for the patient. I have heard him decry the syndrome of "acute remunerative appendicitis." He liked the atmosphere at Hunterdon, "the idea of the full-time men, of the academic association, going over to New York University. People came from Lenox Hill as residents . . . and I liked it very much from that viewpoint." He also valued being his own boss:

> If you felt that a patient didn't have acute appendicitis and was sent in as such you did not operate. You observed it. I had incidents in Trenton—I remember one where one of the surgeons was away for the weekend . . . and I saw one of his patients who had a bellyache. I didn't think it was surgical. Monday afternoon I met the patient walking the halls and she said, "You almost killed me because I had appendicitis." The other guy operated first thing Monday morning. So I went on to pathology and saw the normal appendix report. Such things as that I didn't enjoy. I did enjoy the fact that at HMC we did surgery when necessary and didn't do it when it was not necessary . . . [and] for the association with such people as Pellegrino and Knocke . . . men of quality whom I felt were above my quality. Therefore I could be confident in what they said and what they referred.

He also liked the convenience he found at Hunterdon: "I went to only one place instead of running all over the state. You could concentrate on what you were doing and do it to the best of your ability. The atmosphere was friendly. Certainly you didn't get rivalry or somebody trying to push you aside, like the case I referred to in Trenton—that sort of garbage."

Katzenbach and Roessel shared a generic examining room. They often did orthopedics when the orthopedist was unavailable, except for patients with broken hips who waited until the orthopedist returned. Both he and Roessel had had extensive experience with trauma. I recall patients with severe trauma where Katzenbach's demeanor and skills enabled the team working with him to pull together to save a patient. On one occasion, around 1960, a girl of six was brought to the hospital with acute epiglottitis. The otolaryngologist was away, but Katzenbach was in the building. We all went to the operating room together. He effectively reassured the mother while we prepared the patient. He kidded the little girl into the operating room, and with Colella jollied her into anesthesia, which he was not administering. He skillfully and quickly performed a tracheostomy, and we then watched her together until she could be extubated.

What he demonstrated to me as a pediatrician was openness and willingness to share opinions and ideas to help decide what to recommend to the child's parents. His integrity was such that he could neither sham nor shirk. He was always willing to help: his primary question was, Does this patient need my thoughts or my treatment; if so, how can I help? His genial, low-key demeanor made it easier for even the most anxious or angry parents to share their feelings with him.

During the 1950s, he took actions that by current standards would be clearly out of order. He tells of operating on a patient who remembered that he had set her broken arm when she was 12 years old. She went on to say: "We tried to get my mother but we couldn't reach her to get permission and you said, 'Oh, I know your mother doesn't want your arm crooked so I'll fix it anyway.'" Also, Roessel and Katzenbach performed pyloromyotomies on infants with pyloric stenosis on a regular basis, with anesthesia of open drop ether administered by Colella. This would not be so handled today. During the first 15 years of HMC all such patients were so treated; all made uneventful recovery free of complications.

After Katzenbach left full-time practice, he continued to assist Felix Salerno, Chief of Surgery, with whom he had developed a close personal and professional relationship. He noted increased emphasis on income during the 1960s; he agreed HMC's salaries were low. But the medical care, he felt, continued to be of high quality. In contrast, the personal, friendly atmosphere and the academic association of the early years did not continue. After retiring from surgery, he volunteered, helping operating room staff organize their days. He died on 26 March 2002.

FREDERICK KNOCKE, M.D.

Fred Knocke died in 1995. Information is obtained from his former wife, Lazelle ("Bobbie") Knocke,[44] HMC records and from my personal experience. Fred Knocke grew up in New York City, attended Horace Mann School, Princeton University and Cornell Medical School. He met Bobbie while on a two-year rotating internship at Lenox Hill Hospital. She was then head nurse on the women's surgical floor. Fred was always an active, energetic individual. He was an avid skier; in medical school he would ski all weekend and travel all night to get back in time to work the next day. Residency at New York Orthopaedic Hospital was interrupted by service in World War II. In the 12th Evacuation Hospital (see Grant's profile for more details about this hospital), he worked with Carl Roessel and Edward V. Grant. Fred and Bobbie married just prior to the war, and Bobbie gave birth to twins while Fred was overseas. He did not see them for over two years. He returned to New York at the end of 1945, and became Chief Resident at New York Orthopaedic Hospital, where Bobbie was instructor in nursing.

In 1948 Knocke entered private practice. He became busy; the family saw less and less of him. At Lenox Hill, he ranked as one of the more junior members of the orthopedic department, with years to wait before attaining significant rank, despite good relations with the chief of service. He had a "Park Avenue" practice, which meant having a nurse accompany him on house calls at one elegant penthouse after another. Bobbie recalls the advice he received: "It's ridiculous, but if you don't charge them an arm and three legs, they don't respect you . . . His office nurse said, 'Fred, be sure you make the bill plenty big.'" By 1952, Knocke was sharing an office on the Upper East Side of Manhattan near Lenox Hill Hospital, where he had privileges, with surgeon Carl Roessel and a pediatrician. Roessel learned about HMC through his contact with a patient, HMC Board member George Bushfield. Bobbie said Roessel was "just glowing with the stories of how wonderful it was," and he urged Fred to "come on out and take a look and see what you think of the community and its possibilities." Bobbie's response was, " Oh, Fred, New Jersey! Awful, you know' . . . and he said 'come on out and take a look' . . . So we came on out [in 1952] and visited and I went to the County Superintendent of

Schools to see what horrible school system this probably was . . . It turned out they had a super school system."

Knocke's immediate positive reaction to HMC was a response to the degree of community involvement, much easier commuting to work (compared to New York City), the possibility of seeing more trauma patients and the opportunity to teach and work with the family physicians. Part-time orthopedist Albert Accettola was helpful, a surgeon of fine quality and would cover one day a week when Knocke went to NYU. At Hunterdon Knocke would immediately be the chief of service, a contrast to the slow wait at Lenox Hill. The community was charming; the life style attractive. The family enjoyed outdoor activities. Despite all of this the family made a careful, measured decision involving several trips back and forth. Bobbie would have to give up teaching at Columbia, where she was finishing her Master's in nursing. Accepting the Hunterdon offer meant a reduction in income of at least 50 percent. Fred had never been attentive to the income side of practice, and it mattered little to him that Hunterdon represented a significant loss of income. As Bobbie noted,

> He just was negative about big fees and the idea of taking a cut did not hit him that hard. We figured it out that if we had the farm, we could manage quite well . . . It was a matter of, could we afford to do this and is the life style worth it? Yes, definitely worth it . . . After World War II and three kids there seemed little to worry about as we were young and healthy—also very naive and unsophisticated about finances.

Fred Knocke was a tall, lean, big-boned fellow who never used more words than necessary. He was a workhorse. Not only did he carry the orthopedic load, day and night, but helped in administration, and gardened seriously on the side. He had a delightful smile, but a serious, reserved manner. Nevertheless, he was quietly, softly, utterly sure of himself and what he did, which allowed him to be candid when he felt uncertainty. As a consultant his explanations were brief; if asked, he could teach clearly and as comprehensively as needed. He was as knowledgeable about bone physiology and bodily mechanics as he was of bone pathology. If he had a shortcoming, it was that at times he did not communicate enough with patients. I remember his coming to check on a patient in traction. He asked the patient how he was adjusting to the traction, and left without comment. He knew that all was

going well, and Fred expected the patient to speak up—and quickly—
if there were questions. He had both a sense of humor—and a
temper! Nurse Jeannette Ash, who worked with him, reports that
he could explode if standards of cleanliness were not maintained
to his satisfaction.

Knocke spoke up when the situation called for it. In meetings,
whether on orthopedic or administrative–political matters, he justified
his opinions with common sense, making his points thoughtfully
and carefully. He was tolerant of diversity and always gave careful
consideration to alternative beliefs and attitudes. But once he made
up his mind, that was the end of it. He was unshakable unless
significant new evidence could be presented. He would go to any
length to fulfill his obligations and duties without rancor or bitterness. Fred was one of those people who did not give offense,
and who did not easily take offense. He had a quiet sense of humor, with a grin rather than a guffaw. His qualities led to his
appointment as Associate Medical Director on 1 April 1955, when
Ed Pellegrino succeeded Trussell to become Medical Director.

I remember first meeting Knocke in 1958, when Hunterdon
was recruiting a successor to pediatrician Andy Hunt. I was then
in private practice in the Germantown neighborhood of Philadelphia and on the volunteer staff at Children's Hospital. Fred phoned
to introduce himself as the Acting Medical Director and asked
whether he might interview me at home. To keep our appointment, he drove through a snowstorm to the apartment where I,
my wife of just over a year, and our month-old daughter lived.
After putting himself out to keep the appointment, he then apologized for intruding on our weekend. His interview was considerate, insightful, and warm. Fred was attentive to the baby while
listening carefully to what each of us had to say. And then, refus-
ing offers of a bed for the night, he drove home in the snowstorm,
and, I am sure, took calls for the remainder of the weekend without complaint.

Fred never hesitated to ask for help and often requested consultation from Accettola, the internist or myself on difficult or
unusual patients. Despite his taciturn demeanor, he was attuned
to the needs and feelings of patients. I remember an athletic adolescent girl who complained of low back pain. Others might have
easily dismissed her complaint as due to her gym team practice,
but Fred was not satisfied and simultaneously called me in to see

her while he arranged for radiology studies. The tragedy was that her pelvis was riddled with sarcoma, and she died soon after. On another occasion, he set a broken arm of a five-year-old boy. He was also not satisfied with the story given by a foster mother. He took off the boy's shirt and discovered bruises elsewhere. He asked me to consult, and we agreed that the boy had been abused. The appropriate state agency was notified, but apparently dropped the ball. The child was not removed from the foster home, and a month or two later, he was back in the emergency room, but this time died of multiple injuries. No one was ever prosecuted, but I am sure he was beaten.[g]

The Knockes made an extensive search for a place to live. They fell in love with a farm not too far from HMC, where they, and now Bobbie, have lived ever since. Fred was a serious gardener and was well known as a breeder of dahlias and iris. Bobbie developed her own career, establishing a public health nursing service known as the Family Nursing Service. She was a horse person since childhood, with extensive experience before coming to Hunterdon. They purchased horses, the children learned to ride, and Bobbie opened a riding academy. When the Family Nursing Service decided on an annual horse show as a fund-raiser, it was held on their property. Bobbie still judges at horse shows.

From 1970 until 1976 Knocke served as HMC's Medical Director. In this capacity he was intimately involved in the unrest and disagreements between many members of the Specialist Staff and the Board. He presided through HMC's most difficult period and attempted to reconcile differences, but the gap between the parties was too wide. He needed and recruited orthopedic surgeons to help him with patient care. One left over disagreement with the structure of the Hunterdon staff; one left because of personal problems. Fred and Bobbie divorced and he moved to Detroit, where he remarried. He practiced industrial medicine until his death in 1995. Fred Knocke gave all of himself—which was a great deal—to care for patients, and to HMC's development and improvement. If

---

[g] At the time I complained bitterly to Lloyd Wescott, then President of the N.J. State Board of Control (NJSBC), the umbrella agency that administered the Division of Youth and Family Services, through which children in need of care were helped. Wescott was clearly disturbed over what had happened and did not attempt to defend DYFS. But he did defend their social workers in general, mentioning the size of their caseloads and the efforts that had been made to find more money to fund more social workers, etc. I believe that Wescott, in his capacity as President of the NJSBC, did the best he could under very difficult circumstances.

he did not succeed in accomplishing all that he wished for HMC, it was due to circumstances far out of his control. If energy, motivation, competence and good will could have preserved the Medical Center as originally conceived, that job would have been done.

ALEXANDER MITCHELL, M.D.

Mitchell was raised partly in North Carolina and Florida and partly in New York. His soft voice still reveals his southern roots.[45] He took his A.B. degree and first two years of medical school at the University of North Carolina, and finished at NYU. Internship was at Lenox Hill Hospital, followed by two years with the Army in Germany. Training in urology was at NYU–Bellevue. In 1952, he entered practice in New York. That same year he was approached by the Director of Urology at Bellevue, Robert Hotchkiss, who thought that Mitchell might be interested in the new hospital in Flemington. He interviewed at Hunterdon about the time the structural steel was going up, and agreed to work part time; in 1955 he moved to full time. His reasons for making the change were primarily familial. The Mitchells lived with four children in Manhattan. When the Trussells invited them to house-sit for a month one summer, the Mitchells enjoyed the opportunity to get out of the city. Mitchell was impressed by the quality of physicians already engaged as department heads. He saw an opportunity to build a practice and was tired of multiple hospitals and the stress of city travel.

Allie Mitchell is a fair-skinned man of medium build, precise in speech and action, and gentle in demeanor, soft-spoken, courteous to a fault, and rarely appears upset or angry. His easy manner contrasts with typical surgical decisiveness. When he harbored any doubts, he was always ready to discuss or reconsider how a patient should be handled or next steps. But when he believed he was on the right track, Allie would go ahead regardless of circumstances. Mitchell recalls enjoying the relationships at Hunterdon, the easy accessibility of colleagues whom he respected, and communication with family physicians. He mentioned as an example a call he received from a family physician who thought he might have a case of testicular torsion in his office but wasn't sure. Mitchell replied that he would drop by on the way home and see the patient, something that you wouldn't see happening in New York

City. Too quickly he became busy, limiting his ability to supervise the family physicians.

Of all the specialist staff interviewed, Mitchell expressed the greatest concern over what he felt was HMC's failure to fulfill its obligations to the specialist staff. He cited the absence of a retirement program until Herman Rannels initiated the idea, reneging on a sabbatical he had been promised, crowded office space, and very low salaries compared to peers elsewhere. He also felt that HMC's structure did not motivate all specialists to the same degree; some worked much harder than others. These and other points rankle to this day. The professional aspects of practice are what he remembers with greatest satisfaction; the administrative and business side with least.

The Board minutes for 22 January 1954, some months after Mitchell began part-time work, made provision for disability pay out of the Professional Service Fund, tenure in the event of military service, at least six months' notice of termination of employment, one month of vacation a year, prorated, and to initiate an analysis with a view to providing death benefits and a retirement program. I found no reference anywhere in the minutes to a sabbatical year, although I, too, recall this being mentioned to me when I was negotiating to work at HMC.

The Mitchells enjoyed country life and lived as far out from the Medical Center as they dared. They bought a working farm, which they shared with a farm family, and lived in a large old farmhouse. There was an array of sheep and other animals. Both Mitchells are quite musical. He plays the viola and his wife plays the piano. When their children were grown, they moved to a smaller home in the area, eventually retired, and moved to upstate New York where they live now.

EDWIN OLMSTEAD, M.D.

Edwin Olmstead died several years ago. Information for this profile was obtained from his son, Christopher, an attorney in Atlanta, Georgia.[46] Olmstead was born in South Worcester, New York, about 50 miles west of Albany. According to Catherine Tantum, a lab technician who worked with Olmstead, he described himself as "a poor farm boy who never failed to return each Memorial Day to place flowers on the graves of his parents."[47] He received his B.A. from the University of Pennsylvania. From ROTC, he joined the Army Reserve. Olmstead graduated from the University of Pennsylvania Medical School in 1936, entered active duty with the Army in 1942 as a battalion surgeon and served in the Pacific with an anti-aircraft unit. He left the service in 1946 with the rank of major. Before the war he practiced family medicine in Edmeston, New York, a small upstate rural community. After the war, he trained for two years as a pathologist at the Bronx Veterans Hospital and for a year with the Division of Laboratories and Research at the N.Y. State Department of Health, where Ray Trussell had also worked. Olmstead held other positions and published scientific articles prior to coming to Hunterdon.

Olmstead's son, Christopher, describes what motivated his father to come to HMC: "I think my dad also got tired of being paid with live chickens." The exigencies of practice helped him make up his mind. One snowy evening he received a call from a farmer who said his wife was very sick. "Despite the hour and the weather, my father got in his car and drove several miles to the farmer's home. When he arrived, the husband would not let my father in the home, telling him that his wife was asleep." Family physician John Lincoln related another story Olmstead told him. One winter night Olmstead made a house call to a man with a probable heart attack. Ed wanted to get the patient to the hospital as quickly as possible, and the easiest way was to drive him there himself. On the way, they got stuck in a snow drift. Olmstead was intently rocking the car when he noticed that the seat beside him was empty. His patient had slipped out to push the car. "He had many stories like that."[48]

Jack Fritz, a well-known family physician in Flemington and a medical school roommate of Olmstead, was responsible in great part for bringing Olmstead to Flemington. Board records show that he was appointed in December 1952, six months before HMC opened. A story in the *Hunterdon County Democrat* quotes Fritz: "I remember Ed not only as a great roommate but a fine student who made his mark at Penn . . . I've kept in touch with him off and on through the years and have every confidence that the Board could hardly have picked a better man for the position."[49] Olmstead's son said his father was always proud of what he and the other "founding fathers" accomplished at HMC.

The dedication, loyalty and camaraderie among the original group was phenomenal . . . None of the original physicians associated themselves with the Hunterdon Medical Center because they felt they were going to make a lot of money . . . Things were considerably different in 1975 when he retired than they were . . . when he arrived. Attitudes concerning the practice of medicine had changed.

Christopher Olmstead says, "I also know my father worked too hard. He was the only pathologist for many years and was lucky to be able to locate a visiting replacement so that he could take one week off each year as a vacation." John Lincoln, who assisted with postmortem examinations while building a practice, said of Olmstead:

> Ed was a quiet man with dry wit underlying serious demeanor. He was meticulous and conscientious. He had a good reason for everything he did. He taught constantly. I can remember a number of occasions in the morgue as he performed a post-mortem, listening to his discourse on what he was seeing, and observing how he brought together information from the clinical course, the gross findings, and his storehouse of medical experience. The anatomic pathology service that he managed fulfilled its ideal function as an engine for the study of disease at our hospital.[50]

Kate Tantum notes that he hired a pathologist Louis Cruz to do cytology. Cruz was wheelchair bound, and Olmstead made special arrangements for Cruz that enabled him to do his job—this long before equal opportunity legislation. Olmstead was involved in community sports, scouts and other activities, and started a program in women's health centering on regular examinations.

Olmstead kept all of his slides permanently. I can remember the excitement with which he and I traced the death of an infant which had occurred years before. A first cousin, born years later, proved to have Ivemark syndrome (absent spleen and situs inversus). He reconsidered the earlier death, and was able to show, with knowledge born of later years, that the microscopic study did indeed suggest that the infant had died of sepsis.[h] Ed Olmstead was like that. The fact that he had not identified this years ago was less

---

[h] Congenital absence of the spleen impairs immunity and predisposes to serious bloodstream infections (sepsis). When it is combined with reverse position of the heart (situs inversus), it is called Ivemark syndrome.

important than the fact that we were now able to understand what had really been going on. He was happy that his increased skills enabled him to be more productive.

WALTER A. PETRYSHYN, M.D.

Walter Petryshyn was born in 1922, raised in New York, attended Columbia College of Columbia University, and graduated in 1945 from Long Island College of Medicine (now Downstate division of the State University of New York).[51] His surgical internship was at Lenox Hill Hospital. There Petryshyn performed his first appendectomy—a rite of passage for any surgeon—under supervision of Carl Roessel, the surgical resident. Petryshyn's military service was spent at Sendai, Japan, in the medical detachment at IX Corps headquarters. In 1948 he returned to Bellevue for residency and special training in otologic pathology. In 1951, he was offered an academic appointment at NYU, and joined John Daly, the chief, in practice. Petryshyn feels he was fortunate to have served in a remarkably fine residency, where he trained in head and neck surgery, endoscopy, and micro-otologic surgery, in addition to standard otolaryngology work.

In 1953, Clarence de la Chapelle, who had asked Daly to recommend a suitable consultant at the new Hunterdon hospital, approached Petryshyn. The proposal sounded so interesting and appealing that Petryshyn agreed to consult two days a week. His first impression of the hospital was that it looked as if it was designed by a hotel architect because of the large picture windows in all the patient rooms, fine for a view but leaving patients gasping in the summer heat.[i] After a year Roessel asked him to come full time. Although Petryshyn earned more in New York than at Hunterdon, he chose the "Hunterdon experiment."

De la Chapelle approached Petryshyn at the right time. He and his wife were starting a family and had doubts about city life. The specialist team was impressive and exciting. His old colleague, Carl Roessel, was Chief of Surgery. His multiple subspecialty skills would be in demand and useful at Hunterdon, and he would be able to continue his academic affiliation at NYU–Bellevue, teaching oto-

[i] At the time of construction, the Board decided for financial reasons to forego air conditioning. Years later individual units had to be installed at much greater expense.

logic pathology. At HMC he would see a diversity of problems, such as the head and neck injuries from collisions at the stock car racetrack on the Flemington Fair grounds.[j] The experience provided him with material for a thesis that gained Petryshyn an award and entry to the American Tri-Otological Association, the honor society of his field.

Walter Petryshyn was a precise, careful, hard-working, thorough and assured surgeon. He considered each patient and their options in detail and made his recommendations in a manner of commanding authority. He loved the special areas of interest to him, maxillofacial reconstruction following trauma, micro-otologic surgery, and endoscopy. After requests to Roessel, Trussell and Wescott, Petryshyn was provided with all the equipment he needed—no mean feat in July 1954, when HMC had no working capital or cash flow because everything had been spent on building. Petryshyn covered many fields and performed procedures done today by subspecialists, but at the time the area lacked subspecialty services.

The birth of a third child moved financial needs to the forefront of Petryshyn's thinking. Everyone at HMC made the same salary, but Petryshyn generated sizable fees, for which he received no bonus. In 1958, he spoke to the Board treasurer about this, suggesting that salaries should be based on productivity. No change occurred. When he left Hunterdon, in 1960, his salary was $21,000, corresponding to $124,500 in 2001 dollars. Petryshyn had received offers to become the chief of otolaryngology at Stanford and Case Western Reserve medical schools. A former professor at Bellevue, James Shannon, offered a practice in Montclair, New Jersey, and simultaneously Petryshyn became Chief of Otolaryngology at Seton Hall–New Jersey College of Medicine on a voluntary basis. He also became research director and later Medical Director of the Deafness Research Foundation in New York City and started a temporal bone bank at Mountainside Hospital. He retired from practice in 1986.

[j] The Flemington Agricultural Fair, the last in New Jersey, ceased to exist in 2001. This annual event was a major attraction in Hunterdon County. The grounds, on route 31 between HMC and Flemington, are highly desirable for development. A private corporation owns the land; for many years Lloyd Wescott and Kenneth Myers, of HMC's Board, were very active in this group. Because the fair was only a week a year, to provide income for maintenance, taxes and other expenses, stock car races were held each summer Saturday night. The sound from these noisy affairs spread for miles. Some years ago when patients complained about the racket on hot summer nights, an agreement was negotiated that races would end no later than 11 p.m.

HERMAN RANNELS, M.D.

Herman Rannels died in 1996. His second wife, Nancy, provided much information for this profile.[52] Both were born and raised in Lancaster, Pennsylvania. He attended local schools, obtained his B.S. at Dickinson College in nearby Carlisle, Pennsylvania, in 1934, and his M.D. at the University of Pennsylvania in 1938. He interned at Chestnut Hill Hospital in Philadelphia; specialty training was at the Kensington Hospital for Women in Philadelphia and the New York Post-Graduate Medical School and Hospital in New York City. He served in the Navy during World War II and was stationed in Okinawa and Quantico. After the war he returned to Lancaster, where he was Chief of Obstetrics at St. Joseph's Hospital from 1947 until he came to Hunterdon in 1953.

According to Nancy, Herman said he wanted to leave St. Joseph's Hospital because he felt rigid attitudes there were not conducive to what he considered quality care. It was attractive to him to be able to set up a new service as he desired. Trussell added that Rannels joined the specialist staff at the last moment, on his own initiative, apparently advised by others to look into the opening. His first marriage was breaking up and he decided to leave Lancaster with Nancy. They met for the first time when she was asked to scrub with him. Learning from the other nurses that he was ambidextrous, she prepared needle holders for both hands and asked which he preferred to use. "He jerked to attention at that."

Attitudes in maternity and gynecological care shifted in the years just before Rannels came to Hunterdon. The pioneering work of Grantly Dick-Read was extended to a general community hospital and a university hospital, and publications on enhanced cooperative efforts between obstetricians and general practitioners also appeared.[53] Rannels' new service reflected these changing attitudes. He wanted a program of systematic prenatal education. In 1954, with the participation of Hunt, Parmet, and Margaret Wiles, the Associate Director of Nursing, who had a background in public health, he developed the program.[54] Eight sessions, two hours each, were held evenings so that fathers might attend. Instruction included methods of relaxation advocated by Dick-Read. Parents toured the inpatient unit and were encouraged to ask questions; family physicians were also involved. Rannels emphasized the role of the family physician, while recognizing his responsibility for education and supervision to assure quality of care given by all physicians to patients on the service.[55]

The quality of care in the new service was impressive. Rannels compiled statistics through 1956. During the first two-and-a-half years there were 2,279 deliveries at HMC. Of these 2,008, or 89 percent were performed by family physicians; 1,695 deliveries were spontaneous and 584 were operative, or 26 percent. Of those 584, 56 were Caesarean sections, or 2.5 percent. There were 25 perinatal deaths, and 21 stillbirths, for a total perinatal mortality of 20 per thousand. At that time, comparable rates ranged from 25 to 34 per thousand.[56] Two maternal deaths occurred: one due to a pheochromocytoma that had not been detected before the mother arrived in labor[57] and the other a patient who arrived from another hospital moribund due to exsanguination from an unrecognized placenta previa.

Rannels was forced into a running struggle with the N.J. Department of Health. When HMC first opened, gynecological, some surgical patients and obstetrical patients were mingled on the fourth floor, because of insufficient nursing staff. Integration continued because the number of maternity cases was low compared to the number of beds. This conflicted with obstetrical teaching of the times, descended from Ignatz Semmelweis, that maternity patients must be strictly isolated from all others—what some might call, from a later perspective, the "medicalization" of normal perinatal care. Rannels obtained temporary permission to mix obstetrical and gynecological patients, provided he did an outcome study. This study was performed, and published in 1962, after Rannels had left the Medical Center.[58] The unequivocal results—low morbidity, high occupancy and only a slight increase in nursing hours per patient—did not convince N.J.'s Health Department; conflict continued, ending only when the obstetrical occupancy rate rose and the duration of hospital stay for all patients fell.

Nancy Rannels' comments on her husband's accomplishments, and the references in the literature, differ from comments made by his colleague and successor, Gerald Barad (see Barad profile). I am unable to reconcile the difference.

Recollections of Herman Rannels by other staff whom I have interviewed are more varied than those concerning any other member of the early staff at Hunterdon. Some regarded him as highly competent, while others felt he did not respect tissue as a surgeon should. Some saw him as blunt and arrogant and others found him sensitive to patients' feelings. My own contact with him lasted less than a year, and we were not close, so I can add little. It is correct to say that he relied on obstetrical anesthesia to a greater extent than his successor and that he generated strong opinions, pro or con, in others. There is reason to believe that his style was authoritarian. See Barad's profile for his critique of Rannels. What follows is a sampling of other opinion.

Jeannette Ash, a nurse who worked with Rannels in the office, says:

> He was fun, he taught me all the time. You were learning all the time, because he would teach the patient and teach the nurse as well. If somebody had a complaint he would tell them why he felt it was that or wasn't that, whatever. He would explain in great detail what he was going to do. He never did anything unless he told the patient explicitly what he was doing and why he was doing it . . . He had a lot of prenatals and had a day set aside for them. That was a fun day. Patients either liked him or didn't like him. His approach was "this is the way it is." There was no middle ground. Fact was fact. Yet he was very compassionate if someone was really upset. He was popular. He was always on time, in contrast to Pellegrino, who tended to be late.[59]

Trussell said that:

> He dealt with the local practitioners in a somewhat different way than the other men did but I don't think there is any question that he did a competent job. I think that the problem there in part was that the local practitioners were used to delivering normal pregnancies and probably not asking for help as much as they should. I remember one argument he had with one of the local doctors who had a patient in active labor and who wasn't there. He expected Herman to be in there covering and Herman made it clear to him that it was his job.[60]

Pellegrino explained that:

> Herman's challenge was that the GPs were doing obstetrics and he had to somehow carry out his responsibilities as Chief of Obstetrics for the quality of care of all patients. Herman [was] a bit irascible and a little stubborn. But he was able to move in and out of the delivery room [on short notice to

back up the family physician]. Herman was always there. Somehow, he would appear out of somewhere to be available if difficulties arose. That was more difficult than my task in medicine because his is a "hands-on" specialty. He was a good obstetrician–gynecologist to the extent that a non-expert can judge that. We chose John Bambara and not Herman to deliver our children. That was a matter of personalities. My wife did not want to be treated like a "little mother," which was Herman's approach. I had great respect for him.[61]

Family practitioner John Bambara described Rannels as not "endearing." He was "gruff and tough and somewhat arrogant."[62] Administrator Edward Grant found Rannels "very straightforward. He pulled no punches . . . [and was] utterly competent in what he did."[63] Arno Macholdt, a family physician, served a four-month residency in OB–GYN under Rannels. Macholdt and his wife saw him as "very straightforward, a diamond in the rough. You always knew where you stood with him." With his patients, said Macholdt, "He got along surprisingly well. Sometimes he would be kind of gruff, yet when he was dealing with individual patients it always surprised me how smoothly he got along with them." Rannels delivered two of the Macholdt children.[64] Trudy Macholdt said, "As a patient I found him very sensitive . . . He could say, look, this is the way it is going to be. But if he could see that this was upsetting to you, then he would back off."[65] The two families got on very well; Rannels gave Macholdt one of his beloved collie dogs.

Herman and Nancy Rannels were married in the Mt. Pleasant Church. Andrew and Lotte Hunt stood up for them at the ceremony. Nancy subsequently had their first child here; their second was born after they left the area. They bought a farm near Mt. Pleasant. It was important to them because Herman raised prize collies and sheep. Nancy says: "It was his hobby but my full-time job." Herman's devotion to his dogs was legendary. Once he brought a champion show dog to the morgue, where he operated to remove a lump from its side. On another occasion he brought one of his collies into the Radiology Department to x-ray a suspected fracture, which triggered a shouting match with Steve Dewing, the radiologist. Rannels was very active in the early days of the Family Nursing Service, founded the local Lutheran church, the Kennel Club and several breeding associations.

Rannels resigned in fall of 1959. Nancy Rannels says Herman

"told me he thought his job there was done." I believe he wanted to be Medical Director; this disappointment led to his decision to leave. From Hunterdon he became Medical Director and Chief of Obstetrics and Gynecology at the Miners' Memorial Hospital in Man, West Virginia, from 1960 till 1964. They moved to California, where he held administrative positions at the University of California, Irvine. He ended his clinical career at the Williamsport Hospital, in Williamsport, Pennsylvania, where he founded a residency in Family Medicine. Rannels died in June, 1996.

CARL ROESSEL, M.D.

Carl Roessel was born in Brooklyn, New York, attended private schools, received his B.A. from Princeton in 1935, and graduated from Columbia College of Physicians and Surgeons in New York. It was the Depression era, and even though Roessel was awarded financial scholarships, during his first two years at medical school he waited on tables. According to Buck Katzenbach, "Carl and his roommate were with the *New York Times*. They [were allowed to live at the *Times*] . . . to treat any . . . injuries or sickness and acted as the physicians."[66]

He served a two-year rotating internship and surgical residency at Lenox Hill Hospital in New York City. Walter Petryshyn, a junior resident with him, describes him as "very serious . . . very knowledgeable, he was conservative, and a very good teacher. I liked and respected him."[67] In World War II Lenox Hill Hospital formed a military unit from staff, the 12th Evacuation Hospital. Roessel volunteered, along with Fred Knocke and Ed Grant. They served overseas, in the European theater, for 36 months. (Grant's profile describes in greater detail this experience.) Roessel served as Chief Surgeon on a landing craft during the Normandy invasion. He made four crossings of the Channel, performing surgery on the return trips.

After completing military duty, Roessel returned to New York and in 1947 opened practice in an office shared with Fred Knocke. He married Barbara ("Bobbie") Roessel the same year. He was well established when he heard about a new hospital in Flemington. By now, immersed in the realities of a New York City practice, both Roessel and his family were feeling the stress. They moved to Riverdale, which meant a long commute to the office, and he was

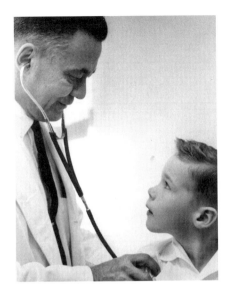

Carl Roessel, the first surgeon at HMC, examining a child on the pediatric floor.

on the staff at three different hospitals. Bobbie Roessel says: "It was hard on him to get around, come home, and then be called back again in the middle of the night. So, he always kept his ears and eyes open for anything that might sound more suitable . . . We didn't want to leave both of our families."[68] George Bushfield, a post-operative patient of a colleague, proved to be the link to that opportunity. Bushfield, who was on the Board of that new hospital in Flemington, alerted Roessel to the opening. Roessel applied for the job and began work in April 1953, organizing the operating suites and surgical floors in cooperation with the nursing supervisors, Jean Moleski on the surgical floor and Ruth Ent in the operating area.

The Roessels were taken with Hunterdon for several reasons. Roessel liked being in charge of a new service. It was near the extended families on both sides. They were pleased with the schools and the area's agricultural character. They also liked the idea of community contact with patients. Bobbie Roessel says, "it gives me great satisfaction when I go into the drug store or someplace and someone comes to me and says, 'Oh, your husband did an appendectomy.'"

Roessel was a slender fellow of just below medium stature, trimly built, with a calm, serious expression. With professional decisions he could be quite concise. Ed Grant, who was a tent mate throughout their service together with Patton's Third Army in Europe, said: "Carl was a very quiet, introspective type of guy. He was very straightforward. He could, like a surgeon, cut right to the point . . . When we were together, it was friendship and then it was also professional."[69]

Roessel was glad to serve as a resource and consultant for the primary care physicians. When a patient was admitted by a family physician or pediatrician, he would consult; if the diagnosis and plan of care were in doubt, he recommended that the patient be followed by the primary care physician until the issues were resolved. He looked in as often as needed, in his supportive and friendly way, making suggestions, but at the same time keeping the lines of responsibility clear between patient, family, and physician.

Roessel was a prototype of the even-tempered surgeon in charge who evaluated situations and acted on them when ready, and not before. Pauline Goger saw him as an "infinitely fair and a good doctor . . . Not only a good doctor, but a surgeon . . . He had a certain dignity about him . . . He didn't mince any words."[70] He was also the Chief Surgeon—the rest of the staff paid him the highest respect and did not hesitate to seek his help with problems far removed from a general surgeon's purview. He was a conservative surgeon, who operated only when he thought he should. Roessel set a pattern of conservative treatment not only in surgery, but also for hospital care in general at Hunterdon, which persisted long after his death—I would say to this day. Family physician John Lincoln described him as

> no nonsense . . . He didn't waste words. If he thought the patient needed to be operated he'd say, "Let's go." If he thought the patient didn't need to be operated, he simply said "nope."
> I remember one time he took a pencil and paper and drew a funny little face and said "that's what a pain looks like. Do you take out a pain?" The point was you don't operate on somebody just because they hurt.[71]

I recall being in the Emergency Department by chance when a man injured in a head-on automobile collision was brought in. Breathing was labored. Color was poor. The steering wheel had struck the front of his chest, breaking ribs. Each time he tried to take a breath, the ribs caved in, preventing air intake. Roessel arrived quickly and immediately recognized the problem: a flail chest. He asked for a toothed clamp. Without a word except to the patient to reassure him, Roessel quickly injected a local anesthetic, and clamped the center chest skin and cartilage and then lifted it straight up in the air, stabilizing the ribs, giving the diaphragm muscle something to pull against, and instantly improving the patient's breathing efficiency. Color and condition improved dramatically. Roessel stood there imperturbable as he held the clamp in place, while issuing a stream of orders about what the next actions should be. His orders were obeyed quickly, and the patient pulled through.

With children he was kind and friendly, considerate and solicitous. He would not act until he was sure of himself. I remember several occasions when he and I observed a child with abdominal pain, possibly acute appendicitis. Carl listened carefully to the patient's history, performed his own examination, and if not convinced he should operate, would articulate reasons why, and leave it to me as pediatrician to observe and call back when needed. That did not mean that he left the case—typically he would look in again as often as needed, until all were satisfied that either the child could be left alone or it was time for surgery. He very rarely failed to operate when he should, and, more importantly, did not often operate unnecessarily.

I also remember becoming very frustrated with him over a child with abdominal pain. In my opinion, she had an acute abdominal condition that should be treated surgically. Carl was not convinced, and when Carl was not convinced, he would not operate. The girl of about ten years had minimal complaints and findings, but I was not comfortable sending her home. We hospitalized her for observation. That evening, no change. The next morning, perhaps slightly more discomfort on palpation. Carl finally decided to operate and indeed she had an inflamed appendix. Only after surgery did we learn from her mother that her daughter never complained and that she didn't react to things. Even the mother couldn't tell if she was upset or uncomfortable. And so one temperamentally mild reactor took in another.

Carl's unflappable approach included himself. Once he told me that he had been bitten by a yellow jacket. I knew he was allergic to stings. "What did you do?" I asked. He said either he would have an anaphylactoid reaction and die, or it would not be so bad, but, in any case, he was alone at home and there was no time to summon help. "So I sat down on a stone for 15 minutes to see what would happen. Since I was not dead, I came over for a shot of epinephrine." I only recall seeing him nonplussed once. We were in the dining room exchanging jokes about medicine. Carl mentioned some surgical advance in the treatment of cancer, and Harry Woske, then Head of Internal Medicine, joked, "Carl, two more new drugs and you'll be back in the barber shop."

Carl Roessel died suddenly in 1964 of a heart attack. He had chest pain, went on his own to the ECG department, and collapsed while a tracing was being taken. He could not be revived.

FREDERICK WOODRUFF, M.D.

Fred Woodruff grew up in Roselle Park, New Jersey, and his wife, Carol, was raised nearby. Woodruff's father, who had a chronic spinal cord disorder that limited movement, operated an insurance business from home. He was young Fred's trusted adviser. After graduating from the local high school, Woodruff volunteered for the Navy college program in 1943 and was assigned to Princeton. He finished six semesters, worked at St. Albans Naval Hospital, and was then sent to Syracuse University Medical School, now SUNY Upstate Medical Center. After his first year of medical school, he financed the remainder through the GI Bill and worked nights as an ambulance driver at the hospital, for room, board, laundry and $25 a month.

He graduated in June 1949 and married Carol the next day. After graduation he took a general internship at the Navy Hospital in Portsmouth, Virginia, followed by a year of family practice residency at Muhlenberg Hospital in Plainfield, New Jersey. He was not at all sure that he had a specialty in mind. He very much enjoyed the clinics of various specialties, which he attended every afternoon. Just as he was accepted for a radiology residency at the VA Hospital in Pittsburgh, Pennsylvania, the Navy notified him to expect to be recalled "at some time." Woodruff's responded by driving down to the Navy Department in Washington, and said: " I am here to tell you I want to get going.' They went into shock."[72] His forthrightness brought him his choice of duty. He was first stationed in Bainbridge, Maryland, and then spent 15 months aboard a ship in the Pacific. After release, he went to the Bronx VA Hospital as a radiology resident.

In 1955, Woodruff's final year of residency, his mentor, Max Poppel, of NYU School of Medicine, one day mentioned Hunterdon. Steve Dewing, who had taken the same training program earlier, was looking for someone to cover for him. Woodruff agreed to work a day a week for 10 weeks, moonlighting by using up vacation days.

Woodruff says:

> When I came here I found a different world than I had known in the past as far as x-ray was concerned. My exposure had been in Plainfield, New Jersey, where I spent a year as a family practice resident. The fellows [at] the radiology group . . . were of a standard type . . . where you read films and left things behind, and ran to an office, ran back to the hospital, that sort of thing.

In-hospital radiology practice and intimate discussions with referring physicians were new to him. He began full-time work in 1957, after Dewing convinced the HMC Board of the need for a second radiologist. Although he had several opportunities, having seen and actually worked at Hunterdon he had no question where to go. "I could talk to the attending physicians. We would discuss the case. We could set up the x-ray a little by what we both thought . . . I could adjust studies because I would be here all the time." He also wanted to innovate, and saw this as a major plus. In addition, Hunterdon would allow both him and his wife to remain near their families. The area attracted them very much as a place to raise their two children. The salary at that time was competitive with what he was offered at other positions: $12,000 a year, equal to $78,000 in 2001 dollars.

For Woodruff, the important thing was the ability to try something new, to create a new way of doing: "I saw that we could build an x-ray therapy [unit] . . . and nuclear medicine . . . and I could present new ideas and move things along. So, I came here because it was a new kind of practice for radiology." He also found he could learn from his colleagues. Woodruff had little experience in orthopedics, but Fred Knocke proved to be an excellent instructor. Discussions with Knocke led to ongoing improvements in techniques and methods. Woodruff was interested in nuclear medicine, and this type of work increased greatly after his arrival. His mentor at NYU–Bellevue was Nobel Prize winner Rosalyn Yalow, a leader in the field. Woodruff spent a day a week there for years during a period when nuclear medicine was rapidly developing.

Woodruff seemed to know everything about every gadget in the entire department. It was not unusual to find him with his sleeves rolled up, working with the developing machines, or adjusting their liquid, in an era when a "wet reading" meant reading a film still wet from the developer. When the first automatic developers came out in 1963, he obtained one, keeping his own supply of spare parts on hand. Once when the machine failed over a weekend, he darkened the entire room and developed the films by hand, hanging them on a clothesline. Another area he enjoyed was radiation therapy. Dewing had a state-of-the-art machine for the period and had written a text standard in the field. Woodruff treated skin cancers, bursitis and tendonitis, conditions which would not be so treated today in light of present knowledge.

Woodruff opened a school for x-ray technicians. Many techs in the department trained there in a two-year course. An example of his can-do ethos concerns completion of the application forms: "I had a little trouble getting [Henderson, the Medical Director] to sign the papers, so I just signed them myself and mailed them in." What was probably most important to Woodruff was that "I could move in directions that I saw a need for and would get support and a chance to do it. I didn't have to raise a huge argument, go through 18 committees to get the school started." He looked for ways to educate himself in all facets of his field, attending courses on management and planning of radiology departments.

In general, Hunterdon lived up to Woodruff's expectations. He would confer on rounds with the internists daily. There was an interchange about diagnoses, and how to order films. He opened a very successful program with Gerald Barad, whom he had known at Bellevue, for treating cancer of the cervix with radon implants. Both had training with the same therapist at Bellevue who was in charge of gynecological radiation. With David Greenbaum, whom he had also known at Bellevue, a very close relationship sprang up: one went to see the fluoroscopies, and the other to see the sigmoidoscopies.

Two other ventures were atypical for a radiologist. He became chairman of the House Staff Committee, and in that capacity for a time managed the Family Practice Residency program. I served on the committee at that time, and in my view, he managed it very well. His other venture was becoming Hunterdon's electroencephalographer. Hunt and others felt that because he did well with images, he should be able to read galvanometer records. Woodruff agreed to take it over, and learned on his day a week in New York from the NYU EEG reader at the psychiatric hospital next to Bellevue.

The Woodruffs lived a quiet life in Flemington in the same home since arrival. Ever a hands-on man, Woodruff supervised the design and construction of it. He died in 2001.

CHAPTER 21

The People

Family Physicians

There were 26 family physicians in practice in Hunterdon County when the movement for the new hospital began. Of this group, John Bambara, Ray Fidellow, M. L. Looloian and Leonard Rosenfeld could be interviewed on the events of the time. Several others were chosen for interview who could make helpful contributions. Family medicine of those days was exemplified by the comment made by Ray Fidellow about his colleague Loo Looloian: "He always felt that he took care of people who were his friends."[1] The interviews have reminded me how hard-working and competent these men were.

A. JOHN BAMBARA, M.D.

"Dr. B." was 87 years old in June, 1996, when he was interviewed. Bambara grew up in Brooklyn, New York. From the age of 13, he worked in a pharmacy after school and on weekends, studying at night until early morning hours, and leaving him little, if any, social life. His goal was always to be a doctor.

> While I was working in the drug store . . . I saw a truck hit a six or seven-year-old girl who was walking her dog . . . When she was picked up, she was brought to the sidewalk in front of the drug store because the druggist didn't want the store to be dirtied with all her blood. She was placed down on the ground with her bloody clothes, and I just saw her take two deep breaths and she expired. And while she was doing that, I just kept saying, "What can I do? What can I do?" And so that started it. And then a few years after that, I came across a picture and the title of the picture was, "The Doctor"[a] . . .

[a] By Sir Luke Fildes. A physician is portrayed, seated, serious and reflective, hand on chin, beside a bed in which a little girl lies.

When I saw that picture, I said, "That's what I want to do"
. . . I wanted to be a family doctor, take care of the kids, take
care of the family . . . That led me into medicine in the first
place, and led me to Flemington in the second place. And the
work in Flemington was something that I had dreamed about
. . . I enjoyed every bit of it.[2]

Bambara graduated from Columbia College of Columbia University and Columbia University School of Pharmacy, with a B.S. and PH.G. After obtaining his M.D. at the New York Medical College in Valhalla, New York, in 1937, he entered a two-year rotating internship at Muhlenberg Hospital in Plainfield, New Jersey. In 1939, as he completed internship, a nurse who lived in Flemington suggested that even though it was a small town, four of the five physicians there were over 65, and it might be a good place to open a practice. Bambara "visited each one of the doctors, and they all said I should not start my practice in Flemington . . . Not wanting to go back to Brooklyn where I came from, . . . I started 1 July 1939, the year that I finished my internship."

Bambara was called to active duty from the Army Reserve in February 1941, just as he was really getting started in private practice. He served for five years—first in the southern United States, then England, France and Belgium with the 25th General Hospital—until discharged in March 1946. Bambara "precepted" for a year with the head of radiology at Muhlenberg Hospital, but received little instruction and felt ill trained, insecure, and "incompetent" in radiology. In 1947 he returned to his practice in Flemington.

Bambara learned of the new hospital from the newspaper and from Lloyd Wescott. Ray Trussell also visited him. Bambara's reaction was positive:

God knows, I was for it because my maternity patients were
very difficult to handle in terms of deliveries . . . It was right
up my alley in terms of having a medical facility nearby . . .
and then when the hospital started and there was a staff, a
bunch of human beings, likable people, well-trained. I felt
great.

In 1939, Dr. Bambara felt confident to charge $2 for an office visit and $3 for a house call, instead of the $1 and $2 the older physicians charged. He says:

I had a patient the first day [with] a fractured arm and I had
to send him to Plainfield to get an x-ray of his arm and, of

> course, I took care of it just from the dictation that I had
> gotten from the x-ray man without seeing the x-ray at all.
> After that the patients kept coming gradually.

His income for the entire first year was less than $1,000 ($12,600
in 2001 dollars). Before entering service, Bambara performed at
least a dozen office tonsillectomies. "I had the equipment and used
an experienced nurse anesthetist whom I knew from Muhlenberg
Hospital." He did not perform any after he returned from the
service, because he was then extremely busy with a large maternity
practice. That was difficult because he delivered his patients at
Somerset Hospital 25 miles away on a two-lane road. On many
occasions he drove patients to the hospital. "I [ran] myself ragged
working 16, 18, 20 hours a day. That's including Wednesdays and
Sundays. I'm ashamed to say it but the remuneration was not enough
for the amount of work that I was doing." Bambara served a term
as President of the Hunterdon County Medical Society and was
well respected. Ray Trussell asked him to treat his family.

"Dr. B." was the nickname used by all. When Bambara was
selected as the central character of an NBC documentary about family
physicians, this became the title of the film. Two points are clear
from the video.[3] First, he was very interested in behavioral aspects
of health care. Many vignettes in the film testify to his concern for
the mental health of his patients. He found a psychosomatic component in 90 percent of his patients. His interest dated to adolescence:

> Older people [used to] talk to me, even as a kid of 15 or 16
> years old, while I was behind the counter . . . Sometimes they
> would talk to me about some of their problems . . . family
> stuff, husbands and wives, kids . . . [Later] when a patient
> came to me I took time . . . [and would] sit there and wait for
> them to talk. Or at least I'd ask a question . . . I would take
> half an hour, or 45 minutes and get $2 or $3 for a visit.

Second, he worked very long hours, which limited his time with
his own family. It is evident from the video that he felt sad about
this, just as it is evident that he enjoyed his work very much. On
one of the rare occasions when he was dining with his family,
Mrs. Bambara said, "Jack [his son] is going to be 13 tomorrow."
The doctor replied, "Jack? Who's Jack?" He says, "Of course, I
was being facetious, but nevertheless it struck me right in the heart.
That added to my need to do something about myself and my
family."

Wescott felt strongly that the film concentrated on Bambara while neglecting the contribution of the Medical Center.[4] It was a film about a particular physician rather than about a family physician at a particular hospital, a position supported by my review of the film. Bambara says the filming distorted reality. He is shown interviewing many patients, but examining none. There was undue emphasis on conflict between family physician and specialist, when, according to Bambara, the two were not at all at odds. As a result of his complaints, he states that the script was changed to lessen the appearance of conflict. On interview Bambara said to me that the filmed case conference was misleading. The patient had an ulcer. Bambara felt as if the discussion was leading toward the specialists taking care of all peptic ulcers. He said to himself:

> What the hell. They don't have to take care of all the ulcer patients. When the general practitioner finds himself in a bind, he can then call a specialist but there is no reason why I couldn't give the patient a diet and the medication if they needed it. That's why I came up with, I can take care of it. Do I have to give my patient to a specialist because he's got a gastric ulcer? I didn't give it to the orthopedic man because the guy broke his arm.[b]

The conditions of practice were different then. Bambara recalls a house call "one winter night with snow two feet high on the roads.

> I was called to see a patient at a farm about five miles away. I barely reached the gate at the farm when the farmer met me. His house was about 300 to 500 feet from the gate and it would have been impossible for me to get through in my car . . . so, he had obtained a long wooden plank, and attached it to the harness of his horse, and I stood up on the plank, bag in hand, the other hand used to keep my balance and I was pulled standing up. I felt like George Washington crossing the Delaware.

"Dr. B." recalled another house call to a farmhouse one night because an elderly woman had tripped on the stairs and "hurt" her shoulder. As he examined her in a dimly lit room, illuminated only by a kerosene lamp, he realized she had dislocated her left

[b] See Pellegrino's concerns over balancing competing values—the responsibility of the Chief of Service to secure quality of care for all patients on his service, whether the Chief was the attending for that patient or not, and respect for the autonomy, confidence of, and relationship with, the family physician who had admitted the patient or requested a consultation.

shoulder. He had her lie down and moved the kerosene lamp to the opposite side of the room.

> I gave her open drop ether for light anesthesia and restored the humerus to its proper position. I was very frightened using the ether with an open flame around. Morphine would have taken longer to act. She was frightened because of the injury and I had to comfort her somehow.

Bambara, who is Catholic, recalls hearing of religious prejudice in central Hunterdon. In 1939, while scouting a practice location, he was told that in 1938 a cross was burned by the Ku Klux Klan on Thatcher's Hill above Flemington.[c] Although the environment for a newcomer was not always friendly, he personally experienced no prejudice. Soon, most of the ministers in the area were his patients, perhaps because when he made a house call on an elderly person living alone, he would ask if the patient wanted the minister to call.

Eventually his work pace took its toll. Jack Fritz, another family physician, had a heart attack and decided to take a residency in dermatology. Bambara heeded the message and in 1959 entered training as a psychiatrist. Pellegrino helped him win a three-year residency at the University of North Carolina Memorial Hospital in Chapel Hill. Peter Rizzolo, at that time a resident in family medicine at HMC, recalls a different story, of a very abrupt departure on an emergency basis for gall bladder surgery.[5] The man had just burned out. Living expenses were aided by a federal stipend for generalists who entered mental health full time. Bambara became Medical Director of the Somerset County Mental Health Center, retired in 1977, and has since worked part time as a volunteer.

LOUIS DOYLE, M.D.

Doyle was raised in West Lafayette, Indiana, where his father was on the faculty of the Graduate School of Veterinary Medicine at Purdue University. Although Doyle had learned a good deal about veterinary medicine from his father, he always knew he preferred human medicine. At Indiana University Medical School he met his wife Beryl, an occupational therapist at the state mental hospi-

---

[c] In the Depression years the Klan's headquarters were in what is now a church on N.J. routes 31-202 near Ringoes, according to Don Shuman. Interview, 9 April 2000. Shuman file, HMCA.

tal. After graduation in 1945, he took a military internship at Fort Lewis, Washington. He served in the military for 12 years. His final posting was in Baltimore at the Air Force Air Research and Development Center, caring for some 2,000 personnel, family, and retirees. The Doyles wanted to leave Baltimore when his tour was up to practice family medicine. Lou saw John Lincoln's advertisement, which seemed attractive, so they made three trips to Flemington. In 1958 Doyle joined Lincoln in the first dual practice in the county. Driving the decision to locate in Flemington was its location between New York and Philadelphia. The area's economics showed relatively high per capita income: "It looked like a place you could move to and probably never have to leave."[6] Doyle did not want to be a solo practitioner, on call 24 hours a day. HMC's structure and its family practice program were not primary considerations.

Doyle found the community, local citizens, practice, hospital and other physicians all he hoped for. HMC encouraged the highest quality medicine of which he was capable. Consulting support, the teaching program, and, above all, the collegiality were particularly gratifying. He could call on a number of people if he had a problem. On the financial side, working with Lincoln required adjustment for both. Doyle explained:

> I was an employee for two years . . . I had access to the books, the cost and the expense and what I was taking home and what he was taking home. It was not what he had represented before even though we were busier and busier. So we went to a medical partnership attorney in New York . . . three or four times; he accepted the attorney's recommendations.

See Lincoln's profile for his perception of the relationship.

Doyle appears low-keyed, relaxed and flexible, but is actually far more intense and holds far stronger opinions than surface appearances reveal. He is a very tall, large-built man with a deep voice, a languid manner, and a wry sense of humor. While he enjoys people and their stories, there was no time in practice to offer counseling.

Doyle described good relations with the specialist staff, except for Gerald Barad. Barad, he felt, did not believe that family physicians should be providing obstetrical care, and his attitude "bordered on hostile." In contrast, Doyle always got on very well with

Herman Rannels. An incident that Doyle found particularly gall-
ing occurred on Christmas Day, 1964. He delivered two of Barad's
patients because the obstetrician was snowbound, as well as several of his own. "I spent all day there this Christmas, with three
young boys at home without a father. It was fine because it wouldn't
happen every year." But then there followed an enormous article
in the local paper. "It never mentioned the nurses or me. It was all
about Barad and how he had come in the next day and delivered
one baby." Doyle found all the other departments and specialists
very supportive and pleasant to deal with. Eventually the practice
gave up obstetrics because of requirements to deliver a minimum
number of patients per year, and also because a new partner did
not want to do obstetrics.

Doyle left private practice in 1986 to work at the Port Authority of New York and New Jersey and at a women's prison in
Hunterdon County. He retains relationships with colleagues, refers to local consultants, and attends the Hunterdon County Medical
Society meetings regularly.

Raymond E. Fidellow, m.d.

Ray Fidellow grew up in Brooklyn and began college at Cornell in
1932. After one semester there was no money to continue. He worked
at odd jobs—clerking at Woolworth's, cleaning, as a grease mon-
key at a gas station, and from 1934 to 1936 as an attendant at a
state hospital. He was able to return to school, at NYU, graduating
with a b.s. in education in 1940. In 1941 he entered the Army, rose
to a commission via officers' candidate school, and went overseas
in January 1942, where he met Buck Katzenbach whom he later
re-encountered at Hunterdon. After three years in New Guinea,
he returned to the United States as executive officer of his antiair-
craft unit. He married soon after, and with the aid of the GI Bill,
he rounded out his b.s. in education with a b.a. in biology, working overtime and doubling up on courses. Fidellow graduated from
NYU School of Medicine in 1951. While there he met Pauline Goger
who was then a year ahead of him. He served a two-year residency
in general practice at Brooklyn Methodist Hospital.

Fidellow responded to an advertisement placed by Trussell, under
the sponsorship of Seward Johnson, to attract a physician to Oldwick,
in northern Hunterdon County, where Johnson lived. He inter-

viewed in March 1953 with Trussell, Bambara, Pellegrino, Hunt and Parmet. Trussell then drove him to Oldwick to meet Johnson, who proposed to let a house he owned to a physician: "He was the one who was going to select who would come here. There were quite a few of us who had applied."[7] Fidellow was accepted and opened his office in July, 1953, just when HMC opened.

In accepting the offer, Fidellow was looking for three things: a place where he was needed, a nice place to live and raise his family, and an area with a good hospital. HMC was "just opening, but their philosophy sounded very good . . . They gave me an idea of what they were trying to do and it clicked with me right away." The housing arrangements were very attractive, too: "We had two children at the time. Imagine going through medical school with two children. It was rough . . . We went right into this house. And of course we didn't have enough finances to buy it at the time. Seward Johnson treated us very well and I am eternally grateful to him."

Ray and Elise Fidellow love where they live. Oldwick consisted of a few houses surrounded by farms. The area was stable, safe, orderly and comfortable. Seward Johnson, influential in bringing them, continued to assist. He rented a home to them for three years, and then allowed the rent to be counted against the purchase price. He encouraged his farm employees to obtain preventive health care and paid the bills. Johnson's influence brought them patients from the community whose inhabitants included many families of wealth and position. Loo Looloian, known to all as "Dr. Loo," who practiced in the nearest town, Whitehouse Station, also helped. Loo, who had a large maternity practice, made immediate arrangements for coverage, and a month after the Fidellows arrived, Loo left on vacation. Loo's style of practice initially left the Fidellows overwhelmed:

> We were swamped. We didn't know what to do with all the people . . . We had cars lined up in the driveway because Loo never made appointments. So they would just come, and they would sit out in the yard, they would bring us vegetables and we were overwhelmed with vegetables and food the first year.
> It really wasn't in payment, it was just generosity.

Initially, obstetrics was a major component of Fidellow's practice. After five years he gave it up because he found it tiring and time-consuming to deliver the 50 babies a year from his own practice and perhaps 10 from Loo's. When he received a call that birth was imminent, he had to leave his office, attended the mother perhaps all day and into the night, and then return to see office appointments. He averaged ten 30-mile round trips to HMC a week. Finally, he turned his maternity patients over to Loo and other physicians and concentrated on office and inpatient practice.

Use of the telephone was idiosyncratic.

> We had an old party line and the main operator was down in the Main Street here in a house in Oldwick. If we wanted to go visit someone, we would tell her where we would be and she would automatically call that number, and, of course, if there were any accidents, she would track us down [to] go out on the call . . . The telephone company . . . was in a private house . . . I asked the person in charge if they would give me an easy number to remember and they gave me the number Oldwick 100 . . . I remember one night I got a call from the hospital, a maternity patient that was there, and [later] I wanted to find out how things were going . . . This is maybe 2:00 or 3:00 or 4:00 in the morning, I called the Oldwick operator but I couldn't arouse her. You know when you rang down there and they had a bell that would wake them up. But she was so fast asleep, I dressed quickly and went down there and awakened her so I could get my call through to the hospital.

Residents in family medicine and medical students from Rutgers Medical School were invited to Fidellow's office and accompanied him on his hospital rounds. Patients rarely objected. Fidellow emphasized clinical observation and behavioral transactions in his teaching. One snowy winter night someone came to Fidellow's home to request help for a relative living on a nearby hilltop. Off Fidellow went with the relative, who owned a Jeep, because the roads were too steep and slick for a conventional automobile. When they arrived at the home, they found that the patient had died. After pronouncing death, Fidellow called a reluctant undertaker to come out and pick up the deceased. When this effort failed, he and the relatives loaded the corpse onto the Jeep. With Fidellow holding on, they drove to the undertaker's. "I remember holding on to it because it was slanted down so far it almost slid off." On other occasions a patient would show up at his office saying she was ready to deliver the baby. He would drive her to the hospital—if he had time!

In retrospect, Elise and Ray Fidellow would do it over again: "The camaraderie was very good. Our social life was excellent." Elise Fidellow adds: "We were all young together." Ray says that he and the specialists

> had similar philosophies aimed at building a community health center. The specialists . . . were always very, very helpful. It was an ongoing education because you would meet someone in the hall and you would bring the problem up right then and there, somebody you might just have seen and asked yourself, what do I do? But I had opportunity to further my own ability to handle people by being able to talk to such a diverse group of specialists.

John F. Fritz, Jr., m.d.

Jack Fritz was a much loved and popular family physician, later turned dermatologist, who lived and worked in the Flemington area for most of his professional career.[8] Jack's square jaw was topped by straight hair parted in the middle, 19th century style. He had a gentle, quiet demeanor, and a warm, soft speaking style. He offered patients careful explanations in lay terms, followed by treatment options and explanations of what to expect. Talking with him in social and professional settings made it easy to understand why he was so popular with his patients.

Fritz grew up in nearby Hopewell, attended Mercersburg Academy in Pennsylvania, and the University of Pennsylvania and its medical school, graduating in 1932, during the depths of the Depression. He interned at Abington Memorial Hospital in suburban Philadelphia, and after several years of practice in West Trenton, Cape May and Stone Harbor, New Jersey, came to Flemington a few years before World War II.

Fritz practiced general medicine, but had a special interest in children and served as Chief of Pediatrics at Somerset Hospital in Somerville about 25 minutes away, although the record shows no special pediatric training. He was county physician for three years, a position now always held by the Chief of the Pathology Department. One measure of the respect with which he was held by his peers, both personally and professionally, is that in March 1953, when the Medical Staff of the soon-to-open Medical Center held its organizing meeting, he was elected President. In February 1957 he suffered a myocardial infarction, left practice to recuperate, just in time to help John Lincoln start his own practice. Fritz took a dermatology residency at Bellevue and returned to the community in 1958 to practice for a number of years as a specialist on HMC's staff.

JOHN FUHRMANN, M.D.

John Fuhrmann's ancestors came from Trenton.[9] His father, Barclay Fuhrmann, also a physician, moved to Flemington directly from medical school, where he practiced until his death in 1953, the year the hospital opened. John attended Hahnemann Medical School in Philadelphia, graduating in 1942. He was in the Army during his last year, serving as a physician on hospital trains. After completing military service, he went into practice with his father. Fuhrmann maintained primarily an office-based practice. He was a social person and close to his patients. He was also very involved with the Medical Society of New Jersey. He served as the perennial Treasurer, Keeper of the Keys, and expert on parliamentary practice of the Hunterdon County Medical Society, a stickler for ensuring that the Society's business was carried out properly. He did not hesitate to use his encyclopedic knowledge of Robert's Rules of Order to steer a meeting the way he felt it should go or to table what he saw as an undesirable resolution. Few felt as strongly about the business of the regular meetings as John Fuhrmann. He was very active at the state level, served on or chaired many committees, was a member of the Council, but never attained his goal of state President. This hurt personally, but he also felt that it was a consequence of Hunterdon being one of the smallest counties, without the clout to elect a President.

According to his wife Jane, John's response to the new hospital was very positive. His sick patients and obstetrical patients were sent to Somerset Hospital, which took much time away from his office, and was one reason he decided to give up obstetrics. So both he and his father really jumped on the HMC bandwagon and were very, very excited about the idea. In particular, both were pleased that all general practitioners would be included on staff and would be able to follow their patients in the hospital. "There was none of this business of saying farewell to your patients at the door of the hospital."

Arthur M. Jenkins, m.d.

Born and raised in Dover, New Jersey, Art Jenkins attended Springfield College, Massachusetts, majoring in history and physical education.[10] He graduated in 1926 and secured a position at Frenchtown High School teaching history and coaching basketball, baseball and soccer decades before it became a popular sport.[d] He roomed with the town physician, Dr. McDonough, who offered advice on athletic injuries. They became close friends, and Jenkins determined on a medical career. He graduated from Duke Medical School and did his residency training at Richmond Memorial Hospital in Richmond, Virginia, and at Union Memorial Hospital in Baltimore. There he was exposed to many Johns Hopkins academic physicians, because clinical faculty often hospitalized their patients at Union Memorial for its somewhat more comfortable amenities. At Union Memorial he met his future wife, Peggy, a private duty nurse; they married in 1937.

Jenkins opened his own practice in Frenchtown in 1938, a sleepy river town ten miles west of Flemington, barely able to support a physician. He was the school physician for many years and loved the job, faithfully attending every school event. He opened a full general practice, including obstetrics, but gave that up because of the disruption of both his professional and private life. Instead he chose ophthalmology as a special area of interest and obtained special training on a part-time basis in Philadelphia. For the remainder of his career he performed office refractions, but not surgery.

Art was a small, wiry, active, genial man, easy to know and get on with. His daughter describes a wonderful sense of humor. Indeed he preserved his optimistic spirit and outlook on life even when his final illness had been diagnosed. Jenkins, who smoked incessantly at a time when many physicians did, died of lung cancer in the early 1960s.

Prior to hmc's opening, Jenkins hospitalized his patients at Warren

---

[d] In those days each small community had its own high school; larger regional institutions came to Hunterdon well after World War II.

Hospital, in neighboring Phillipsburg, Warren County. When HMC opened, he transferred staff membership and allegiance. Jenkins got on well with his peers, and at the organizational meeting of the Medical Center staff in March 1953, he was elected Vice-President. His support for the new hospital was quite helpful, because he was respected for his mixture of thoughtfulness and country canniness.

I am sure that were he alive, Art Jenkins could relate many anecdotes similar to those told by John Bambara, Ray Fidellow and Loo Looloian. He had a country practice among a group of patients not accustomed to city-style care. As Ray Trussell said, he was the "main man" in his community, and, from this foundation of influence, was very able to further acceptance of HMC in the western portion of Hunterdon County, which had a long tradition of care at Warren Hospital.

JOHN A. LINCOLN, M.D.

Lincoln, born in Texas, lived in California and northern New Jersey, where he met his future wife, Betty, when he was 12 and they both played on the same baseball team: "She was the only girl on the team and probably the best athlete."[11] After high school, he briefly attended college and then joined the Navy. Following service, he returned to Syracuse University, then went to medical school at NYU, graduating in 1952. After a rotating internship at Temple University Hospital in Philadelphia, he served in the Army in Massachusetts on the obstetrical service. He recalls one dramatic experience there:

> The first time I did a C-section I did it not because I knew how but because I had to. The real obstetrician was away. I called a general surgeon and asked him to help me. He said "Why are you asking me, I've never done one." I said, "Well, I've never done one either, but I'd like someone who's been in an abdomen before with me." So we did it together and it went well, fortunately.

Early in 1954 the Lincolns were exploring practice opportunities around Philadelphia. Although he had planned pediatrics, he decided to practice family medicine; if it did not work out, he would seek additional training. Looking at northwestern New Jersey, they stopped for lunch in Flemington. Both found the town attractive. A casual encounter on the street led them to the hospital, where the next day an interview was held with Trussell. They decided to open a practice.

The country atmosphere, friendly community, hospital structure and relationships between family physicians and specialists were the principal reasons for settling here. Trussell was very encouraging and attempted to convince them to open an office in High Bridge or in Milford further from HMC, because of greater need for a family physician, but Lincoln chose Flemington. Several people "gave me some considerable assistance at this time because I needed to find a place to live and a place to use as an office and I had no money." Leo Selesnick, a dentist in Flemington and the brother of a medical school classmate, helped with advice and an invaluable lesson about close-knit, small-town relationships:

> I mentioned to Leo that I met a man who was a local [official] and my impression of him was that he was terribly honest but not terribly bright. Leo said "Well, you're partly right; he is terribly honest but he is also terribly bright and he is my cousin."

It took time to get his practice off the ground: "The practice started off with me seeing one, maybe two patients a day and just gradually grew." Ed Olmstead, HMC's pathologist, hired Lincoln to assist with postmortem examinations for five dollars per hour. It turned out to be a very useful experience, not only because of its educational value, but also because it led to closer relationships with the other physicians. Practice in Flemington was quite competitive; the community was growing, but not very rapidly. Other physicians guarded their practices jealously.

> I met everyone I could and I joined just about every organization . . . I was president or vice president of everything but the WCTU [Women's Christian Temperance Union] . . . After a year it looked as though we were going to be able to make it and we started to look around for a house.
>
> The local power structure helped. A bank official introduced the Lincolns to a businessman who sold them his home in town, large enough for home and office.

Lincoln soon learned that the locals did not always rush to the doctor with symptoms of illness:

> I vividly remember one of my first patients. It was a woman who came in and said that she must have had the virus last

week, and now she'd noticed that when she drinks water it
tends to run out her nose. This woman had acute bulbar po-
lio and of course was quickly sent to the hospital. They had a
big iron lung outside her room at the hospital.[e] She made a
full and complete recovery without any problems at all.

After Jack Fritz left because of a heart attack, Lincoln suddenly
found himself busy. Lou Doyle joined the practice in a year or so.

That worked out extremely well from our standpoint. I was
an ambitious hardworking guy. Lou was very flexible and easy-
going and we got along beautifully. We shared a practice with
basically the same office hours and we never kept track of
who brought in what or if one of us had more work than the
other. We kept the hours the same and divided the income.

Doyle's memory of their relationship differs.

Lincoln became involved in medical education, training family
practice residents. In 1970, he left private practice to become the
first Director of the Phillips–Barber Family Health Center in
Lambertville, HMC's first satellite Health Center. In 1972 he opened
a new residency program in family medicine at the University of
Washington. By 1980 he felt he had done what he could do and
decided it was "more fun starting something than running it," so
he re-entered private practice with a large group in the Seattle
area, remaining there until 1991, when he retired at the age of 65.

M. W. LOOLOIAN, M.D.

Dr. Loo was raised in Stewartsville, in Warren County, New Jersey, now about 30 minutes drive from Whitehouse Station, where
he practiced. His father was a Presbyterian minister. He vividly
recalled the difference between how medicine was practiced in his
youth and how it is practiced now. He fell and dislocated his left
elbow at the school just up the street from his house.

[e] The iron lung, or more properly the Drinker respirator, was one of the first pulmonary
function support devices. The patient was placed in an iron tube, with his head projecting from
one end. Seals, either plastic or leather, prevented air leakage. At the other end, a bellows was
activated by a noisy motor and a complex set of levers. About 30 years later, long after the
device had become outmoded, the HMC administrator asked me whether it was still needed. I
was one of the very last physicians on the staff who had personal experience and was able to use
it. With some feelings of nostalgia, I acknowledged that there was no good reason to keep it.
But considering the variety of objects that become "collectibles," perhaps we should have held
on to the half-ton, six-foot long device.

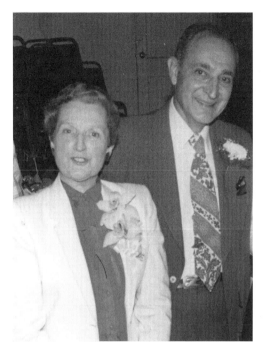

Dr. and Mrs. Looloian
(Loo and Dotty Loo)
at their retirement party.

> Today they call the ambulance and they would give oxygen
> and intravenous and I don't know what else. All that was
> done with me was one of the teachers got me by this arm and
> we walked down the street, about a quarter of a mile to [the
> doctor's office] and he took one look at it and grabbed it and
> jerked it back in place.[12]

Loo also remembered 13 stitches after a laceration without local
anesthesia.

He attended Maryville College in Tennessee, expecting to become a chemical engineer, but switched to medicine, receiving his
M.D. in 1943 from the University of Pennsylvania. After a nine-
month general internship at Orange Memorial Hospital in Orange, New Jersey, Loo entered the Marine Corps in January 1944,
with the rank of Captain. He was stationed briefly at St. Albans
Naval Hospital, Camp Lejeune, was with the Fleet Marines at Tinian
and Saipan, Okinawa, and then was with forces occupying Nagasaki
after the war, where, incidentally, no attention was paid to residual radiation. His last post was near Norfolk, Virginia, for six

months. The Looloians married in 1946 and have a son and a daughter.

After discharge Loo took a general practice residency at Samaritan Hospital in Troy, New York. He responded to an ad of a practice for sale in Whitehouse Station, near where he grew up. The incumbent physician had developed a problem with substance abuse. Dr. Loo purchased the real estate, practice and equipment for $13,000 (the equivalent of $102,300 in 2001 dollars). The family moved in on 15 June 1947. The seller remained with them for two weeks to introduce them to his patients. The house became a combination home and office.

Loo could not remember exactly how he first heard about the new hospital—whether from newspaper articles, the activities of Rose Z. Angell, or at meetings of the Hunterdon County Medical Society.

> We always had monthly Medical Society meetings, and it was a very closely knit society at that point. We would talk about it briefly . . . Specialists were going to be coming into the county and there had never been any specialists before but there certainly was no animosity about it that I was ever aware of.

Loo was a handsome fellow with a resonant baritone voice, a prominent chin, and an assured manner. He also was a man of integrity. I respected him as much as any physician I have ever known. It is not that he knew more than others—he did not and would readily say so himself. It was rather his willingness to call things as he saw them, right or wrong, argue his point of view as forcefully as he could, and adopt that of his colleague, if he came to see that it was better. He was sensitive to the attitudes of his patients, but realistic about their needs, and what he could accomplish. Ray Fidellow said: "If he told me that the sun had come down out of the sky and was going in circles around the house, I wouldn't have even bothered to look out to see, I would know it was so."[13]

Prior to HMC's opening Loo sent his patients to Somerset Hospital. He continued to do so for the first year or two of HMC's operation. He had close working relations with specialists at Somerset, which were not easy to terminate. He did not get on well with all Hunterdon specialists. On one occasion in the summer of 1953, he brought a specialist from Somerset to HMC to see a patient of his because he felt that the Hunterdon specialist had not responded appropriately. Loo first, last and always acted on his perception of what was in the best interests of his patient. If he disagreed with a consultant, it was not over Loo's prerogatives, or Loo's interests, but over quality of care or the process of care.

Loo ran his practice in an idiosyncratic but effective fashion. Dorothy Looloian, his wife, a nurse, known to all as "Dotty Loo" and to her husband as "The Madam" or just "Madam," managed the office and spoke with patients. Her husband did not deal with patients on the telephone. She scheduled all his activities. In the morning, patients who needed house calls were accustomed to telephone early so that Dotty Loo could line up a schedule. Loo would leave for HMC early, often before dawn; en route, or returning, he made house calls. He averaged approximately 20 house calls a week. He felt he always learned more about people on house calls, and in addition it was more fun.[f] There are certain patients—the disabled, the chronically ill or those very sick with high fevers—who should not have to travel to the doctor's office. The majority could be handled at home with simple equipment in the doctor's bag, or, in 2001 by telemedicine apparatus. He was aided by Dotty Loo's careful scheduling to minimize travel time. She knew the people, the community and the geography, and made his trip efficient without sacrificing patient needs. Two stories from the *Hunterdon County Democrat* add spice to the record.

> Dr. Looloian of Whitehouse Station went to a patient's home on a snowmobile Sunday afternoon. "He just put his instrument case in a plastic bag and saddled it on the snowmobile," says his wife . . . Their next door neighbor says "It was quite an ordeal. The snow was still falling and blowing in our faces and we ran into several snowdrifts. The doctor asked me to go with him on my snowmobile because he had trouble with his. He hadn't had it too long . . . we traveled 5 and half miles each way. It took us one hour and five minutes to get there and back.[14]

On another wintry house call, he promised a patient that he would

> be back Monday. But on Monday of this week the road was blocked by six-foot snowdrifts and none of the other family members could even get from the house to the road. So, when

[f] My experience is the same. I made house calls for four and a half years in Germantown, before moving to Flemington. These visits taught me about normal children and families.

a knock came at the door and the doctor appeared, the patient asked in some wonderment, "How did you get through to get here?" "Snowshoes," said the doctor. And everybody laughed . . . [until they] peered out the window, and there, disappearing over the slope on snowshoes, was Dr. M. W. Looloian.[15]

In the office, there was no appointment schedule, but rather office hours, flexible so that those who needed more urgent attention received it. "The Madam and I really enjoyed medicine. It was a joint endeavor and I never had anybody in my office. We always just took people as they came. We never had appointments. I took my own blood pressures, my own temperatures and my own histories. The Madam helped me with what was necessary. I had no receptionist, no nurse. We enjoyed it." Dr. Loo developed a large obstetrical practice—about 60 deliveries a year. His fee was $75 for prenatal, perinatal and postnatal care (about $490 in 2001 dollars). He did several unintended home deliveries, two in bathtubs and one in a haymow. After 18 years, he gave up this portion of his practice because it was so time-consuming.

Ray Fidellow noted that

> Loo was a stickler for cleanliness in the hospital. He used to go around and if there were any dust balls under the bed, he would let housekeeping know. Loo today feels that medicine has become too much of a business. Patients have become numbers. Doctors take care of diseases rather than patients. He always felt that he took care of people who were his friends.[16]

Loo was not one for organizational activities. He was repeatedly offered an opportunity, which he just as repeatedly declined, to serve as President of the Medical Staff. He came to every meeting, and did not hesitate to speak his mind, but could not see himself in an organizational function. "I'm just not a politically motivated person to get involved in Board meetings and conferences and I didn't have enough time, either." David Greenbaum described Loo as

> first class, who would sometimes bug us and say, "why?" . . . Loo would challenge [us]. "Why do you want to order this?" And it is sort of the thing now that is very appropriate to ask. "What is the outcome?" He was I think in many ways ahead of his time in addition to being a very decent guy.[17]

On his retirement in 1982, the Hunterdon County Medical Society devoted its quarterly meeting to honor the man and his work. Speakers representing specialist and family practice staff and hospital administration offered praise and respect. When Loo was asked to respond, what he said—out of modesty, not churlishness—was: "If I had known you were planning to do this I would not have come." I believe that was the feeling of the man and best expresses what he was and is. One story he related also displays his wry sense of humor:

> In 1954 there was a problem with flies getting into the operating room. No one seemed to do much about it. So, after an appendectomy, I caught a fly and with Carl Roessel's assistance tucked the fly into the lumen of the appendix and sent it off to the lab. No abnormal path report ever appeared.

Another story he told on himself:

> I'd finished telling my patient . . . that I thought Dr. Stover's [an orthopedic surgeon who had worked on developing the air cast] "air splint" was a fraud. Looking over my shoulder, Connie [Stover] was . . . standing in the doorway. Obviously, I was wrong, since "air splints" of various kinds are still widely used.

After retirement from general practice in 1982 the Looloians moved to Maine, where for many years they had maintained a summer home. Until very recently, Dr. Loo worked in emergency rooms and walk-in medical clinics. Dotty Loo died after a lingering sickness, leaving Loo feeling very much alone. His vigor, alertness and attitude to medicine were unchanged. Dr. Loo died 26 July 2002.

ARNO MACHOLDT, M.D.

Arno Macholdt grew up in Nyack, New York. Unsure about a career, he took the advice of a friendly scoutmaster who suggested nursing since Macholdt liked working with young people. He earned his R.N. at Rockland State Hospital, a mental institution with a separate children's unit, not far from his home. Before World War II, he was called up from the Naval Reserve to serve as an enlisted man on a supply ship plying the Atlantic. His R.N. was of no help to Macholdt in obtaining a commission. An early form of gender discrimination existed at the time; had Macholdt been female, he would have entered the service as a commissioned officer.

After three years at sea and six months at Cornell in health care training for the ensign program, he was sent to Guam with the 3rd Marine Division, which was scheduled to make the first landings to invade Japan. With war's end, he entered Columbia University in 1946, went on to College of Physicians and Surgeons, and obtained his M.D. in 1952. He spent two years as a resident at Roosevelt Hospital. Macholdt decided he needed additional training in OB–GYN. HMC offered training of flexible duration. Believing that this was preferable, Macholdt drove to Flemington in June 1954 to interview with Herman Rannels, Chief of Obstetrics.

The first impression was "the nicest hospital in the middle of a cow pasture I had ever seen."[18] Macholdt liked what he heard in his interview. The program consisted not of didactic lectures, but day-to-day and person-to-person experience, working with Rannels and performing procedures under direct supervision. In this intimate atmosphere the two of them "got along quite well." When Macholdt's mother needed a hysterectomy, he asked Rannels to operate, suggestive of their closeness and mutual confidence. A positive attitude toward Huntington was fortified during four months of residency because of many kindnesses shown by many people. Arno and his wife, Trudy, were newly married, and she was employed in New York. Neither was comfortable in the city. Soon the commute was too much. When Trussell heard of the problem, he promptly offered her a position in Medical Records. They took furnished rooms in Clinton, house-sat for the Trussells for a month, and finally rented half a farmhouse south of Flemington from Helen Jaworsky, who later became secretary to the Medical Director—in Hunterdon County all circles close. Soon after, Dr. Baker, of High Bridge, in northern Hunterdon County, offered his practice and home for sale. The Macholdts bought the practice and moved in. Dr. Baker remained for several weeks to introduce his patients and local styles of practice.

Baker had been on staff at Somerset and Warren hospitals, but Macholdt decided he much preferred to be on staff where he had been working already. His practice grew quickly, averaging 50 maternity patients a year. Despite his youthful interest in working with children, he did not attempt to care for sick children and usually requested HMC's pediatrician to take over any unusual conditions. As with Loo, Macholdt's office was managed by his wife, Trudy. She quickly learned medical office management skills and became his "right hand from then on . . . She's better than most nurses and all my patients swear [by her]." Arno faithfully attended staff meetings and served his time on committee work. "I've never been very political as far as the hospital goes . . . I really couldn't get upset or make any negative comments on anybody. I just did not feel it was my place or that I knew enough to do that." He still practices in the same office that he purchased in 1954.

PETER RIZZOLO, M.D.

Peter Rizzolo's early years were difficult. He was the youngest in a family of seven children living in urban north Jersey. His parents separated when he was four years old, and his father did not help support his family. Life was harsh—they survived on what his mother, who spoke only Italian, and the older children could bring home. Peter was the only one who went past 12th grade. He attended one year of college on money earned in high school; thereafter he worked full time and finished college at night. He graduated from Creighton University Medical School in 1955, his schooling financed through a government program. Rizzolo's motivation to become a physician stemmed from the death of a beloved older sister, who died of tuberculosis after a long illness. He interned at Orange Memorial Hospital, then spent two and a half years in the Navy. His training focused on submarines and deep-sea diving, and he was charged with teaching recruits how to escape from a sunken submarine. All of this was somewhat stressful because he could not, and did not, learn how to swim. Despite the stress of submarine service, Rizzolo preferred it to his only alternative assignment, two years of examining recruits in Albany, New York.

While serving in the Navy, a friend encouraged Rizzolo to look at HMC. She was a medical student of Ed Pellegrino's: "He's unbelievable," she told Rizzolo. "You round with him [and he drops] pearls all over the place."[19] Her description sounded like a family doctor's dream come true. Rizzolo and his wife, Alyce, drove to Flemington for an interview, which took place in the penthouse.[g] He felt overwhelmed by the group interview with most of the spe-

g The "penthouse," a room with a table and seats for up to two dozen, was located up a flight of stairs (definitely *not* accessible for motorically challenged persons) near the center of the original building. It had a view out over the countryside, whence the name. It was dismantled during the 1966 addition for ambulant care services.

cialist staff, recalling that he was "peppered" with questions, but, in any case, was accepted for residency, beginning in September 1958.

In the residency, Rizzolo said he didn't get much teaching from the family practice physicians because they were in and out of the hospital so quickly. They would come in very early, write orders and leave, which the residents didn't appreciate: "Most of the family doctors were just not available at the critical time when we were admitting a patient and needing to talk with them." But Rizzolo felt that having the full-time staff available was like having specialty residents there. Many people said you can't train in a place without other residents, but "the full-time staff met that need and they were more experienced than supervising residents would have been. So I got a lot out of it . . . I enjoyed practice so I must have built up my confidence somehow."

During residency, the Rizzolos decided to remain in the area and spoke with John Bambara about joining his practice. One Sunday late in June, Bambara telephoned saying he had to go to the hospital and have his gallbladder removed and would be laid up for weeks. According to Rizzolo, Bambara said:

> "I have 30 people with appointments tomorrow and my appointment book is scheduled a month in advance. I have 15 ladies that are pregnant and will be having their babies this month. I have people in the hospital. Can you take over tomorrow morning?" Rizzolo said, "What!" and Bambara replied, "I'll be out for about six weeks and then I'll join you."

(See Bambara's profile for a somewhat different telling of the story— no medical emergency and a more leisurely decision about a change of practice.) Rizzolo agreed, pending approval by HMC, with which he had a one-year contract that did not end until the following September. Approval was granted, because the Residency Committee thought there was no other way to provide patient care without delay.

For Rizzolo, it was "like a bomb going off." He spent most of his time with obstetrical patients at HMC. His family never saw him. Bambara was not quick to return. Many of his patients experienced complications, and Rizzolo was able to obtain the necessary help from the specialist staff. He remains grateful to them for their support and teaching. A hard worker, Rizzolo began hospital rounds at 6:30 in the morning, often before the patients had awakened. Typically, he was seeing three to five postpartum women and their babies, as well as patients on the medical floor. If he was on schedule, house calls followed rounds, office hours began at 1 p.m. and lasted until 10 or later at night. Rizzolo found practice under these circumstances to be much more stressful than his residency.

The Rizzolos lived in Hampton, about 30 minutes from HMC while he was a resident and during the first few difficult months in practice. The night their third child was born, Peter was a resident working in the delivery room. Alyce decided she was in labor and drove herself to the hospital. Because it was snowing, she had to stop the car every so often to clear the windshield. By the time she arrived she was in active labor. "I passed him in the delivery room and said, 'I'm here.' So we waved to each other."[20] By the time Peter looked from one delivery room to the other, he saw Barad pulling out their baby.

Both Rizzolos acknowledge the stresses of private practice in the form of fatigue and loss of family time. Peter reflected on those days: "I think it was very bad on Alyce not to have me around very much . . . She was home full time but I felt guilty . . . I wanted to be with the kids more . . . I enjoyed being home evenings and having time to play with the children." Alyce "thought he enjoyed the practice. Life didn't seem that hectic to me. I don't know why. We had fun when he came home and the kids gathered round."[21]

By 1974, the Rizzolo family numbered six growing children, and Peter decided that a life style change was in order. He left private practice to head HMC's residency program. In 1978 he joined the University of North Carolina at Chapel Hill in a comparable position. Subsequently he was granted a Fellowship in Geriatrics and remained at UNC as the head of that division. In 2000 because of cardiovascular disease, he retired to pursue full time a career as a writer of fiction. He has already published one book.

LEONARD ROSENFELD, M.D.

Rosenfeld grew up in Spotswood, a small New Jersey town. After graduating from Rutgers College, he joined the Air Force, but could not pursue pilot training because he was subject to airsickness. He served with a depot supply group in Guam. In 1950, he graduated from Hahnemann Medical School and interned at Newark Beth Israel Hospital. Rosenfeld opened his practice in Hunterdon County in 1951. A Flemington dentist, Leo Selesnick, who trained with him invited him for a visit. Rosenfeld fell in love with the area. He was also familiar with the community, through his future wife, Hope, who was employed by the Wescotts. As Rosenfeld scouted for a place to open his practice, he visited various physicians in practice, all of whom were more interested in protecting their turf than anything else, reflecting the same attitudes encountered by John Bambara and John Lincoln. Ultimately, Rosenfeld selected Ringoes, in south Hunterdon.

When Rosenfeld began practice, he charged $3 for an office visit and $4 for a house call. In his area a house call meant substantial travel because Ringoes was, and still is, a small community, little more than a crossroads, scattered among farms (and now residential developments) on all sides. The nearest towns of any size were Lambertville and Flemington, each a half hour from Ringoes. Because patients felt it was worth the extra dollar for a house call, Rosenfeld found himself spending increasing amounts of time in travel. Accordingly he took the bold step of raising house calls to $5.

Before HMC opened, Rosenfeld's inpatients were treated at Somerset Hospital in Somerville or at Helene Fuld near Trenton. Rosenfeld says he had little to do with planning the new Medical Center, although he was in communication with specialists even before joining the staff. When he asked a specialist for a consultation a typewritten report would be ready within a few hours, "and the charge, as I remember, was $15."[22] After HMC opened, when Rosenfeld referred a patient to Roessel, he was invited to assist at surgery. Soon young students and residents were given the work of assisting, and Rosenfeld felt pushed further and further away from the operating table.

> My nose was out of joint for a while there. I can understand it better now. I've mellowed with age . . . It was for the betterment of medicine, the residents got trained. I would end up holding the retractor or maybe snipping a couple of ligatures. I got over it. I got to be the second assistant or maybe the third assistant. I only assisted on my own patients.
> I never volunteered to come in on anyone else's.

Leonard Rosenfeld was always serious, hard working, and aware of his own limitations, perhaps too much so. He wanted to do the right thing, and his primary question was always, What is the best quality care that can be delivered? He did not engage in community, hospital or medical politics, but was content to leave that to others, although he did not hesitate to raise questions when he thought he should. He was a solo practitioner until 1959 or 1960, when he took a partner, but their goals and style differed sharply and the associate left to practice in another part of the county.

Initially the Rosenfelds always enjoyed the area, and Hope was deeply immersed in volunteer organizations, the school board, and many other activities in the community. During World War II, she was, at the age of 18, a member of the Women's Land Army on the Wescott farm in Union Township, northern Hunterdon County, an area now buried under the huge Spruce Run reservoir. She milked cows, trained calves, mucked out stables, and supervised the Wescott's daughter, then a toddler. Wescott "was charming and wonderful and made me part of the family. I would have dinner with them every night."

Eventually, the Rosenfelds tired of the community, quite likely from overwork and overexposure. Small-town politics, solo practice and the call schedule weighed on them. He took a salaried position in California where he remained until 1992. In the fashion of the era, he was told that the health plan for which he worked "no longer needed his services." The plan carried out a computation on the hours he worked, the money he produced, and what it cost to pay and maintain him. He was not a profit center. "They asked me to retire. I haven't regretted it. I'm kind of glad. I might still be in my working shoes." Leonard Rosenfeld died 15 September 2002.

CHAPTER 22

The People

House Staff

Planning for the teaching program was initiated early. On 18 December 1952, the same meeting at which the Director of Nursing, Miss Lela Greenwood, was appointed, the Executive Committee approved a procedure for appointing residents and students, and limited their number. I was able to identify one resident and one medical student at the time HMC opened.

AARON R. RAUSEN, M.D.

Aaron Rausen was raised in Manhattan. He became interested in medicine, particularly pediatrics, when a sibling died of meningitis during World War II at a time when sulfonamides were already available. After graduating from New York City schools, he worked during the summer of 1947 at Columbia University College of Physicians and Surgeons. There a faculty member befriended him and directed Rausen to Dartmouth College. After three years there, he was awarded a scholarship to enter Downstate Medical School. Rausen had finished his third year of medical school in 1953 when he saw a notice inviting volunteers to rotate to HMC. Rausen was taken with the idea of the specialist staff acting as consultants, because the only pediatricians he saw in his training to date were generalists. He also thought he would like to experience rural life. Rausen found himself at Hunterdon the first week the hospital opened; he was assigned to Pediatrics because he planned to enter that field.

Rausen was a student body of one that summer and recalls Hunt as extremely solicitous and kind. He had no contact with the family doctors, but lived in the hospital day and night. Rausen said that he would often go to the Emergency Room to

hang around and watch what was going on. I vividly recall
some of the patients that I saw. One of the first that I recall
[seeing was] a lady that was brought in with postacidotic or
alkalotic tetany who was hyperventilating and had carpopedal
spasm . . . It was either the ambulance driver or one of the
assistants in the Emergency Room who very quietly put a
paper bag over the lady's face and had her breathe and her
carpopedal spasms subsided instantaneously.[1]

Rausen graduated from Downstate in 1954, trained at Bellevue
and completed his residency at Mt. Sinai with the eminent Horace
Hodes. He is now the Director of the Hassenfeld Children's Center for Cancer and Blood Disorders at NYU's School of Medicine.
His experience at Hunterdon with Andy Hunt led him to favor a
pediatric practice that would be somewhat more scientific and yet
offer "the kind of considered approach to people like Andy Hunt
and probably others I had been exposed to along the way." During his chief residency year at Mt. Sinai he made a decision that
led to an encounter typical of pediatric training at that time.

The unconscious weighing of the two attitudes [general vs.
academic] . . . prompted me then to go to Horace Hodes . . .
and say "I've decided not to be a general pediatrician. I want
to be a hematologist" . . . Hodes . . . yelled at Zeppe [Helen
Zepp], who was his bacteriology assistant [and sounding board,
confrere and supportive associate in almost every aspect of his
work], "Get me Lou in Boston." [Louis Diamond, who died
in 1999, was the pediatric hematologist at Harvard, and if not
the leading, one of the leading scholars of that field.] And she
got him on the phone while I was sitting there in his office
and he said, "I have somebody for you." And that was basically the selection process. I was informed by Dr. Hodes that
Dr. Diamond expected to see me in his office at around 10 or
11 the next morning and I told Dr. Hodes that I was on call
that night. He said, "I'm in charge, you're not on call." My
interview consisted of Dr. Diamond getting up from behind
his desk and extending his hand to me and welcoming me as
his 32nd Fellow in Pediatric Hematology. That literally was
my interview . . . that's why the fact that I had been the first
student at the Hunterdon Medical Center, obviously without
having orchestrated it, accounted for a career path.

DAVID SANDERS, M.D.

David Sanders was born in Paterson, New Jersey, on 27 June 1926 and raised in Brooklyn, New York. He attended public schools and then Columbia College, where he was in the Navy V-12 program during World War II. In that program one had to choose between being a doctor, dentist or engineer. He chose medicine and in 1949 graduated from what is now SUNY Downstate Medical Center. Following a pediatric internship at Flower-Fifth Avenue Hospital, including four months of adult medicine, Sanders went to Bellevue.

After a year's residency at Bellevue, Sanders served two years with the Air Force in Alaska, at a small station hospital with a large dependent population. He established a rooming-in program with six or seven women and their babies in one large room. Despite the crowding, the program was successful. As his service was drawing to a close, he wrote to L. Emmett Holt, Chairman of Pediatrics at Bellevue, inquiring about further training. Holt suggested a six-month residency at Hunterdon, followed by another six months at Bellevue. That sounded "moderately interesting"[2] to him, but then he received a letter from Andrew Hunt describing the program "in a very exciting way." They "hit it off well"; without further ado, Sanders decided on Hunterdon, which, he says, "changed my life." His residency began on 1 July 1953, two days before HMC opened. Sanders believes that chance plays a big part in life. Had HMC not had an "arrangement with NYU, and had I not been thought of by Emmett Holt, I would not have had my psychiatric training at Columbia and would not have ended up [where I am]."

Sanders describes his time at Hunterdon with warmth and satisfaction: "We were all young and idealistic." His relationships with staff were salubrious, and Sanders speaks of the time with the same glow as that of many others present at the creation. HMC's first patient, a boy with appendicitis, was met by the entire staff and was "probably the best-taken-care-of patient we ever had." Sanders was delighted at the opportunity to help Hunt get the Pediatric Department started. Besides seeing patients, Sanders worked with nurses to set up the Pediatrics Department, develop procedures, design charts, create routines and regulations. Sanders set up the parent-visiting program and rooming-in for newborns. In addition, he also did examinations for the Chronic Illness Survey, but was not involved with planning or writing up the results. After he finished his six months at Hunterdon, he moved on to Bellevue to complete the year in Pediatrics. The following summer, he returned to Hunterdon for a month to relieve Hunt, who was on vacation. During this time,

> Ray [Trussell], being Ray, could not have been more friendly and helpful. [He would meet with me] every morning, we would have coffee, and he would say, "How are things going on the ward?" and he would come checking up on me but in a very friendly helpful way . . . It made it much better for me.

For Sanders, one of the most rewarding aspects of being at Hunterdon was his relationship with Hunt, who treated him as a colleague rather than as a student. Sanders felt his residency was more like a personal tutorial with the head of the department. Hunt's influence was one of the key reasons why Sanders, two years later, left pediatrics and entered psychiatry. They became close, and socialized frequently. The Hunterdon experience was very different from Bellevue and the military. Sanders says that he was closest to Hunt, Pellegrino and Trussell. He found Hunt charming, flexible and down-to-earth; Pellegrino brilliant, intense and a magnificent teacher; and Trussell focused, determined and extraordinarily effective.

After leaving Hunterdon, Sanders finished his year at Bellevue, and entered private practice in Manhattan as a pediatrician. At the same time, he held several other positions: teaching at Flower-Fifth Avenue Medical School, working for HIP's group practice and part time with the New York City Department of Health, at that time led by the distinguished Helen Wallace. It was during this period that Sanders decided on psychiatry. He happened to meet Trussell again about that time, which led to Sanders becoming the first trainee in Columbia's new program offering joint training in Psychiatry and Public Health. Subsequently he was a member of the Columbia faculty for six years, served as Chief of Psychiatry in the New York City Department of Hospitals, and then became Assistant Director of Psychiatry at Cedars-Sinai Hospital in Los Angeles. He was also active with the American Psychiatric Association. He is now retired.

CHAPTER 23

The People

Administrative Staff

EDWARD V. GRANT

Grant was raised in Jersey City, New Jersey. After graduating from parochial school in 1937, he was a messenger by day while taking night school courses. In 1939, he worked at the New York World's Fair and then obtained a job as elevator operator at Lenox Hill Hospital. Over three years he rose through the ranks, serving in purchasing, personnel, and accounting. At 21 he ran successfully for public office against a representative of the Hague administration in Jersey City.[a] When World War II began, Lenox Hill Hospital formed a 750-bed evacuation hospital. At least 100 physicians and nurses joined. Grant became officer in charge of supply, transportation and utilities. In England for 19 months the hospital moved six times and was principally involved with wounded Air Force personnel. Grant's tentmate was Carl Roessel. At the invasion of Normandy the unit was sent to the beaches, taking the wounded directly from the LSTs that evacuated them. The unit went to France to support Patton's Third Army, at times within two miles of the front. After discharge from service with the rank of major in November, 1945, Grant returned to Lenox Hill as an assistant administrator in charge of professional services relating to the medical staff. He found it to be "a great learning experience."[1]

Ed Grant then lived in Levittown, Long Island. A neighbor, Shorty Johnson, was an inveterate outdoorsman and canoeist. Shorty moved to Hunterdon County and invited Grant to join the an-

---

[a] Frank Hague was the longtime, old-style political boss of Jersey City. When questioned about the legality of a proposed action, his response was, "I am the law."

nual canoe ride down the Delaware, which still takes place every year. Grant met Jack Little (a well-known caterer and businessman), John Nevius (owner of a regional department store chain, and later HMC Board member), and George Parker (a real estate broker very active in fund-raising for HMC). Mrs. Mame Little showed him the hospital site—a large hole in the ground.

In the interim, Grant was hearing how wonderful the institution was from two HMC specialists, Carl Roessel and Fred Knocke, who had served in the military with Grant. In 1955 Clarence de la Chapelle of NYU told Grant of administrative changes at Hunterdon. Grant had been instrumental in helping a son, Norman de la Chapelle, begin a career in health care administration. With Trussell's departure, Pellegrino became Medical Director, and a new post of administrator was created. De la Chapelle told Grant he thought it would be good if he went out for an interview and, if selected, to take the position. One professional administrator, Joseph Williamson, had already left over the severe financial problems that emerged in 1953 and 1954. From then, until Grant's appointment, Trussell and Miss Lela Greenwood performed all senior administrative duties.

Grant was very taken with Pellegrino's integrity and philosophy of life and medicine, and felt they would "click." Pellegrino made it very clear that he did not want to be administrator. "His philosophy, his feelings, his lifelong ambition . . . were in medicine and not hospital administration . . . He wanted someone who would run the hospital with him and for him." The Hunterdon position was an opportunity to go from being No. 2 in administration at Lenox Hill to being the boss, a point that was particularly persuasive to Grant, since his career at Lenox Hill had started at the bottom of the ladder. Moreover, this was not just any hospital, as Clarence de la Chapelle told Grant: "There is nothing like this setup in the United States or Canada." Finally, Grant wanted to raise his children in Hunterdon County and be involved in the community.

Grant was appointed Associate Director for Administration on 25 March 1955, coming to Flemington one day a week and becoming full time in May. Murray Rubin had already been hired as Business Office Manager. Grant and Rubin got on well together, and Rubin was soon promoted to Assistant Administrator. They remained a team until both left for other positions. When Grant arrived, he found hospital finances in serious, if not critical, condition. The operating loss the first year was $186,000.[b] Grant had reservations about HMC's financial viability. There was a huge mortgage, and business office affairs were in a shambles. Bills for patient care that should have been mailed were piled in boxes. Receivables were so large that if they could be collected, it would be possible to keep the institution going. Grant asked Staff and Board, who were very supportive, to do all they could, legitimately, to increase in- and outpatient utilization. Grant and Rubin worked out a budget. At the end of their first year, reality was only two-tenths of a percent off projection, which Grant attributes to Rubin. He said members of the Board would kid them about "fudging the books."

There were expensive problems with boilers, sewage disposal, air conditioning in the operating room, labor and delivery rooms. Sealed, windowless rooms on the third and fourth floor were extremely uncomfortable in warm weather. In 1956 and 1957 Grant and Rubin obtained $43,400 from the Ford Foundation to provide air conditioning. Care of the indigent was aided with the help of Lloyd Wescott, the Freeholders, and the Large Foundation. By 1957, when occupancy rose to over 85 percent, and 1958, when it was over 95 percent, the deficit was eliminated. For the first time, HMC was on a firm financial footing.

Ed Grant is friendly, outgoing, warm and sociable. Of medium height, fair complexion, bright blue eyes, and ready smile, he describes himself as an "Irish storyteller." He may charm people, but he does not rely on charm alone, but backs it up with sound thinking and good sense. Grant has a knack for describing situations in a direct, straightforward manner, while not giving offense. He is able to criticize or disagree while maintaining trust and confidence. His social network is vast, helped by frequent parties at his home attended by Board, specialist staff, family physicians, nurses and friends. At a certain point in the evening out would come his accordion, and there would be music. Sometimes guests brought their own instruments. Grant also plays piano, violin, banjo, guitar and sings.

For years, HMC used old Checker cabs for transport. Grant ex-

---

[b] Trussell wrote: "No hotel can break even the first year," on a draft manuscript of this book.

plains why. He had gone to a party at Bea and Harry Silver's, owners of a taxicab business in New York City. Bea asked whether he would like a taxicab for the hospital.

> I said, "Gee, I'd love it but . . . I won't take it unless I can get a meter in it." I was joking and Bea called upstairs to Harry and said, "Harry, Eddie wants a taxicab, but he won't take it unless you put a meter in it." Harry said, "He can have one."
> We got seven taxicabs altogether before they were done.

Grant's tenure at HMC, together with that of Murray Rubin, was invaluable, for I am not sure the institution would have survived without them. This does not take away from the achievements of other Medical Center pioneers, but none had the background in hospital administration and finances, and none claim to have been ready to deal with the problems emerging in this area. I look back on Grant's stay as a time in which the sinews of HMC were strengthened, enabling it to tolerate the stresses of later years.

In 1967, Grant became the first male Administrator of the New York Infirmary.[c] While there he was approached by Ray Trussell to assume a faculty position and to take residents in administration from Columbia. Grant said, "Ray, I've never even gone to college." Trussell, he said, replied, "You have all the qualifications and experience we need." Grant retired in 1983 to Florida and continues to pursue his life-long interest in music.

LELA GREENWOOD, R.N.

Miss Greenwood—it would never occur to me to call her or even think of her as other than Miss Greenwood—shares, with a few others, the distinction of being one of those key professionals whose role was central to the Hunterdon Medical Center. She set the highest standards for personal and professional care, recruited a nursing staff of the finest caliber and was a major administrative support to everyone around her.

Miss Greenwood was born in 1906 on a 160-acre farm near the village of Oxford, Indiana.

[c] The hospital was founded by Dr. Elisabeth Blackwell, the first accredited woman graduate from a medical school. The tradition of female preponderance at the hospital continued. When Grant accepted the position there, its Board was predominantly female and there were approximately three hundred female physicians on staff.

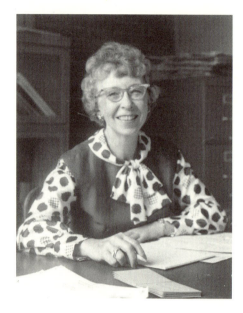

Miss Lela Greenwood, the first Director of Nursing, in an uncharacteristic place—at her desk.

> My grandparents came in a prairie schooner from New England and . . . settled on this farm . . . about 50 miles from . . . the Illinois state line. I went to Oxford school, a little country one-room school. I went there for four years in a hack for grade school. In the meantime we moved into town. My father sold the farm because of ill health.[2]

She attended Indiana University, earned a degree in Romance languages and remained fluent in French and Spanish. Miss Greenwood had wanted to be a nurse since the age of four, when she visited her mother in a hospital after surgery and was fascinated by the nurses and their work. At the suggestion of her family doctor, she entered Bellevue Hospital School of Nursing, from which she graduated with honors, despite a prolonged bout of sickness in the form of scarlet fever, erysipelas and pneumonia. Her physician was Clarence de la Chapelle. In those days, this very serious disease had a high mortality rate. Her ability to throw this off while maintaining academic standards illustrates her robust constitution.

At Bellevue Hospital, Miss Greenwood quickly rose to the position of Nursing Supervisor of the Medical Building. In this role she was in charge of 13 wards of a 500-bed building, with dual responsibility for administration, instruction and liaison with representatives of the three medical schools who provided staff. She collaborated as co-author of two nursing texts, one of which became a standard textbook on pneumonia and its nursing care. She was in charge of the Medical Nursing Service throughout World War II, carrying on with short staff. In 1947, she earned a master's degree from Teachers College at Columbia University. In 1950 she became Supervisor of Clinical Instruction of NYU's School of Nursing.

Clarence de la Chapelle, who had remained close to Miss Greenwood, called her in December, 1952, to discuss her thoughts on nursing care. He arranged an appointment for her with Ray Trussell. On the appointed day, Trussell came to New York with J. Seward Johnson and Lloyd Wescott to see her. Asked if she would like to be a Director of Nursing, she replied: "I've never been a Director of Nursing." Trussell responded: "And I've never been a Director either." Initially, she was not impressed, preferring to continue teaching, which was a major focus of her work. However, "I went home and I started thinking about it. And, I thought, it was in the country. I was born in the country. I loved the country, and I thought, why not?" She visited Flemington on the Lehigh Valley Railroad from New York, to meet with Trussell, Pellegrino, Parmet and Hunt. She accepted the position because of the challenge of directing the entire nursing service, opening a new service and setting new standards, as well as the quality of the physicians whom she had met. To reflect and prepare herself for a completely new undertaking, she returned to her roots in Oxford for a month.

Miss Greenwood was asked to create a nursing staff out of thin air. On her arrival 1 April 1953, there were a total of five applications for positions. Salesmanship was called for.

> They were all very dubious. They didn't know me. They didn't know what kind of person I was going to be. They didn't know the hospital, whether it was going to flourish or not. It was very tough going. I figured that I had to have 28 nurses around the clock to staff the hospital, day, evening and night.

Trussell said Miss Greenwood spent hours on the telephone recruiting with a "very friendly professional voice."[3] Soon there was a waiting list, but Board minutes of mid-June 1953 note the difficulty of obtaining nurses for evenings and nights.[4] Differential pay was offered, but lack of housing played a major role in nursing recruitment. When the hospital opened on 3 July 1953, Miss Greenwood had assembled a staff of 53, 34 registered nurses plus practical nurses, nurse's aides and clerks.

The caliber of HMC's nursing staff, then and to this day, is nothing short of phenomenal in professionalism, kindness and patient care. Much of this undoubtedly is due to the character of local residents, the stock from which nurses come. But much of this is also due to the culture created by Miss Greenwood, who set the standards adhered to ever since.

HMC's opening was delayed by two days because supplies, stored in warehouses all over the county, were not in the building and ready for use. Miss Greenwood's staff was ready 91 days after she arrived. However, the opening of the fifth and second floors could not take place because there were no nurses available to staff them. By 24 July 1953, Miss Greenwood reported to the Board that there were only one crib and two beds for women open, and the third floor was filled with critically ill patients.

Miss Greenwood provided inestimable administrative support for the new Pediatric Service opened by Hunt. HMC was also one of the first hospitals in the country to offer routine rooming-in for mothers. Clara Anthony, head nurse on Maternity, said of Miss Greenwood, "The patients always came first. She set up this place so that new patients would get first attention and immediate attention when they needed it."[5]

Her administrative experience was of great value to Ray Trussell. They would meet over a cup of coffee every morning to review the status of patients and the events of the previous 24 hours. She was an unofficial assistant administrator, making suggestions about problems at all levels. These conferences, Trussell says, were like a course for him on hospital administration. He had come to Hunterdon with an extensive background in Public Health and Epidemiology, but with limited experience in institutional administration. Miss Greenwood describes him as "sympathetic . . . with me every minute."[6] Pellegrino said:

> Lela was not aggressive, yet firm, willing to listen to other people. She was a person of intelligence. She knew how to "handle" doctors in the way the older nurses knew how to handle them. Those nurses were in charge and we knew it. She was a lady in the best sense of that word. Women don't like to hear that today, but there is a distinction . . . She was also a good leader. The other nurses respected her. She knew how to handle them too. She learned from the problems at

Bellevue. Nothing flustered her. That was typical of a Bellevue nurse—a good Bellevue nurse.[7]

Bobbie Knocke said:

> We softened her up a little bit. When she got sick one time, we decided Lela should have a cat. She had this new house and so she should have a cat. So, we got together and bought a little cat carrier and put a little baby pussycat in it, and we brought it to the hospital and said, "Lela, we just brought you a companion for the day that you would like to talk to." She said, "Ah, a cat in the hospital. They're not allowed. Dogs and cats are not allowed." And we said, "Well, as long as *you* are breaking the rules!" Well, she fell in love with that kitty cat and it made all the difference in the world for her. She suddenly became very warm and said, "Imagine, sneaking that in here and sneaking it out. How will I do that?"[8]

One nurse, Jeannette Ash, said of Miss Greenwood: "She was very direct. She knew what she wanted. You could talk to her. She was different from other administrators I have known, not austere; you didn't have to go to her in fear and trembling."[9] There was a sense of community, in which she was included, throughout those early years. On her retirement, Miss Greenwood summed up her experience:

> All of us who came in the early days were so anxious to have this place function as the community wanted it to . . . I would have done anything under the sun to make a success of this hospital—to make it what the community wanted it to be, and what they had given so much to get . . . This attitude got to . . . all of us . . . It was the spirit of the place.

Miss Greenwood, who came to Hunterdon in her late forties, remained single. On her retirement in 1973, she continued to live in the home she had bought not far from Annandale. When she became frail, she moved in 1990 to an assisted living community where she died on 13 December 1997 at age 91.

MURRAY J. RUBIN

Murray Rubin was born in 1926 in Brooklyn and raised on Staten Island, attending public schools. During World War II he served in the Army Air Force for two years in the United States. Before

the war, he hoped to become a physician, but found this impracti-
cal. From a magazine he learned that accounting was a desirable
profession, so he entered NYU's School of Commerce, graduating
in 1949.

In July 1954, his accounting firm, McNichol Johnson & Co.,
assigned him to perform the annual audit for Hunterdon Medical
Center. The audit was difficult: "We put in a lot of overtime because the place was a financial mess."[10] For six months, six days a
week, 10 to 12 hours a day Rubin made the long commute from
his home on Staten Island. The task was "monumental." He found
a closet full of boxes containing bills that had not been sent out to
patients, third party payers or governmental agencies. HMC's business office, it seemed, had been too busy to bill. On my arrival at
HMC, six years after it opened, I can recall patients telling me that
medical, nursing and other professional care was tops, but the business
office was, charitably, difficult.

Rubin worked to correct the situation by trying to hire people
with a knowledge of accounting.

> Everyone in the community had a friend who needed a job,
> and they all wanted to work at the Medical Center. But we
> needed qualified people . . . bookkeepers, accountants and
> the like . . . There weren't that many people in the commu-
> nity with that kind of training. So, we were training people
> on the job while we were trying to get the work done. One of
> the most difficult parts of the project was getting bills sent to
> the appropriate agency, insurance company, or third-party payer
> so that we could collect some money. There was literally no
> cash flow. The Board spent all the funds on building and
> equipment and there was no money left for working capital
> . . . To make matters worse, people were aware that our bill-
> ing system was inaccurate and therefore, didn't pay . . .
> Hunterdon came close to closing after being open for just a
> year.

HMC's first Annual Report, released midyear 1954 before Rubin
could reorganize the business office, consisted of estimates, because hard numbers were not available. The Board would point a
finger at William Lamont, an executive at Riegel Paper and Board
Treasurer, and say "get in there and find out what's going on; he
spent a great deal of time in the business office, like an unpaid
employee, but very dedicated." In September of that year, shortly

before Rubin was hired full time, Trussell reported to Commonwealth an optimistic picture of specialist finances—they were within a few thousand dollars of being self-supporting, adding in grant funds from Commonwealth and Kress, which were a small part of the total.[11] In two years' time, the financial situation was alleviated. The third annual report showed a deficit of only $41,000 and was accurate.

Murray Rubin is an affable gentleman who wanted to do his job, do it right and well, and also please and satisfy people. When he could not accomplish all these goals for a given situation, his priority was a careful and honest job. Because he was anxious to please, a number of physicians did not always grant him the respect he deserved. Although Rubin often remained quiet unless asked a direct question, in the eight years we were on the staff together I never was aware of anything he did less than rock solid and straight up. If he had a failing, it was that he was not as knowledgeable about managing medical practices as he was about hospital finance and administration. By the time he left, the specialists' practices had become a big business, and physicians were more and more closely scrutinizing the state of their finances. A legendary story is the time that Rubin kept the entire business office staff into the night, because there was a discrepancy in the books of ten cents. His reason was that while this amount was trivial, it could mask large errors both plus and minus, which had almost but not quite cancelled out. Rubin says, "Every month, I insisted on balancing the accounts so we could have a basis to start from . . . I would buy them pizza and keep them there until 10, 11, or midnight."

In 1967, when Ed Grant left, Murray Rubin felt he should become administrator, as he had been promised. A series of negotiations took place, with the result that he was not offered the position. He resigned to become Executive Director of Memorial General Hospital in Union, New Jersey. He remained there until 1979, when he went to St. John's Riverside Hospital in Yonkers, New York, staying until 1991, when he retired.

Joseph A. Williamson

Joseph Williamson came to Hunterdon from the post of Assistant Administrator of Sharon Hospital in Pennsylvania. He became ad-

ministrator of HMC in December, 1951, responsible for the business office, the physical plant and non-professional employees. He
served as an infantryman in Europe during World War II and
spoke German fluently. Further information on his background is
not available. HMC's Board minutes were signed by him from 1952
until late 1953. At that time, in the face of the mounting financial
problems and the operating deficit already mentioned, he resigned.
Rubin has already commented on fiscal management. Board minutes indicate that they were quite upset and suggest Trussell was
also dissatisfied with Williamson's work. Trussell wrote that
Williamson was hired by Louise Leicester, fired by Lloyd Wescott
and never had a chance to do his job.[12]

CHAPTER 24

The People

Nursing Staff

M any fine nurses have worked at the Medical Center, and a number of the original nursing staff are still in Hunterdon County. Two with whom I am acquainted were selected as representative. This in no way suggests that the other members of the nursing staff would be less able to contribute to this volume.

CLARA ANTHONY, R.N.

Clara Anthony was born and raised in Mount Carmel, Pennsylvania, a small mining town known for tough high school football teams. After she received her R.N. in 1938 at Geisinger Memorial Hospital in central Pennsylvania, she completed a six-month course in obstetrical and gynecological nursing at the Pennsylvania Hospital for Women in Philadelphia. During World War II she was employed at Geisinger, teaching military nurse cadets. Anthony took a postgraduate course that featured an obstetrician from Grace-New Haven Hospital speaking on their rooming-in program. "It just really knocked me over . . . when I found out the attitude that the obstetrician [at Yale] took about having the babies with their mothers."[1] She determined to put this into practice because she was at that time head nurse in the newborn nursery at Geisinger.

> My favorite children were the little bitties, the preemies . . . I used to go in when the other nurses would have their lunch and I would sneak in there. It was a little cubby hole and that little box was where they had the baby in. You went in and you fed the baby, gave it medication, and that's all you were supposed to do with the baby. Well, I didn't think that was fair. I would pick it up and hold it, talk to it. I just did it on my own and behind backs.

➤ 401

Miss Anthony was very disappointed at the reaction she received from the head of obstetrics at Geisinger when she talked about the Yale program. He dismissed it as a fad.

Many close friends were deciding to work at Hunterdon, and Anthony herself developed "itchy feet." She had progressed as far as she could at Geisinger, and the salary scale was lower than at other hospitals. More importantly, Anthony found an affinity of interest with Miss Greenwood in family-centered maternity programs. Hunterdon represented an opportunity to put into action ideas that had long interested her, including teaching for, and greater participation by, parents. Anthony was offered the position of Maternity and Newborn Supervisor and came to Hunterdon in June 1953.

On arrival, Anthony found "a big building with not all the furniture in it." Patients from internal medicine were often placed in the obstetrics area, because of a need for beds. Equipment in the labor and delivery suite was minimal. There was a delivery bed and a

> little basket lined with blankets and, when necessary, some electric bulbs to keep the baby warm . . . We had to go all over the county to get all the equipment together because they had stored things for the OB floor . . . I guess it must have been two years before we finally had all the [equipment] in the area.

Despite the somewhat chaotic conditions, Anthony was very happy there. She says: "I would go back and work all over again if I could . . . That's just my field and I just wanted to help to get it all set up . . . I felt that I had found my niche."

Anthony continued and expanded an educational program for prospective mothers begun by Margaret Wiles. After five years, the program was expanded to include the then new alternative Lamaze method, as well as other programs of distraction in labor. She increased fathers' participation in the perinatal process, first by bringing them into the labor room. Family physicians, who did most of the deliveries, were quite comfortable with this innovation. The next year, one of the family physician, Vladimir "Arch" Ctibor, asked why couldn't fathers be allowed in the delivery room. Anthony remembers Ctibor as "a wonderful person [who] treated his patients like they were his own children." Because the father had been masked and gowned for the labor room, all that was needed were a few pillows on the floor in case the father fainted.

In 1980, under a grant obtained by the Department of Pediatrics for a Lactation Consultation Service, breastfeeding was taught by a lactation consultant. It required all of Anthony's tact to incorporate the Lactation Service into the existing education program, because the nurses who taught patients breastfeeding felt that they were doing a perfectly adequate job. It was not easy for them to accept that a specially trained Lactation Consultant might offer additional expertise, but Anthony recognized early the potential benefits of such a program and was a vital supporter.

Rooming-in came to Hunterdon with Anthony as well as Hunt. If they brought the seed, the Board had provided fertile ground four years earlier before any of the physicians, or even Trussell had arrived. In a request for proposal from architects, Clifford E. Snyder, Chairman of the Committee on Architecture, specifically asked that a new relationship between maternity and nursery spaces be considered. From the time the hospital opened, rooming-in was allowed, rather than not recommended. Almost half of new mothers took advantage of the opportunity. Rannels endorsed the program and a number of the family physicians, particularly Fritz, Bambara and Looloian, were heartily in favor of it. Hunt favored rooming-in on maternity, but he did not emphasize it.

Anthony enjoyed providing premature infants with appropriate stimulation decades before the advent of neonatal intensive care units. At Hunterdon, she said,

> I would go in and help take care of the babies when they were getting their bath, getting some treatments . . . watching the oxygen . . . [We had] a teeny weeny baby we revived so many times. She was the smallest one we ever had there . . . They were local people . . . Maybe three or four times in an hour I would go in there and give some loving care to that baby and help clear its respiratory system . . . She came out all right and when she was a year old, her mother brought her up to the hospital and we had a little party. And I still see her mother every now and then in the grocery store and this little one is going to have her second baby.

Miss Anthony was always devoted to the best quality of care that could be obtained. She was not an abrasive person but she could be relied on to assert herself for what she felt in the best interest of patients. Her staff was devoted to her, and she remained as Supervisor on the maternity floor until her retirement. She continued to live in Flemington until her death in 2000.

JEANNETTE E. ASH, R.N.

Jeannette Ash was raised on her father's Ayrshire cattle farm in Raritan Township. Her father, Oliver Everitt, who knew Lloyd Wescott well through agricultural activities, would debate with him the merits of different breeds of cattle. Ash graduated from Flemington High School in 1936, and received an R.N. in 1939 from the Presbyterian Hospital School of Nursing in Newark, New Jersey. She was employed there as an obstetrical nurse, married and returned to Hunterdon County 10 years later. Ash remained a Medical Center employee for 35 years, retiring in 1988. Her husband died of a cardiac arrest in 1980. She continues to live in a home built on land that was part of her father's farm.

Ash and her family lived near Ringoes in 1950. They were involved with the fund drive for the Medical Center. She was at home with two small children, but knew she would need employment for financial reasons. In 1953 she answered an advertisement for nurses at the new hospital. As one of the first nurses hired she was given a choice of assignment and specified days, because she had children at home. Two-and-a-half months before HMC opened, Ash was asked to start work early, because Ed Pellegrino needed help with his office consulting practice. By then the Diagnostic Center building was open for use, but there were no linens or equipment. She had to explore cellar storage rooms for needed material. "It was lots of fun."[2]

In Ash's previous employment at Presbyterian Hospital, her relationship to physicians was in the tradition of "handmaiden to the gods." In her new position, everyone worked together on more equal terms, and she found this new spirit very enjoyable and satisfying. Everyone took turns going to the Circle Diner to pick up lunches, and family physicians and specialists were both seeing patients in the Diagnostic Center.

Ash worked with nurse Grace Peterson and a volunteer in the Emergency Room. Arrangements were somewhat casual. The room was small, but equipment was in easy reach. They depended at times on noticing when a car drove in. There were only three stretchers, one in the main room, one at the side, and one for casting. If a nurse felt uneasy about the judgment of a house officer, she would retreat to the little office and call the appropriate specialist, always receiving a prompt response: "You had the feeling it wasn't all your responsibility. You had someone to back you up." House officers wondered how specialists always seemed to turn up exactly when needed.

Ash sums up the atmosphere for those early years:

> Everything just had to be right. He [Trussell] just wanted things right. I think [all] the early people felt that it would either live or die. They were responsible in other words for making a go of it. If it didn't go it was their fault . . . I don't care whether they were doctors, administrators or what. Because they had been given the chance to try this and so therefore it was everybody's responsibility . . . They were all in it together. And it was broadcast all over so . . . if you fell on your nose, everybody would know it. It was very real. Everybody felt that way and everybody was working at their best. They just had to. It was really something. And it didn't matter who you were . . . Even the people who were cleaning . . . had input also . . . They would come and tell you . . . something was wrong. It was not just the higher echelon that had the say-so, it was everybody in it together. It was all one. It was a group thing that everybody had to work on and it was really a very fine place to work.

Notes

◆ PREFACE

1. Trussell RE. *The Hunterdon Medical Center: the story of one approach to rural medical care.* Cambridge, MA: Harvard University Press, 1956.

◆ INTRODUCTION

1. Evans LJ to LB Wescott, Chairman of the Board of Trustees, HMC, 30 August 1976. Wescott file, HMC archives (hereafter cited as HMCA).

2. Keenan T. "A foundation perspective on Community Access to Child Health (CATCH) Program." *Pediatrics* 1999 Jun; 103 (6 Pt 3): 1428–9.

3. Minutes, open meeting, HMC Board of Trustees, 1 December 1949, Board of Trustees file, HMCA.

4. Confidential Report Submitted to the Hunterdon County Board of Agriculture, 3 July 1946 by the committee chaired by LB Wescott, Board of Agriculture file, HMCA.

◆ CHAPTER I: *The Community and People*

1. *Hunterdon County Democrat,* 16 July 1953.

2. *Hunterdon County Democrat,* 23 July 1953.

3. Kovi LV. *As ye sow.* Flemington, NJ: Hunterdon County Board of Agriculture, 1980, pp. 28 et seq.

4. Moreau H., quoted by G Smith of Commonwealth Fund in memorandum, 14 September 1951. Commonwealth 1951 file, HMCA.

5. Ginsburg E., Director, Division of Mental Health Services, Commonwealth. Draft of proposal for mental health services in Hunterdon County, 28 February 1951, Commonwealth 1951 file, HMCA.

6. Data from Departments of Labor, and of Housing, and the U.S. Census, reported in *Hunterdon County Democrat,* 24 April 1997.

7. McIntyre WG. Interview by author, 8 April 1996. Unless otherwise indicated, transcripts of all author interviews, whether of audiotapes or handwritten notes, can be found in the Hunterdon Medical Center archives of this project filed by interviewee's name.

8. Schmidt HG. *Rural Hunterdon: an agricultural history.* New Brunswick, NJ: Rutgers University Press, 1946.

9. Lance W. Interview by author, 23 May 1995.

❧ CHAPTER 2: *People and Organization*

1. Hunt EW to Commonwealth Fund, 23 June 1926. Phillips–Barber file, HMCA.

2. Southmayd HJ to EW Hunt, 26 June 1926. Phillips–Barber file, HMCA. Eventually, Commonwealth supported the creation or improvement of 15 rural hospitals.

3. Ackerman CW to G Smith, Commonwealth Fund, 23 July 1930. Phillips–Barber file, HMCA.

4. Angell RA. Personal communication 28 July 1996. Robert Angell has served as a member of HMC's Board.

5. Angell RZ. Director's Report, Hunterdon County Welfare Board, 1942. Board of Chosen Freeholders, Hunterdon County archives.

6. Angell RZ. Director's Report, Hunterdon County Welfare Board, 1941. Board of Chosen Freeholders, Hunterdon County archives.

7. Editorial, *Hunterdon County Democrat*, 1 July 1951.

8. 1968 eulogy by Dwight Babbitt, a former Hunterdon County Agricultural Agent. Memorial brochure, Louise Bonney Leicester. Leicester file, HMCA.

9. McIntyre WG. Interview by author, 8 April 1996.

10. Kovi LV. *As ye sow*, p. 60.

11. Tantum C. Interview by author, 16 October 1996.

12. Evans LJ. 1968 eulogy. Memorial brochure, Louise Bonney Leicester. Leicester file, HMCA.

13. Bushfield G to LB Wescott, 20 February, 1956. Leicester file, HMCA.

14. For this, and other personal information about Ann Stevenson, I am indebted to Carol Baker. Telephone interview by author, 20 April 1997. Ann Stevenson file, HMCA.

15. Kovi LV. *As ye sow*, p. 59.

16. For this information, and much other vital data on the development of HMC, I am indebted to Marguerite L. (Mrs. Harry) Moore, the first HMC employee. Although not involved until 1948, she made extensive notes based on first-hand discussion with participants; in 1971 she made a systematic compilation, in a series of files labeled with her name, now in the HMCA.

17. Angell RZ to BC Smith, 19 May 1942. the Rockefeller Archives Center; Commonwealth 1949 file, HMCA. The bulk of the research for this project on the Commonwealth Fund was carried out in the Commonwealth Fund archives, housed in the Rockefeller Archives Center in N. Tarrytown, New York (hereafter cited as RAC, CF). Permission was granted to reproduce documents from this collection that were used in this project and they can now be found in the archives of the Medical Center.

18. Southmayd HJ to RZ Angell, 21 May 1942, Commonwealth 1949 file, HMCA.

19. Angell RZ to L Leicester, 11 December 1945. Angell file, HMCA.

20. Minutes, County Board of Agriculture, 2 January 1946. HMCA.

21. Minutes, County Board of Agriculture, 6 February 1946. HMCA.

22. McIntyre WG. Interview by author, 8 April 1996.

23. Kovi LV. *As ye sow,* p. 60 et seq.

24. Handley HE, in his report of the first site visit by Commonwealth to Hunterdon, 8–10 February 1950, quotes Snyder's comment to him in almost the same words. RAC, CF; Commonwealth 1950 file, HMCA. In addition Snyder mentioned how surprised he was by the report returned by the special committee.

25. Kovi LV. *As ye sow,* pp. 19–20.

26. McIntyre WG. Interview by author, 8 April 1996.

27. Ibid.

28. Wescott LB to D Davis, President, HMC, 10 November 1986. Wescott file, HMCA.

29. Wescott LB to C Snyder, 20 January 20 1953. Wescott file, HMCA.

30. Wescott LB to C Snyder, 13 July 20 1966. Wescott file, HMCA.

31. Miller JA to L Evans, 14 February 1946. RAC, CF; Commonwealth 1949 file, HMCA.

32. Obituary, James Alexander Miller. *Bull NY Acad Med* 1948; 24(2): 744–45.

33. De la Chapelle CE. Memorial tribute to Mrs. Leicester, 1968. Leicester file, HMCA.

34. Evans LJ. Memorandum, 1 March 1946. RAC, CF; Commonwealth 1948 file, HMCA.

35. See the magisterial study of the Fund by Harvey AM, Abrams SL. *For the welfare of mankind: the Commonwealth Fund and American medicine.* Baltimore: Johns Hopkins University Press, 1986.

36. Kovi LV. As ye sow, p. 60 et seq.

37. Confidential Report submitted to the Hunterdon County Board of Agriculture July 3, 1946, by the following committee, L. B. Wescott, Chairman. Board of Agriculture file, HMCA.

38. Ibid.

39. Minutes, Executive Committee, County Board of Agriculture, Court House, Flemington, 3 July 1946. HMCA.

✦ CHAPTER 3: *Lloyd Wescott*

1. Van Ness E. "Lloyd Wescott and the power of giving." *Trenton Sunday Times* 4 January 1976.

2. Clark DW (Wescott's daughter). Interview by author, 20 June 1997. Transcript of audiotape, Wescott Family file, HMCA.

3. Wescott audiotapes; Wescott LB to C Snyder, 13 July 1966. Wescott file, HMCA.

4. McIntyre WG. Interview by author, 8 April 1996.

5. Wescott LB to Editor, *Hunterdon County Democrat*, 2 November 1969. Wescott file, HMCA

6. Myers KB. Interview by author, 12 July 1995.

7. Ibid.

8. Wescott LB. Memo on proposed Mental Health Center to other Board members, 30 January 1968. Wescott and Board of Trustee files, HMCA.

9. Hotchkiss B. Joint interview with D Wescott Clark by author, 20 June 1997. Transcript of audiotape, Wescott Family file, HMCA.

10. Trussell RE. Interview by author, 9 November 1995.

11. Clark DW. Interview by author, 20 June 1997.

12. Personal communication, mid 1970s.

13. Wescott LB to FJ Knocke on the occasion of Wescott's resignation, 3 November 1976. Wescott file, HMCA.

14. Lance W. Interview by author, 23 May 1995.

15. Wescott LB to W Rockefeller, 11 April 1952. HMCA.

16. Clark DW. Interview by author, 20 June 1997.

17. Trussell RE to LJ Evans, 6 September 1950. RAC, CF; Commonwealth 1950 file, HMCA.

18. Wescott L letter of resignation to HMC Board, 1 June 1978. HMCA.

❧ CHAPTER 4: *Ferment of Ideas*

1. The Committee on the Costs of Medical Care published 22 studies on the economics, the adequacy and the availability of medical care. Reference might also be made to Lee RI, Jones LW. *The fundamentals of good medical care*. Commission on the Costs of Medical Care; 1933 Report No. 22. Chicago: University of Chicago Press, 1933; reprinted by Archon Books, Hamden, CT, 1962.

2. Richmond JB. *Currents in American medicine: a developmental view of medical care and education*. Cambridge, MA: Harvard University Press, 1969.

3. Committee on the Costs of Medical Care. *Medical care for the American people. Final report*. Chicago: University of Chicago Press, 1932: 59–65, 109–10.

4. Galdston I, ed. *Medicine in the changing order. Report of the New York Academy of Medicine Committee on Medicine and the Changing Order*. New York: Commonwealth Fund, 1947

5. Bryant JH, et al. *Community hospitals and primary care*. Cambridge, MA: Ballinger, 1976.

6. Commission on Hospital Care. *Hospital care in the United States, conclusions and recommendations*. New York: Commonwealth Fund, 1947, pp. 1, 6 et seq.

7. De Kruif PH. *Kaiser wakes the doctors.* New York: Harcourt Brace, 1943.

8. Wilson R. "Health center." *Mod Hosp* 1944; 63: 53–5.

9. Esselstyn CB. "Group practice with branch centers in a rural county." *N Engl J Med* 1953; 248: 488–93

10. For this and subsequent information I am indebted to Caldwell B. Esselstyn, Jr., who gave generously of time in a telephone interview, 30 November 2001.

11. Garland JE. *An experiment in medicine; the first twenty years of the Pratt Clinic and the New England Center Hospital of Boston.* Cambridge, MA: Riverside Press, 1960.

12. Anonymous. Bingham program accomplishments. For this and other information on the Bingham program I am indebted to Chris Fischer, Member Service Representative, American Medical Association.

13. Consultative Council on Medical and Allied Services, Ministry of Health of Great Britain. *Interim report on the future provision of medical and allied services.* London: H.M. Stationary Office, 1920.

14. For information about Bassett I am indebted to Jane Schlesser, Bassett's Public Information Officer (telephone interview March 1997), and Dr. Clinton van Zandt Hawn, retired Pathologist-in-Chief (telephone interview 24 March 1997), as well as Hawn's article provided by Ms. Schlesser: *The Mary Imogene Bassett Hospital,* a pamphlet published by the New York State Historical Society in Cooperstown, the Village, ed. LC Jones, 1982.

15. Hawn C. *The Mary Imogene Bassett Hospital.*

16. MacKenzie GM. "The social functions of the modern hospital." *Westchester Medical Bulletin* 1942 Dec: 7–11, pp. 74.

17. Ibid., pp. 7–11.

18. Ibid.

19. Coddington DC, Moore KD, Fischer EA. *Making integrated health care work. Case Study No. 3: Bassett Healthcare.* Englewood, CO: Center for Research in Ambulatory Health Care Administration, 1996.

● CHAPTER 5: *The Countywide Committee Swings into Action*

1. Minutes, Executive Committee, County Board of Agriculture, 6 November 1946.

2. Southmayd HJ. Memorandum of meeting, 19 March 1947. RAC, CF.

3. Evans LJ. Memorandum of meeting, 8 October 1947. RAC, CF.

4. Evans LJ and HJ Southmayd, Memoranda. RAC, CF.

5. Evans LJ. Memorandum of interview with L Leicester, 10 March 1948. RAC, CF.

6. Evans LJ and unknown individual. Memorandum of transmittal, 10 March 1948. RAC, CF.

7. Lewinsky-Corwin's biographical sketch derived from his obituary, *New York Times*, 9 May 1953, and an unsigned document (Corwin file, HMCA).

8. Lewinsky-Corwin EH. *The American hospital*. New York: Commonwealth Fund, 1946.

9. Lewinsky-Corwin EH to L Leicester, 2 December 1948. Corwin file, HMCA.

10. Lewinsky-Corwin EH. Report of survey of health and hospital needs in Hunterdon County, New Jersey, January, 1948. HMCA.

11. Bortz EL. "The hospital and the physician." *Hospitals* 1948: 22; 61–132; Parran T. "Voluntary hospital looks to the future." *Mod Hosp* 1946; 66: 73–5; Wilson R. "Health center." *Mod Hosp* 1944; 63: 53–5; Gregg A. Benefits of group practice. The Kingsley Roberts Memorial Lectures Series. New York: Medical Administrative Service, 1949; Bayne-Jones S. "The hospital as a center of preventive medicine." *Ann Intern Med* 1949; 31: 7–16.

12. The three reports can be found in the Corwin File, HMCA.

13. Ibid.

14. Fitz R. "The non-teaching hospital and medical education." *Conn State Med J* 1944; 8: 814–7.

15. Means JH. *Doctors, people and government*. Boston: Little, Brown, 1953.

16. Snyder C and LB Wescott to EH Merrill, Jr., President of the Hunterdon County Medical Ass'n., 28 January 1949. Corwin file, HMCA.

17. Evans L. Memorandum, 1 February 1949. RAC, CF. Commonwealth 1949 file, HMCA.

18. Myers KB. Interview by author, 12 July 1995.

19. Trussell R. Interview by author, 9 November 1995.

20. *Hunterdon County Democrat*, 25 June 1953.

➤ CHAPTER 6: *Carrying Out the Plan*

1. First draft of the proposed Constitution and By-laws for the Hunterdon Medical Center. Date and author unknown. Board of Trustees file, HMCA.

2. Minutes, HMC Board, 12 April 1948. Board of Trustees file, HMCA.

3. Minutes, HMC Board, 1948, month and day unknown. Board of Trustees file, HMCA.

4. Evans LJ. Memorandum to unknown recipient, 11 January 1949. RAC, CF. Commonwealth 1949 file, HMCA.

5. Smith G, HJ Southmayd and HE Handley. Internal memoranda, 12 January 1949. RAC, CF. Commonwealth 1949 file, HMCA.

6. Lewinsky-Corwin EH to LJ Evans, 13 January 1949. RAC, CF. Commonwealth 1949 file, HMCA.

7. Evans LJ. Memorandum of meeting with L Leicester and EH Lewinsky-Corwin, 1 February 1949. RAC, CF. Commonwealth 1949 file, HMCA.

8. Moore M. Notes on founding of HMC, document undated but referred to events that occurred in 1948. Moore file, HMCA.

9. Trussell RE. *The Hunterdon Medical Center: the story of one approach to rural medical care.* Cambridge, MA: Harvard University Press, 1956, p. 34.

10. Confidential memorandum to EA Salmon, 3 May 1949. RAC, CF. Commonwealth 1949 file, HMCA.

11. Bushfield GI to LB Wescott, 20 January 1956. Leicester file, HMCA. As of the time this letter was written, Bushfield's comparison may have displayed tact with respect to Wescott.

12. Leicester LB. Revision of memorandum to Dr. Trussell and Mr. Wescott, discussed with them May 1951 and "revised for clarification and brevity, not for content, Jan. 1952." Leicester file, HMCA.

13. Leicester LB. Memorandum to R Trussell, undated and stapled to explanatory note of 28 December 1951. Leicester file, HMCA.

14. Author's review, Commonwealth Fund archives for 1950 at Rockefeller Archives Center.

15. Leicester LB. Memorandum of resignation, with cover commentary by William Lamont, 7 June 1956. Leicester file, HMCA.

16. Furnas JC. "We fetched ourselves a medical center." *Harper's Magazine* 1952 Jun: 54–60. See also LB Wescott in many documents and notes, HMCA, and Trussell RE. *The Hunterdon Medical Center: the story of one approach to rural medical care.* Cambridge, MA: Harvard University Press, 1956.

17. *Hunterdon County Democrat*, 20 March 1952.

18. Trussell RE. Interview by author, 9 November 1955.

19. Gebhardt WR to HJ Southmayd, 17 February 1948. RAC, CF.

20. Tarantola I. Multiple letters to LB Wescott et al. HMCA.

21. Lazarus H to C Snyder, 29 November 1949. RAC, CF. CF file 1949, HMCA.

22. Fisher L to LB Wescott, 27 July 1953. Wescott file, HMCA.

23. Crane AD. "Our health is our wealth." *American Agriculturist* 1960 October 15: 36, 41.

24. Wescott LB, quoted from his obituary, *Hunterdon County Democrat*, 24 December 1990.

25. Evans LJ. Memorandum to M Aldrich, 4 September 1951. RAC, CF.

26. Smith G. Memoranda on Visits to Hunterdon County, 13–14 September 1951. RAC, CF.

27. Wescott LB to M Aldrich, 22 October 1951. Board of Trustees file, HMCA.

28. Lance WL. Interview by author, 23 May 1995. Lance file, HMCA.

29. Wescott LB to MP Aldrich, 12 September 1951. Commonwealth 1951 file, HMCA.

30. Schley R Jr. to MP Aldrich, 24 October 1951. Fund-raising file, HMCA.

31. Wescott LB. Interview 24–25 January 1982, interviewer unknown. HMCA.

32. These discussions are summarized by Trussell in *The Hunterdon Medical Center,* chapter 4, pp. 34–51.

33. Minutes, open meeting of Board of Trustees, 1 December 1949. Board of Trustees file, HMCA.

34. Leicester L to LJ Evans, 6 January 1950. Commonwealth 1950 file, HMCA.

35. Handley HE. Memorandum of visit to Hunterdon, 10 February 1950. RAC, CF.

36. Evans LJ. Memorandum of visit to Hunterdon, 16 February 1950. RAC, CF.

37. Evans LJ. Memorandum of visit, 29 November 1950. RAC, CF.

38. Handley HE. Memorandum of meeting, 1 March 1950. RAC, CF. Commonwealth 1950 file, HMCA.

39. Randolph CR. Memorandum of site visit, 28 September 1950. RAC, CF. Commonwealth 1950 file, HMCA.

40. C Snyder to L Evans, 8 March 1950. RAC, CF and HMCA. Copy annotated by L Leicester: "What constitutes comprehensive care? . . . How can we obtain it? How can we pay for it?"

41. Smith G. Memorandum, interview with LB Wescott and L Leicester, 20 April 1950. RAC, CF. Commonwealth 1950 file, HMCA.

42. Evans LJ. Transcript of speech, 22 May 1950. RAC, CF. Commonwealth 1950 file, HMCA.

43. Spence JC. *The purpose and practice of medicine.* London: Oxford University Press, 1960, pp. 273–4.

44. Evans LJ to MP Aldrich, 23 May 1950. RAC, CF. Commonwealth 1950 file, HMCA.

45. Harvey & Abrams. *For the welfare of mankind,* pp. 220–1.

46. Evans LJ. "The rural hospital." *J Am Med Assoc.* 1938 Mar 26: 945–8.

47. On community health centers, see Evans LJ. "The place of a small community hospital in postwar medical education." *J Assoc Am Med Coll* 1944; 19: 97–104. Pellegrino ED. Interview by author, 27 November, 1995.

48. Wescott LB. HMC Notes, 14 June 1979. Wescott file, HMCA. These were private papers Wescott maintained in preparation for a book on Hunterdon that he never wrote.

❧ CHAPTER 7: *Ray E. Trussell*

1. Trussell R. Interview by author, 9 November 1995, transcript, annotated by the interviewee. Trussell file, HMCA.

2. Handwritten note on draft of manuscript for this book.

3. Smith G. Supplementary Notes, 6 March 1950. RAC, CF. Commonwealth 1950 file, HMCA.

4. Wescott LB to RE Trussell, 16 March 1950. Trussell file, HMCA.

5. Trussell RE. Interview by author, 9 November 1995.

6. Trussell RE to L Wescott, 1 May 1950. HMCA.

7. Trussell RE. Interview by author, 5 December 1995.

8. Trussell RE. Interview by author, 9 November 1995.

9. Ibid.

10. Rubin M. Interview by author, 4 March 1996. Rubin file, HMCA.

11. Wescott LB to L Evans, 24 December 1953. Wescott file, HMCA.

12. Grant E. Telephone interview by author, 6 February 1996.

13. Trussell RE. Interview by author, 9 November 1995.

14. Trussell RE. Memorandum to Executive Committee, 24 November 1952. Board of Trustees file, HMCA.

15. Sanders D. Telephone interview by author, 22 October 1996.

16. Rausen AR. Interview by author, 29 February 1996. Ash J. Interview by author, 3 December 1996.

17. Pellegrino ED. Interview by author, 27 November 1995. Pellegrino file, HMCA.

18. Wescott LB to RR Henderson, 13 August 1965. Wescott file, HMCA.

19. Sanders D. Telephone interview by author, 22 October 1996.

◆ CHAPTER 8: *Building a Medical Center*

1. Snyder C. Letter circulated to candidate architects, 1 December 1949. Architect file, HMCA.

2. Minutes, HMC Board, 6 January 1950. Board of Trustees file, HMCA.

3. Jordan R. Memorandum of meeting, 10 January 1950. RAC, CF.

4. Handley HE and CR Randolph. Memorandum of meeting, 1 March 1950. RAC, CF. Commonwealth 1950 file, HMCA.

5. Trussell RE. Interview by author, 9 November 1995.

6. Evans LJ. Memorandum to M Aldrich, 23 May 1950. RAC, CF. Commonwealth 1950 file, HMCA.

7. *Hunterdon Republican* [a newspaper], 24 August 1950.

8. Minutes, Board of Trustees, 28 July 1950. Board of Trustees file, HMCA.

9. Trussell RE. Minutes, Board of Trustees, 7 July 1950. Board of Trustees file, HMCA.

10. Handley HE. Memorandum, 13 July 1950. RAC, CF. Commonwealth 1950 file, HMCA.

11. Trussell RE. Report of the Director, July 5–July 31, 1950, marked received 9 August 1950; initialed LJE (Evans). RAC, CF. HMCA.

12. Ibid.

13. Trussell RE to LJ Evans, 4 August 1950. Commonwealth 1950 file, HMCA.

14. Ibid.

15. Evans LJ. Memorandum to M Aldrich, 25 September 1950. RAC, CF. Commonwealth 1950 file, HMCA.

16. Aldrich MP to LB Wescott, 27 September 1950. Commonwealth 1950 file, HMCA.

17. Trussell RE. Considerations Governing the Hunterdon Medical Center Staff Appointments and Organization, 1950. Medical Staff file, HMCA.

18. Jordan R. Memorandum of meeting, 10 January 1950. RAC, CF.

19. Smith G. Memorandum of Interview with L Wescott, L Evans and G Smith, 17 November 1950. RAC, CF. Commonwealth 1950 file, HMCA.

20. Unsigned Report of the President and Staff to the Directors of the Commonwealth Fund, 11 January 1951. Commonwealth 1951 file, HMCA.

21. Trussell RE to LJ Evans, 30 January 1951. Commonwealth 1951 file, HMCA.

22. Leicester L to LJ Evans, 16 February 1951. Commonwealth 1951 file, HMCA.

23. Trussell RE to LJ Evans, 10 April 1951. RAC, CF. Commonwealth 1951 file, HMCA.

24. Summary Statement of the Objectives of the Hunterdon Medical Center and the Major Principles and Agreements Governing the Center's Organization, Administration and Program, 11 January 1952. HMCA.

25. Explanation of Request for Funds to Initiate Integrated Community Health Program, n.d., but content strongly suggests early 1952 (see page 2, section h). Board of Trustees file, HMCA.

26. Ibid.

27. Trussell RE. Interview by author, 5 November 1995.

◆ CHAPTER 9: *Family Medicine*

1. Spence JC. *The purpose and practice of medicine.*

2. Randolph CR. Memorandum of survey of public health resources, 9 March 1950. RAC, CF.

3. Minutes, Board of Trustees meeting, 16 December 1953. HMCA. Looloian MW. Interview by author, 8 June 1996.

4. Wescott LB. Presentation at the 3rd national AMA–ANA Conference; 1967 Feb 23.

5. As cited in Menges R. "Country doctors get medical center facilities." *Med Econ* 1953 Mar.

6. Lewinsky-Corwin EH. Report of Survey of Health and Hospital Needs in Hunterdon County, New Jersey, January, 1948, p. 19. Corwin file, HMCA.

7. Evans LJ. Memorandum of meeting at Commonwealth Fund, 1 February 1949. RAC, CF.

8. Fund-raising brochure, "The Health of Hunterdon Is the Wealth of Hunterdon," n.d., probably 1949. HMCA.

9. Trussell RE to LJ Evans, 2 May 1950. RAC, CF. Commonwealth 1950 file, HMCA.

10. Trussell RE. Interview by author, 5 December 1995.

11. Trussell RE. Report of the Director, Hunterdon Medical Center, 4–30 November 1950. HMCA.

12. Trussell RE. Interview by author, 9 November 1995.

13. Bambara AJ. Interview by author, 14 June 1995.

14. Trussell RE. Interview by author, 9 November 1995.

15. Nyberg CE. "Survey of general practice in hospitals." *GP* 1951; 4: 95–8.

16. Katcher AL to LB Wescott, 19 April 1961; Wescott LB to AL Katcher, 24 April 1961. Medical Staff file, HMCA.

17. Wescott LB. Family practice and the community hospital. Paper presented at the Association for Hospital Medical Education; 1972 Feb 4; Chicago.

18. Pellegrino ED. "Role of the community hospital in continuing education – the Hunterdon experiment." *J Am Med Assoc* 1957; 164: 361–5.

19. Stevens R. *American medicine and the public interest.* New Haven: Yale University Press, 1971, p. 297.

20. Snope F. Personal communication, 13 January 1997.

21. Zapp J. Personal communication, 12 December 1996.

22. Means JH. *Doctors, people and government.* Boston: Little, Brown, 1953.

23. Freidson E. *Profession of medicine; a study of the sociology of applied knowledge.* New York: Dodd, Mead, 1970.

24. Kasanof D. "Where country doctors learn and teach." *Patient Care* 1978 Jun 30: 118–46. Data from Hunterdon Medical Center records, Hunterdon County Library, American Medical Association, American Academy of Family Practice, and the New Jersey Board of Medical Examiners.

25. Trussell RE to LJ Evans, 21 June 1954. Commonwealth 1954 file, HMCA.

26. Hunt WM. Memorandum to H Simmons and others, 22 October 1976. Phillips–Barber file, HMCA.

☙ CHAPTER 10: *The Specialist Staff*

1. Means, *Doctors, people, and government.*

2. Smith G. Memorandum, 17 November 1950. RAC, CF.

3. Trussell RE to LJ Evans, 10 April 1951. RAC, CF. Commonwealth 1951 file, HMCA.

4. Report of the President and Staff to the Directors of the Commonwealth Fund, 11 January 1951. RAC, CF. Commonwealth 1951 file, HMCA.

5. Trussell RE. Handwritten note on draft of this document.

6. Rannels HW. "Medical care and education in rural areas." *Bull Matern Welfare* 1958; Mar–Apr.

7. Trussell RE. Progress Report to Family Physicians, letter 27 June 1952. HMCA.

8. Committee on the Costs of Medical Care. *Medical care for the American people. Final report.* Chicago: University of Chicago Press, 1932: 59–65, 109–10.

9. Trussell RE. Personal communication, 21 December 1996.

10. Johnson JS to RE Trussell, 5 August 1953. Johnson file, HMCA.

11. Trussell RE to JS Johnson, 10 August 1953. Johnson file, HMCA.

12. Kress RH letter quoted in Minutes, Board of Trustees, 25 October 1951. Board of Trustees file, HMCA.

13. Trussell RE. Personal communication.

14. Jordan R. Summary of Hunterdon Medical Center, 11 January 1950. RAC, CF.

15. Smith G. Memorandum, 17 November 1950. RAC, CF.

16. Minutes, Board of Trustees, 4 June 1951. Board of Trustees file, HMCA.

17. Minutes, Board of Trustees, 25 July 1952. Board of Trustees file, HMCA.

18. Trussell RE. Handwritten note on draft of this document.

19. Parmet M. A child psychiatrist in a rural medical center. Paper presented at the 30th Anniversary Seminar Philadelphia Child Guidance Clinic; 1955 Oct 29; Philadelphia.

20. Minutes, Executive Committee, 27 August 1953. Board of Trustees file, HMCA.

21. Trussell RE. Memorandum to Executive Committee, Board of Trustees, 12 November 1952. Board of Trustees file, HMCA.

22. Trussell RE. Interview by author, 5 December 1995.

23. Rubin M. Interview by author, 4 March 1996.

24. Ibid.

25. Grant E. Telephone interview by author, 6 February 1996.

26. Trussell, RE. Memorandum to Executive Committee, 21 January 1953. Board of Trustees file, HMCA.

❧ CHAPTER 11: *Building Relationships and Opening the Doors*

1. Pellegrino ED. Interview by author, 27–28 November 1995.

2. Fidellow, E. Interview by author, 11 July 1995.

3. Parmet B. Interview by author, 20 January 1996.

4. Katzenbach M. Interview by author, 28 March 1995.

5. Rosswag CT. Interview by author, 7 February 1996.

6. Summary Statement of the Objectives of the Hunterdon Medical Center and the Major Principles and Agreements Governing the Center's Organization, Administration and Program, 11 January 1952. HMCA.

7. Trussell RE. Draft of Considerations Governing the Hunterdon Medical Center Staff Appointments and Organization. Undated, and edited by hand. HMCA.

8. See Balint M. *The doctor, his patient and the illness.* New York: International Universities Press, 1957; Williams TF. "Patient referral to a university clinic: patterns in a rural state." *Am J Publ Health* 1960; 50: 1493–507; Muzzin LJ. "Understanding the process of medical referral. Putting the findings into perspective." *Can Fam Physician* 1992 Apr; 38: 817–21.

9. Fisher ES, Welsh HG. "Avoiding the unintended consequences of growth in medical care: how might more be worse?" *JAMA* 1999 Feb 3; 281(5): 446–53.

10. Pellegrino ED. Telephone interview by author, 4 December 1996.

11. Lincoln JA. Interview by author, 19 July 1996.

12. Trussell RE. Interview by author, 9 November 1995.

13. Trussell RE. Interview by author, 5 December 1995.

14. Pellegrino ED. Interview by author, 27 November 1995.

15. Pellegrino ED. "Role of the community hospital in continuing education – the Hunterdon experiment." *J Am Med Assoc* 1957; 164: 361–5.

16. Pellegrino, ED. Interview by author, 27 November 1995.

17. Rannels HW. "The role of the trained obstetrician in a rural community." *Obstet Gynecol* 1956; 8: 189.

18. Bambara AJ, Hunt AD. "Specialist plus, not versus, family physicians: a setting conducive to effective postgraduate education." *Postgrad Med* 1956 Sep; 20: 305–9.

19. Bambara AJ. Interview by author, 14 June 1995.

20. Pellegrino ED. Interview by author, 27 November 1995.

21. Rausen A. Interview by author, 29 February 1996.

22. Trussell RE. Memorandum to Staff, Hunterdon Medical Center, 18 March 1953. Medical Staff file, HMCA.

23. Medical Staff Minutes, Hunterdon Medical Center, 3 and 24 March 1953. Medical Staff file, HMCA.

24. Ibid.

25. Trussell RE. Memorandum to Staff, Hunterdon Medical Center, 18 March 1953. Medical Staff file, HMCA.

26. Minutes, Board of Trustees, Hunterdon Medical Center, 26 June 1953. Board of Trustees file, HMCA.

27. Pellegrino ED. Telephone interview by author, 4 December 1996.

28. Felch WC, Scanlon D. "Bridging the gap between research and practice. The role of continuing medical education." *JAMA* 1997 Jan 8; 277(2): 155–6.

29. Sorum PC. "Two tiers of physicians in France: general pediatrics declines, general practice rises." *JAMA* 1998 Sep 23–30; 280(12): 1099–101.

30. Wescott LB. "Hunterdon: the rise and fall of a medical Camelot." *N Engl J Med* 1979 Apr 26; 300(17): 952–6.

31. "Miss Greenwood retires." *MiniMag* (Hunterdon Medical Center in-house publication) 1973 Jun; 4: 1–4.

32. *Hunterdon County Democrat*, 30 July 1953.

33. Rubin M. Personal communication, 1996.

34. Herr C. Interview by author, 22 July 1997.

❧ CHAPTER 12: *Affiliation with a Medical School*

1. As cited in Harvey & Abrams, *For the Welfare of Mankind*.

2. Black H. *Doctor, teacher and hospital chief*. Chester, CT: Globe Pequot Press, 1982.

3. Sutton FC. *Hospitals* 1948; 22: 33–5.

4. Park EA. "The pediatrician and the public." *Pediatrics* 1948; 1: 828–9.

5. De la Chapelle C. Talk before Board of Trustees, staff and community at Hunterdon Medical Center, 13 September 1955. HMCA. Sheehan was a consultant involved in Medical Center planning from an early date. See also, de la Chapelle CE, Jensen F. *A mission in action; the story of the Regional Hospital Plan of New York University.* New York: New York University Press, 1964.

6. Gebhardt WR to HJ Southmayd, 17 February 1948. RAC, CF.

7. De la Chapelle C. Talk before Board of Trustees, staff and community at Hunterdon Medical Center, 13 September 1955. HMCA.

8. Trussell RE to LJ Evans, 9 May 1951. Commonwealth 1951 file, HMCA.

9. Remarks by M Begun at Clarence de la Chapelle Memorial Service, 1 July 1987. Text supplied to author courtesy of de la Chapelle's son, Norman F. de la Chapelle.

10. Trussell RE. Interview by author, 5 December 1995.

11. De la Chapelle N. Personal communication, 25 August 1997.

12. Wescott LB. Community hospital–medical school associations. Presented to the Association for Hospital Medical Education; 1971 Sep 11; Atlanta.

13. Haggerty R. Personal communication, ca. 1978.

◆ CHAPTER 13: *Innovation in Mental Health, Pediatric and House Staff Teaching Programs*

1. Robinson GC. "The patient as a person." *Bull Johns Hopkins Hosp* 1940; 66: 390–7.

2. Ripley HS. "Psychiatric consultation service in a medical inpatient department. Its function in diagnosis, treatment and teaching." *Am J Med Sci* 1940; 199: 261–8. Crispell RS. "Extramural and neuropsychiatry in a general hospital." *South Med Surg* 1940; 102: 105–10.

3. Evans LJ to RE Trussell, 5 May 1950. Commonwealth 1950 file, HMCA.

4. Trussell RE to LJ Evans, 21 August 1950. Commonwealth 1950 file, HMCA.

5. Handley H. Memorandum of Site Visit, 27 September 1950. RAC, CF. Commonwealth 1950 file, HMCA.

6. For a useful source on Ginsburg's thinking, see Ginsburg EL. Public health is people; an Institute on Mental Health in Public Health seminar held at Berkeley, CA, 1948. New York: Commonwealth Fund, 1950.

7. Trussell RE. Interview by author, 5 December 1995.

8. Minutes, Board of Trustees, 2 May 1951. Board of Trustees file, HMCA.

9. Trussell RE. Report to Family Physicians, June 1952. Family Practice file, HMCA.

10. Leicester L. Discussion of the Budget Prepared for the Commonwealth Fund. Board of Trustees file, HMCA.

11. Mercer ME. Report on Activities of the Division of Child Development, New York Hospital, 12 November 1952. Archives, Department of Pediatrics, New York Hospital.

12. Trussell RE. Interview by author, 5 December 1995.

13. Mercer ME. Interview by author, 23 July 1997.

14. Ibid.

15. Parmet M. A child psychiatrist in a rural medical center. Paper presented at the 30th Anniversary Seminar, Philadelphia Child Guidance Clinic; 1955 Oct 29; Philadelphia.

16. See Ebaugh FG, Rymer AC. "Psychiatric facilities within the general hospital." *Mod Hosp* 1940; 55: 71–4 and Tarnover SM. "Psychiatry in a general hospital of a small city." *N Engl J Med* 1948; 239: 466–8. Both describe inpatient hospital care of psychiatric patients on open medical floors of a general hospital. An additional discussion of merging psychiatric and general medical care in a general hospital is found in Crispell RS. "Extramural and neuropsychiatry in a general hospital." *South Med Surg* 1940; 102: 105–10.

17. Parmet M. "The role of the full-time psychiatrist in the general hospital." *J Med Soc NJ* 1960; 57: 562–5. Also Parmet M. "The supervisory nurse's role in promoting mental health." *Am J Nurs* 1957; 57: 329.

18. Minutes, Board of Trustees, 26 September 1952. Board of Trustees file, HMCA.

19. Grant E. Telephone interview by author, 6 February 1996.

20. Trussell RE. The Mental Health Aspects of the Hunterdon Program: Their Interrelationships and Continuation. 1953. Mental Health file, HMCA.

21. Minutes, Board of Trustees, 29 December 1954. Board of Trustees file, HMCA.

22. Ibid.

23. Parmet MD. The Mental Health Program of the Hunterdon Medical Center, July 1954–August 1956. HMCA.

24. Pellegrino ED, Parmet M, Henderson RR. Emotional problems in the management of recent myocardial infarction. Paper presented at the Clinical Conference, Hunterdon Medical Center; 1955; Flemington (NJ). Parmet M. "The role of the full time psychiatrist in the general hospital." *J Med Soc NJ* 1960; 57: 562–5. Parmet M, Pellegrino ED. Treatment of the psychiatric patient in an open medical floor in a community general hospital. Paper presented at the Annual Meeting of the American Psychiatric Association; 1960 May; Atlantic City (NJ).

25. Grant E. Personal communication, 1996.

26. Wescott LB to RR Henderson, 24 September 1963. Wescott file, HMCA.

27. Minutes, Joint Conference Committee, 2 July 1973, with attached memorandum from Adams. HMCA.

28. Author's personal experience.

29. Rose JA. "The relation of the family to the hospital." *Med Clin North Am* 1952; 36: 1551–4.

30. See, for example, Senn MJE. "Role of psychiatry in a children's hospital service." *Am J Dis Child* 1946 Jul; 72: 95–110. Klatskin EH. "Choice of rooming-in or newborn nursery." *Pediatrics* 1950; 6: 878–89. McBryde A. "Compulsory rooming-in in the ward and private newborn service of Duke Hospital." *J Am Med Assoc* 1951; 145: 625–8. Moncrieff A., Walton AM. "Visiting children in hospital." *Br Med J* 1952 Jan 5: 43–4. Hay JD. "Self-demand feeding in the maternity unit." *Br Med J* 1952 Nov 29: 1180–2. Jackson K. "Problem of emotional trauma in hospital treatment of children." *J Am Med Assoc* 1952; 149: 1536–8. Illingworth RS. "Self-demand feeding in a maternity unit." *Lancet* 1952 Apr 5; i: 683–7.

31. Hunt AD, Trussell RE. "They let parents help in children's care." *Mod Hosp* 1955; 85: 89–91.

32. Spence JC. "The care of children in hospital." *Br Med J* 1947; 1: 125.

33. Spitz RA. "Hospitalism: an inquiry into the genesis of psychiatric conditions in early childhood." *Psychoanal Study Child* 1945; 1: 53. Bowlby J, Robertson J. "Responses of young children to separation from their mothers." *Courrier2* 1952: 132. Örsten P, Mattson, Å. "Hospitalization symptoms in children." *Acta Paediatr* 1955; 44: 77–92. Campbell K, Blanch M. "Unrestricted visiting in a children's ward. Eight year's experience." *Lancet* 1955 Nov 5; 2: 971–3. Powers GF. "Humanizing hospital experiences." *Am J Dis Child* 1948; 76: 365–79. Bowlby J. "Attachment and loss." In: *Separation, anxiety and anger*, vol. II. New York: Basic Books, 1973.

34. Hunt AJ. Interview by author, 17 December 1995. See the following references for more detail on the program: Morgan ML, Lloyd BJ. "Parents invited." *Nurs Outlook* 1955 May; 3: 256–9. Hunt AD, Trussell RE. "They let parents help in children's care." Hemmendinger M. "Rx: admit parents at all times." *Child Study (NY)* 1956–1957 Winter: 3–9. Hunt AD. "An experiment in teamwork." *Child Study (NY)* 1957 Winter: 9–14. Cavitch B. "Parents assist in care of hospitalized children." *Nurs World* 1959 May; 5: 133. Katcher AL, Grant EV. "Parents help care for their children." *Hospitals* 1961 Mar 1.

35. Hunt AD, Parmet M. "Collaboration between pediatrician and child psychiatrist in a rural medical center." *Pediatrics* 1957; 19: 462–6.

36. Leman E. "Mothers make effective aides at Hunterdon Medical Center." *Hosp Top* 1966 Oct; 44(10): 95–8. Linde SM. "When children need their parents most." *Today's Health* 1968 Jun: 26–9, 66–7.

37. Wolf RE. "The hospital and the child." In: Solnit AJ, Provence SA, editors. *Modern perspectives in child development*. New York: International Universities Press, 1963.

38. Spence, op. cit.

39. Jackson EB. "The initiation of a rooming-in project at the Grace-New Haven Community Hospital. In: Senn MJE, editor. Problems in infancy."

Transactions of the 1st Josiah Macy Conference, 1947. Other articles in the same volume discuss obstetrical, pediatric, nursing, psychiatric and architectural features of the program. See also Jackson EB. "A hospital rooming-in unit for four newborn infants and their mothers." *Pediatrics* 1948; 1: 28-43, which recounts in more detail the genesis of the Yale program and some of the background.

40. Moloney JC. "The newborn, his family and the modern hospital." *Mod Hosp* 1946; 67: 43–6.

41. Montgomery TL. "Bedside care of the newborn by the parturient mother." *Med Clin North Am* 1948; 32: 1699–1709.

42. Richardson FH. "Rooming in: modern medicine goes old fashioned." *South Med J* 1952; 45: 131–7.

43. Sanders D. Telephone interview by author, 22 October 1996.

44. Hunt AJ. Interview by author, 17 December 1995.

45. Martell LK. "Response to change: maternity nursing after World War II." *MCN Am J Matern Child Nurs* 1995 May–Jun; 20(3): 131–4.

46. Katcher AL, Lanese MG. "Breast-feeding by employed mothers: a reasonable accommodation in the work place." *Pediatrics* 1985 Apr; 75(4): 644–7.

47. Trussell RE. Memorandum to Executive Committee, 12 November 1952. Board of Trustees file, HMCA.

48. Trussell RE to LJ Evans, 21 June 1954. Commonwealth 1954 file, HMCA.

49. Pellegrino E. Interview by author, 27 November 1995.

❧ CHAPTER 14: *Efforts to Offer Health and Sickness Care to Those Who Lack Money to Pay*

1. Ginsburg E. Director, Division of Mental Health Services, The Commonwealth Fund, Draft of Report, 28 February 1951. Commonwealth 1951 file, HMCA.

2. *Hunterdon County Democrat*, 10 October 1957.

3. Lance W. Interview by author, 30 January 1997.

4. Herr C., a second cousin of Large, was kind enough to provide copies of these letters.

5. By-Laws, Hunterdon Medical Center, 26 June 1953. Board of Trustees file, HMCA.

6. Pellegrino ED. Interview by author, 28 November 1995.

7. Doyle L. Interview by author, 30 January 1996.

8. The Three Fears, Special Bulletin, American Association for Labor Legislation, 131 East 23rd Street, New York City, NY, February 1919. Prepayment Plan file, HMCA.

9. Cabot RC. "Better doctoring for less money." *American Magazine* 1916 May, as cited by Williams TF. "Cabot, Peabody and the care of the patient." *Bull Hist Med* 1950; 24: 462–81.

10. Rothman DJ. *Beginnings count: the technological imperative in American health care.* New York: Oxford University Press, 1997.

11. Stevens R. *American medicine and the public interest.* New Haven: Yale University Press, 1971.

12. Rorem CR. "Sickness insurance in the United States." *Bull Am Hosp Assoc* 1932 Dec., "Group hospitalization: Mecca or mirage?" *Mod Hosp* 1933 Jan. and "Hospital service plans and private insurance contrasted." *Hospitals* 1940 Jul; 14: 32–5. See also Schenewerk GA. "Group hospital insurance." *Hospitals* 1940; 14: 38.

13. Trussell RE. First Director's Report, 5–31 July 1950. Commonwealth 1950 file, HMCA.

14. Baehr G, Deardorff NR. "What the Health Insurance Plan of Greater New York offers to older persons." *Publ Welfare* 1951 Mar. Reprinted by the American Public Welfare Association, Chicago, Illinois.

15. Smith G. Memorandum of meeting, Commonwealth Fund, 17 November 1950. RAC, CF.

16. Trussell RE to LJ Evans, 20 April 1953. Commonwealth 1950 file, HMCA.

17. Summary Statement of the Objectives of Hunterdon Medical Center. Approved by Board of Trustees, 11 January 1954. Revised 1 February 1952. HMCA.

18. Ibid.

19. Ibid.

20. Trussell RE to LJ Evans, 20 April 1953. Commonwealth 1953 file, HMCA.

21. Nicholas RC. Report of Committee on Third Party Payments, 4 June 1953.

22. Executive Committee Minutes, 27 April 1953. Board of Trustees file, HMCA.

23. Executive Committee Minutes, 1 May 1953. Board of Trustees file, HMCA.

24. Goldfield N. "Truman and the medical profession: replay or lesson for the nineties." *Physician Exec* 1993 Mar–Apr; 19(2): 3–9.

25. Wescott LB to LJ Evans, 24 December 1953. Commonwealth 1953 file, HMCA.

26. Trussell RE to LJ Evans, 21 June 1954. Commonwealth 1954 file, HMCA.

27. Henderson RR to L Wescott, 12 February 1962. Wescott file, HMCA.

28. Trussell RE. Interview by author, 5 December 1995.

29. Mannix JR. "Cleveland likes inclusive rates." In: Bachmeyer AC, Hartman G, editors. *The hospital in modern society.* New York: Commonwealth Fund, 1943.

30. Trussell RE. Interview by author, 5 December 1995.

31. Perloff E. *Report of a Special Committee on the Provision of Health Services.* Chicago: American Hospital Association, 1970.

32. Salerno F. Interview by author, 27 July 1999.

33. Report of the Advisory Panel on Health Professions Education and Managed Care for the Pew Health Professions Commission: *Health Profes-*

sions Education and Managed Care: Challenges and Necessary Responses. San Francisco: UCSF Center for the Health Professions, 1995.

34. McKinsey & Co. Assessing the Hunterdon Medical Center's Impact. 23 May 1977. Prepayment file, HMCA.

35. Reinhardt UE. "The economist's model of physician behavior." *JAMA* 1999 Feb 3; 281(5): 462–5.

36. Davis D. Telephone interview by author, 22 April 1997.

37. Rothman DJ. *Beginnings count.* Shortell SM, Waters TM, Clarke KW, Burdetti PP. "Physicians as double agents: maintaining trust in an era of multiple accountabilities." *JAMA* 1998 Sep 23–30; 280(12): 1102–8.

38. Lamm, R. D., Marginal Medicine. *JAMA* 280: 931–933, 1998.

39. Fisher ES, Welsh HG. "Avoiding the unintended consequences of growth in medical care: how might more be worse?" *JAMA* 1999 Feb 3; 281(5): 446–53.

40. *AMA* News 44:1–2, 13 August, 2001.

41. Wise R. Interview by author, 29 April 1997.

42. Ibid.

43. Grand LN. Personal communication, 11 October, 2001.

❧ CHAPTER 15: *Community and Ambulant Care Facility*

1. Committee on the Costs of Medical Care. *Medical care for the American people. Final report.* Chicago: University of Chicago Press, 1932: 59–65, 109–10.

2. Evans LJ. "The rural hospital." *J Am Med Assoc* 1938 Mar 26: 945–8.

3. Walker WF. "Opportunities in public health programs for community hospital participation." *Hospitals* 1940; 14: 28–31.

4. Cody HJ. "The contribution a hospital may make to its community." *Hospitals* 1940; 14: 13–7.

5. Brown A. "How the children's hospital can best meet community needs." *Hospitals* 1940; 14: 42–5.

6. Trussell RE. Interview by author, 8 November 1995.

7. Trussell RE, Elinson J. *Chronic illness in a rural area. The Hunterdon study,* vol. III chronic illness in the United States series. Cambridge, MA: Harvard University Press, 1959, a report that has become a medical classic.

8. The Commission was a joint effort of the American Medical Association, the American Public Health Association and the American Hospital Association.

9. For a detailed autobiographical essay, see the chapter "City Slums to Sociosalustics" in *Medical sociologists at work*, Elling RH & M Sokolowska, eds. New Brunswick, NJ: Transaction Press, 1978.

10. Elinson J. Interview by author, 7 December 1995.

11. Trussell RE. Interview by author, 5 December 1995.

12. Moore ML. Report to the Medical Center Board of Trustees: "The

Community Serves the Chronic Illness Survey and the Chronic Illness Survey Serves the Community," 1955. Moore file, HMCA.

13. Moore ML. Records of Conduct of Chronic Illness Survey, n.d. Moore file, HMCA

14. Wiles MB. "The nurse on the survey team." *Nurs Outlook* 1957 Aug; 5(2).

15. Ash JE. Interview by author, 3 December 1996.

16. Elinson J. Interview by author, 7 December 1995.

17. Trussell RE. Interview by author, 5 December 1995.

18. Trussell RE. Memorandum to Board of Trustees and Directors of Services: Report by Mrs. Parmet and Mrs. de Rochemont on Community Expectations, 25 March 1953. Board of Trustees file, HMCA.

19. Elinson J. Interview by author, 7 December 1995.

20. Trussell RE, Elinson J. *Chronic illness in a rural area. The Hunterdon study*, p. 55.

21. Elinson J. Interview by author, 7 December 1995.

22. Chmeil JF, Drumm ML, Konstan MW, Ferkol TW, Kercsmar CM. "Pitfalls in the use of genotype analysis as the sole diagnostic criterion for cystic fibrosis." *Pediatrics* 1999 Apr; 103(4 Pt 1): 823–6.

23. Pellegrino ED, quoted in Trussell RE, Elinson J. *Chronic illness in a rural area. The Hunterdon study*, p. 302.

24. Pellegrino ED. Telephone interview by author, 4 December 1996.

25. Terris M. "Joint housing of hospitals, health departments and laboratories." *Am J Publ Health Nations Health* 1951; 41: 319–25, reporting a survey performed in 1948.

26. Randolph CR. Public Health Services in Hunterdon County, N.J., 9 March 1950, Report to Commonwealth Fund. Commonwealth 1950 file, HMCA.

27. Handley HE. Memorandum of Site Visit for Commonwealth Fund, 27 September 1950. Commonwealth 1950 file, HMCA.

28. See Strauss H. "Health education in hospitals and outpatient departments." *Am Publ Health Nations Health* 1945; 35: 1175–8 and Witke IM. "Teaching the public." *Mod Hosp* 1944: 57–8, among others.

29. Johnson JS. to RR Henderson, 17 November 1961. Johnson file, HMCA.

30. Wescott LB to DW Davis, 4 September 1986. Wescott file, HMCA.

31. Wescott LB to JS Johnson, 10 February 1977. Wescott file, HMCA.

32. Trussell RE to LJ Evans, 16 January 1952. RAC, CF. Commonwealth 1952 file. HMCA.

33. Trussell RE. Interview by author, 5 December 1995.

34. League of Women Voters. "Health Services in Hunterdon County," 1961. Document No. 3270, Hunterdon County Historical Commission.

35. John Van Nuys of the Hunterdon County Health Department provided this information. Telephone interview by author, 22 January 1997. Health Department file, HMCA.

36. Minutes, Board of Trustees, 22 July 1966. Board of Trustees file, HMCA.

37. *Easton Express,* 10 July 1967.

38. Grand LN. Interview by author, 3 October 2001.

39. Minutes, Board of Trustees, 13 June 1951. Board of Trustees file, HMCA.

40. Wescott LB to K Myers, 12 January 1954. School Health file, HMCA.

41. Wescott LB to RR Henderson, 24 February 1960. Wescott file, HMCA.

42. "Full Wellness Center," *Hunterdon County Democrat,* 2 April 1998.

43. Leuck M. *A further study of dental clinics in the United States.* Chicago: University of Chicago Press, 1932. See Lischer BE. "Dental service in hospitals." *Hospitals* 1943; 17: 94–6 for a description of the structure and functions of a hospital dental service.

44. Trussell RE. *Hunterdon Medical Center,* p. 142.

45. Beckley J. Personal communication, 18 September 2001.

♦ CHAPTER 16: *Years of Stress and Change*

1. Wescott LB. HMC Notes, 14 June 1979. Wescott file, HMCA.

2. Fisher ES, Welsh HG. "Avoiding the unintended consequences of growth in medical care: how might more be worse?" *JAMA* 1999 Feb 3; 281(5): 446–53.

3. Trussell RE. *Hunterdon Medical Center,* pp.174–212.

4. Trussell RE to LJ Evans, 7 March 1955. Commonwealth 1955 file, HMCA.

5. Minutes, Board of Trustees, October and November, 1958. Board of Trustees file, HMCA.

6. Trussell RE. Development of rules and regulations for staff of Hunterdon Medical Center, 18 March 1953. Medical Staff file, HMCA.

7. Minutes, Medical Staff, 3 and 24 March 1953. Medical Staff file, HMCA.

8. Minutes, Board of Trustees, 16 December 1953. Board of Trustees file, HMCA.

9. Katcher AL memorandum to RR Henderson, 17 March 1966. Henderson file, HMCA.

10. Wescott LB. HMC Notes, 14 June 1979.

11. Statement of Medical Staff Relationships, 10 March 1961. Medical Staff file, HMCA.

12. Rakove JN. *Original meaning: politics and ideas in the making of the Constitution.* New York: Knopf, 1997.

13. Katcher AL to LB Wescott, 19 April 1961; Wescott LB to AL Katcher, 24 April 1961. Family Physician file, HMCA.

14. Wescott LB. Memorandum to Members of the Executive Committee, 11 May 1961. Medical Staff file, HMCA.

15. Minutes, Board of Trustees meeting, 28 June 1963. Medical Staff file, HMCA.

16. Salerno F. Interview by author, 7 February 1996.

17. Wescott LB. Memorandum to RR Henderson, 3 June 1963. Wescott file, HMCA.

18. Summary Statement of the Objectives of the Hunterdon Medical Center, adopted 1 February 1952. Board of Trustees file, HMCA.

19. By-Laws of the Hunterdon Medical Center, adopted 26 June 1953. Board of Trustees file, HMCA.

20. Professional Service Plan of the Hunterdon Medical Center, 24 December 1953. Medical Staff file, HMCA.

21. Statement on Staff Interrelationships, By-Laws, Hunterdon Medical Center, November, 1961, p. 17. HMCA.

22. Henderson RR. Memorandum to Needs Committee members, 12 September 1963. HMCA.

23. Fidellow R. Interview by author, 20 April 1995.

24. RR Henderson to Medical Staff, 8 June 1965. Medical Staff file, HMCA.

25. Minutes, Ad Hoc Committee on Consultations, 2 September 1975. Medical Staff file, HMCA.

26. Lewinsky-Corwin EH. Report of Survey of Health and Hospital Needs in Hunterdon County, New Jersey, January, 1948, p. 19. Corwin file, HMCA.

27. Wills G. *Lincoln at Gettysburg.* New York: Simon & Schuster, 1992, pp. 157 et seq.

28. Minutes, Board of Trustees, 16 December 1966. Board of Trustees file, HMCA.

29. Henderson RR to LB Wescott, 12 February 1963. Henderson file, HMCA.

30. Trussell RE. Interview by author, 9 November 1996.

31. Wescott LB. "Innovation in medical staff organization." *Hosp Med Staff* 1972 Mar; 1: 14–9.

32. Pellegrino ED. Remarks at Board of Trustees meeting, 1975. Board of Trustees file, HMCA.

33. Pellegrino ED. Telephone interview by author, 4 December 1996.

34. Salerno F. Interview by author, 27 July 1999.

35. Wescott LB. Annual Report, Board of Trustees, 25 January 1976. Board of Trustees file, HMCA.

36. Herr C. Interview by author, 22 July 1997.

37. Lillian French, et al., Plaintiffs, vs. Hunterdon Medical Center, et Las. [sic] Defendants, Superior Court of New Jersey, Chancery Division: Hunterdon County, Docket No. C 4463 76. Date not available.

38. Simmons H. Presentation to National Health Forum, March 1978, San Francisco, CA. Medical Staff file, HMCA.

39. Salerno F. Interview by author, 7 February 1996.

40. Herr C. Interview by author, 22 July 1997.

41. LB Wescott to JS Johnson, 6 March, 14 April, 25 April, 15 May and 10 July, 1975. Wescott file, HMCA.

42. Wescott LB. Annual Report to Board of Trustees, 23 January 1976. Board of Trustees file, HMCA.

43. Wescott LB to S Johnson, 1975. HMCA.

44. Wescott LB. Audiotape of interview by unknown interviewer, 24–25 January 1982. HMCA.

45. Wescott LB. Holograph letter to D Davis, 9 December 1980. Davis file, HMCA.

46. Davis D. Telephone interview by author, 22 April 1997.

47. Ibid.

48. Ibid.

49. Katcher AL. Confidential memorandum to R Wise, 29 January 1992. Medical Staff file, HMCA.

❦ CHAPTER 17: *Hunterdon Medical Center up to the Present*

1. Pellegrino ED to LJ Evans, 11 May 1956; LJ Evans to E Pellegrino, 16 May 1956. Commonwealth 1956 file, HMCA.

2. Pellegrino ED to LJ Evans, 4 June 1958. Commonwealth 1958 file, HMCA.

3. Henderson RR. Memorandum to L Wescott, 5 November 1959. Commonwealth 1959 file, HMCA.

4. Passin SM. Memorandum to E Claus, 10 February 1978. HMCA.

5. Wescott LB to CW Herr, 20 June 1980, commenting on Mission Statement. HMCA.

6. *Hunterdon County Democrat*, 19 August, 1999.

7. Vali FM. Access to Primary Care in New Jersey, January, 2001, Health Research and Educational Trust of New Jersey, Princeton, NJ.

❦ CHAPTER 18: *Conclusions*

1. Devries JM et al. "Developing models for pediatric residency training in managed care settings." *Pediatrics* 1998; 101: 753–9.

2. Evans LJ. Presentation to Board of Trustees meeting, 1 December 1949. Board of Trustees file, HMCA.

3. Shortell SM, Waters TM, Clarke KW, Burdetti PP. "Physicians as double agents: maintaining trust in an era of multiple accountabilities." *JAMA* 1998 Sep 23–30; 280(12): 1102–8. Lamm RD. "Marginal medicine." *JAMA* 1998 Sep 9; 280(10): 931–3.

4. Trussell RE. *The Hunterdon Medical Center.*

❦ CHAPTER 19: *Early Members of HMC's Board and Other Important Contributors*

1. McIntyre W to AL Katcher, 29 January 1997. McIntyre file, HMCA.

2. Kovi LV. *As ye sow.*

3. Samson VJ, Rev. Dunbar's daughter. Telephone interview by author, 16 January 1997.

4. Wescott LB. "Should doctors be members of hospital boards of trustees?" Presentation, Public Relations Institute, American Hospital Association, August, 1958.

5. Lance WE. Interview by author, 30 January 1997.

6. Johnson JS Jr. Telephone interview by author, 27 April 1997.

7. McIntyre W to AL Katcher, 29 January 1997. McIntyre file, HMCA.

8. Johnson JS Jr. Telephone interview by author, 27 April 1997.

9. Lance WE. Interview by author, 23 May 1995.

10. Wescott LB to DS Klopfer, 21 March 1960. Wescott file, HMCA.

11. Wescott LB to P Myers, 14 March 1969. Wescott file, HMCA.

12. Johnson JS Sr. to R Trussell, 9 August 1950. Johnson file, HMCA.

13. Johnson JS Jr. Telephone interview by author, 27 April 1997.

14. Johnson JS Sr. to R Henderson, 17 November 1961. Johnson file, HMCA.

15. Johnson JS Sr. to R Henderson, 14 October 1959. Johnson file, HMCA.

16. Johnson JS Sr. to R Henderson, 18 April 1961. Johnson file, HMCA.

17. Petryshyn W. Telephone interview by author, 12 September 1996.

18. Goldsmith, Barbara, *Johnson v. Johnson*; Knopf, New York, 1987, p. 7–10.

19. Lance WE. Interview by author, 23 May 1995. Unless otherwise indicated, all quotations in this profile come from my interview with Lance.

20. *Hunterdon County Democrat.*

21. Shuman D. Interview by author, 9 April 2002. Shuman file, HMCA.

22. McIntyre W. Telephone interview by author, 17 February 1997.

23. Minutes, Executive Committee, Board of Trustees, 23 April 1953. Board of Trustees file, HMCA.

24. McIntyre W. Telephone interview by author, 17 February 1997.

25. Myers KB. Interview by author, 12 July 1995. Myers died shortly after our interview, and a transcript of it was edited by Myers's daughter and a dear friend, Ed Stout, also a well-known local citizen. Unless otherwise indicated, all quotations in this profile come from my interview with Myers.

26. *Legislative Manual, New Jersey,* 1937: 372–373.

27. *Hunterdon County Democrat,* 20 March 1952 and 21 October 1993.

28. Sauerland A. Telephone interview by author, 31 March 1997. Schomp file, HMCA.

29. Zahler DJ. Telephone interview by author, 13 February 1997.

❧ CHAPTER 20: *The Specialist Staff*

1. Hunt AD. Interview by author, 17 December 1995. Unless otherwise indicated, all quotations in this profile come from this interview.

2. Trussell RE. Interview by author, 5 December 1995.

3. Ibid.

4. Park EA. "The preservation of the ideal in a university children's clinic." *Can Med Assoc J* 1952; 66: 478–85.

5. Rausen AR. Interview by author, 29 February 1996.

6. Pellegrino E. Interview by author, 27 November 1996.

7. Parmet B. Interview by author, 20 January 1996. The bulk of the information in this profile derives from this interview. Unless otherwise indicated, all quotations in this profile come from this interview.

8. Ash J. Telephone interview by author, 3 December 1996.

9. Minutes, Board of Trustees, 6 June 1952. Board of Trustees file, HMCA.

10. Parmet B to AL Katcher, 21 May 1996. Parmet file, HMCA.

11. Parmet M. "An added dimension for child guidance services." Presentation, date and occasion unknown, HMCA. Parmet M. "Flexible use of child guidance personnel in a medical center." *Ment Hyg* 1959; 43: 48–52. Parmet M, Hunt AD, Rosen M. "Interdisciplinary organization around the pediatric patient," undated. HMCA.

12. Pellegrino ED, Parmet M, Henderson RR. "Emotional problems in the management of recent myocardial infarction." Paper presented at the Clinical Conference Hunterdon Medical Center; 1955; Flemington (NJ).

13. Parmet M. Personal communication, approximately 1960.

14. Pellegrino ED. Interview by author, 27 November 1995. Unless otherwise indicated, all quotations in this profile come from this interview.

15. Pellegrino ED. *Mod Med* 1971 Oct 4: 18–38.

16. Trussell RE. Interview by author, 5 December 1995.

17. Sanders D. Telephone interview by author, 27 October 1996.

18. Ash J. Interview by author, 3 December 1996.

19. Trussell RE. Interview by author, 5 December 1995.

20. Pellegrino ED. "Role of the community hospital in continuing education—the Hunterdon experiment." *J Am Med Assoc* 1957; 164: 361–5.

21. Rizzolo P. Telephone interview by author, 6 August 1995.

22. Rosenfeld L. Telephone interview by author, 21 July 1996.

23. Rubin M. Interview by author, 4 March 1996.

24. Katzenbach CB. Interview by author, 28 March 1995.

25. Greenbaum D. Telephone interview by author, 20 February 1996.

26. Lincoln JA. Interview by author, 19 July, 1996.

27. Accettola A. Interview by author, 8 May 1995. Unless otherwise indicated, all quotations in this profile come from this interview.

28. Barad G. Interview by author, 24 January 1996. Unless otherwise indicated, all quotations in this profile come from this interview.

29. Rizzolo P. Telephone interview by author, 6 August 1995.

30. Colella E. Telephone interview by author, 18 September 1996. Unless otherwise indicated, all quotations in this profile come from this interview.

31. Dewing ES to AL Katcher, 10 February 1996. Dewing file, HMCA.

32. Woodruff F. Interview by author, 25 April 1995.

33. Goger PR. Interview by author, 9 June 1995. Unless otherwise indicated, all quotations and most of the information on Goger in this profile come from this interview.

34. Bambara J. Interview by author, 14 June 1995.

35. Goger PR quoted in "Doctor you call may be a woman," *Hunterdon County Democrat*, 26 August 1976.

36. Fuhrmann J. Interview by author, 5 February 1996. Rosswaag C. Interview by author, 7 February 1996.

37. Tantum C. Interview by author, 16 October 1996.

38. Ash J. Interview by author, 3 December 1996.

39. Pellegrino ED. Telephone interview by author, 4 December 1996.

40. Hunt AD to AL Katcher, 10 March 1997.

41. Greenbaum D. Telephone interview by author, 20 February 1996. Unless otherwise indicated, all quotations in this profile come from this interview.

42. Roessel C, Greenbaum DS. "Upper gastrointestinal hemorrhage." *Med Clin North Am* 1964; 48: 1493–1502.

43. Katzenbach CB. Interview by author, 14 July 1995. Unless otherwise indicated, all quotations in this profile come from this interview.

44. Knocke L. Interview by author, 2 May 1995. Fred Knocke was deceased at this time; all information was supplied by Lazelle Knocke in interview or correspondence. Unless otherwise indicated, all quotations in this profile come from this interview.

45. Mitchell A. Interview by author. Unless otherwise indicated, all quotations and most of the information on Mitchell in this profile come from this interview.

46. Olmstead CD. Personal communication, 18 September 1995. Unless otherwise indicated, direct quotations and most of the information in this profile come from this interview.

47. Tantum C. Interview by author, 16 October 1996.

48. Lincoln JA. Interview by author, 19 July 1996.

49. *Hunterdon County Democrat*, 15 April 1953.

50. Lincoln JA. Interview by author, 19 July 1996.

51. Petryshyn WA. Interview by author, 12 September 1996. Unless otherwise indicated, direct quotations and most of the information in this profile come from this interview.

52. Rannels N. Telephone interview by author, 7 September 1996. Unless otherwise indicated, direct quotations and most of the information in this profile come from this interview.

53. Roth LG. "Natural childbirth in a general hospital." *Am J Obstet Gynecol* 1951; 61: 167–72. Thoms H, Wyatt RH. "One thousand consecutive deliveries under training for childbirth program." *Am J Obstet Gynecol* 1951; 61: 205–9. Watson BH. "Specialist–general practitioner cooperation in an obstetrical department." *Calif Med* 1951; 75: 261–4.

54. Rannels HW. "Medical care and education in rural areas." *Bull Matern Welfare* 1958; Mar–Apr. Parmet M. "Flexible use of child guidance personnel in a medical center." *Ment Hyg* 1959; 43: 48–52.

55. Rannels HW. "Obstetrics in a rural community." *Postgrad Med* 1959; 25: 180–4. Rannels HW. "The role of the trained obstetrician in a rural community." *Obstet Gynecol* 1956; 8: 189.

56. Ibid.

57. Rannels HW. "Pheochromocytoma and pregnancy." *Obstet Gynecol* 1956; 7: 33–5.

58. Rannels HW. "Combination in a single hospital service of gynecologic and obstetric patients." *JAMA* 1962; 180: 517–20.

59. Ash J. Interview by author, 3 December 1996.

60. Trussell RE. Interview by author, 9 November 1995.

61. Pellegrino E. Interview by author, 28 November 1995.

62. Bambara J. Interview by author, 14 January 1995.

63. Grant E. Interview by author, 6 February 1996.

64. Macholdt A. Interview by author, 28 June 1995.

65. Macholdt T. Interview by author, 28 June 1995.

66. Katzenbach CB. Interview by author, 28 March 1995.

67. Petryshyn WA. Interview by author, 12 September 1996.

68. Roessel B. Interview by author 1996. Unless otherwise indicated, direct quotations and most of the information in this profile come from this interview.

69. Grant E. Telephone interview by author, 6 February 1996.

70. Goger P. Interview by author, 9 June 1995.

71. Lincoln J. Telephone interview by author, 19 July 1996.

72. Woodruff F. Interview by author, 25 April 1995. Unless otherwise indicated, direct quotations and most of the information in this profile come from this interview.

➤ CHAPTER 21: *Family Physicians*

1. Fidellow R. Interview by author, 20 April 1995.

2. Bambara AJ. Interview by author, 14 January 1995. Unless otherwise indicated, all quotations in this profile come from this interview.

3. "Dr. B.," videotape, produced by NBC television, date unknown.

4. Wescott LB to J Nelson, NBC, 12 January 1961. Wescott file, HMCA.

5. Rizzolo P. Interview by author, 6 August 1995.

6. Doyle L. Interview by author, 14 January 1996. Unless otherwise indicated, all quotations in this profile come from this interview.

7. Fidellow R. and E. Joint interviews by author, 20 April and 11 July 1995. Unless otherwise indicated, all quotations in this profile come from Ray Fidellow.

8. Material for this profile was obtained from the files of the *Hunterdon County Democrat*.

9. Jane Fuhrmann, John Fuhrmann's widow, was kind enough to provide information about him.

10. Material for this profile was obtained from the *Hunterdon County Democrat* and from an interview 7 June 1997 with Dr. Jenkins' older daughter, Dr. Lynn Jenkins-Madina.

11. Lincoln JA. Telephone interview by author, 19 July 1996. Unless otherwise indicated, all quotations in this profile come from this interview.

12. Looloian MW. Interview by author, 8 June 1996. Unless otherwise indicated, all quotations in this profile are taken from this interview.

13. Fidellow R. Interview by author, 20 April 1995.

14. *Hunterdon County Democrat*, undated. Looloian file, HMCA.

15. Ibid.

16. Fidellow R. Interview by author, 20 April 1995.

17. Greenbaum D. Telephone interview by author, 20 February 1996.

18. Macholdt, A. Interview by author, 28 June 1995. Unless otherwise indicated, all quotations in this profile are taken from this interview.

19. Rizzolo P. Telephone interview by author, 6 August 1995. Unless otherwise indicated, all quotations in this profile are taken from this interview.

20. Rizzolo A. Telephone interview by author, 6 August 1995.

21. Ibid.

22. Rosenfeld L and H. Telephone interview by author, 21 July 1996. Unless otherwise indicated, all quotations in this profile are taken from this interview.

◂ CHAPTER 22: *House Staff*

1. Rausen A. Interview by author, 29 February 1996. Unless otherwise indicated, all quotations in this profile come from this interview.

2. Sanders D. Interview by author, 22 October 1996. Unless otherwise indicated, all quotations in this profile come from this interview.

◂ CHAPTER 23: *Administrative Staff*

1. Grant EV. Telephone interview by author, 6 February 1996. Unless otherwise indicated, all quotations in this profile come from this interview.

2. Greenwood L. Interview by author, 9 June 1995. Unless otherwise indicated, all quotations in this profile come from this interview.

3. Trussell RE. Interview by author, 5 December 1995.

4. Minutes, Board of Trustees, 11 June 1953. Board of Trustees file, HMCA.

5. Anthony C. Interview by author, 4 March 1996.

6. Trussell RE. Interview by author, 5 December 1995.

7. Pellegrino E. Interview by author, 28 November 1995.

8. Knocke B. Interview by author, 2 May 1995.

9. Ash J. Telephone interview by author, 13 December 1996.

10. Rubin M. Interview by author, 4 March 1996. Unless otherwise indicated, all quotations in this profile come from this interview.

11. Trussell RE to L Evans, 27 September 1954. Commonwealth 1954 file, HMCA.

12. Trussell RE. Handwritten note on draft manuscript of this book.

❧ CHAPTER 24: *Nursing Staff*

1. Anthony C. Interview by author, 4 March 1996. Unless otherwise indicated, all quotations in this profile come from this interview.

2. Ash J. Interview by author, 3 December 1996. Unless otherwise indicated, all quotations in this profile come from this interview.

Bibliography

Anonymous. "Ed Pellegrino." *Mod Med* 1971 Oct 4: 18–38.

Baehr G. Economic aspects of group practice. The Kingsley Roberts Memorial Lecture Series. New York: Medical Administration Service, 1949.

Baehr G, Deardorff NR. "What the Health Insurance Plan of Greater New York offers to older persons." *Publ Welfare* 1951 Mar.

Balint M. *The doctor, his patient and the illness.* New York: International Universities Press, 1957.

Bambara AJ, Hunt AD. "Specialist plus, not versus, family physicians: a setting conducive to effective postgraduate education." *Postgrad Med* 1956 Sep; 20: 305–9.

Bayne-Jones S. "The hospital as a center of preventive medicine." *Ann Intern Med* 1949; 31: 7–16.

Black H. *Doctor, teacher and hospital chief.* Chester, CT: Globe Pequot Press, 1982.

Bortz EL. "The hospital and the physician." *Hospitals* 1948; 22: 61–132.

Bowlby J. "Attachment and loss." In: *Separation, anxiety and anger*, vol. II. New York: Basic Books, 1973.

Bowlby J, Robertson J. "Responses of young children to separation from their mothers." *Courrier2* 1952: 132.

Breo D. "Specialists skirmish with clinic over practice rights." *AMA News* 1977 August 15: 11–3.

Brown A. "How the children's hospital can best meet community needs." *Hospitals* 1940; 14: 42–5.

Bryan JE. "View from the hill." *Am Fam Physician* 1977 Nov; 16(5): 291–7.

———. Hunterdon Medical Center. Part 1, The big picture in a small frame. Place and date of publication unknown.

Bryant JH, et al. *Community hospitals and primary care.* Cambridge, MA: Ballinger, 1976.

Cabot RC. "Better doctoring for less money." *American Magazine* 1916 May.

Campbell K, Blanch M. "Unrestricted visiting in a children's ward. Eight year's experience." *Lancet* 1955 Nov 5; 2: 971–3.

Cavitch B. "Parents assist in care of hospitalized children." *Nurs World* 1959 May; 5: 133.

Chmeil JF, Drumm ML, Konstan MW, Ferkol TW, Kercsmar CM. "Pitfalls in the use of genotype analysis as the sole diagnostic criterion for cystic fibrosis." *Pediatrics* 1999 Apr; 103(4 Pt 1): 823–6.

Clark M. "Miracles and mishaps. Closing the quality gap." *Atlantic Monthly* 1966 Jul.

Coddington DC, Moore KD, Fischer EA. *Making integrated health care work. Case Study No. 3: Bassett Healthcare.* Englewood, CO: Center for Research in Ambulatory Health Care Administration, 1996.

Cody HJ. "The contribution a hospital may make to its community." *Hospitals* 1940; 14: 13–7.

Commission on Hospital Care. *Hospital care in the United States, conclusions and recommendations.* New York: Commonwealth Fund, 1947.

Committee on the Costs of Medical Care. *Medical care for the American people. Final report.* Chicago: University of Chicago Press, 1932: 59–65, 109–10.

"Community hospital of the year." *Architectural Forum* 1952 Jan.

Community hospitals and the challenge of primary care. Paper presented at the Center for Community Health Systems Columbia University; 1975 Jan; New York.

Consultative Council on Medical and Allied Services, Ministry of Health of Great Britain. *Interim report on the future provision of medical and allied services.* London: H.M. Stationary Office, 1920.

Cook FJ. "The ideal hospital – and what it means." In: Cook FJ. *The plot against the patient.* Englewood Cliffs, NJ: Prentice–Hall, 1967: 308–35.

Crane AD. "Our health is our wealth." *American Agriculturist* 1960 October 15: 36, 41.

Crispell RS. "Extramural and neuropsychiatry in a general hospital." *South Med Surg* 1940; 102: 105–10.

De Kruif PH. *Kaiser wakes the doctors.* New York: Harcourt Brace, 1943.

De la Chapelle CE, Jensen F. *A mission in action; the story of the Regional Hospital Plan of New York University.* New York: New York University Press, 1964.

——— . Presentation to the Board, Staff, Community, Personnel of the Hunterdon Medical Center; 1955 September 13; Flemington (NJ).

De Romilly J. *A short history of Greek literature.* Chicago: University of Chicago Press, 1985.

Devries JM et al. "Developing models for pediatric residency training in managed care settings." *Pediatrics* 1998; 101: 753–9.

Ebaugh FG, Rymer AC. "Psychiatric facilities within the general hospital." *Mod Hosp* 1940; 55: 71–4.

Elliott J. "More ways than one. A look at pluralism in health-care." *Lancet* 1969 Apr 5; 1(7597): 715–8.

Esselstyn CB. "Group practice with branch centers in a rural county." *N Engl J Med* 1953; 248: 488–93.

Evans LJ. "The place of a small community hospital in postwar medical education." *J Assoc Am Med Coll* 1944; 19: 97–104.

————. "The rural hospital." *J Am Med Assoc* 1938 Mar 26: 945–8.

Falk D. "Hunterdon Plan termed model for health system." *Fam Pract News* 1977 Oct 15; 7: 1, 78–9.

Felch WC, Scanlon D. "Bridging the gap between research and practice. The role of continuing medical education." *JAMA* 1997 Jan 8; 277(2): 155–6.

Fisher ES, Welsh HG. "Avoiding the unintended consequences of growth in medical care: how might more be worse?" *JAMA* 1999 Feb 3; 281(5): 446–53.

Fitz R. "The non-teaching hospital and medical education." *Conn State Med J* 1944; 8: 814–7.

Freidson E. *Profession of medicine; a study of the sociology of applied knowledge.* New York: Dodd, Mead, 1970.

Furnas JC. "We fetched ourselves a medical center." *Harper's Magazine* 1952 Jun: 54–60.

Galdston I, ed. *Medicine in the changing order. Report of the New York Academy of Medicine Committee on Medicine and the Changing Order.* New York: Commonwealth Fund, 1947.

Garland JE. *An experiment in medicine; the first twenty years of the Pratt Clinic and the New England Center Hospital of Boston.* Cambridge, MA: Riverside Press, 1960.

Ginsburg EL. *Public health is people; an Institute on Mental Health in Public Health seminar held at Berkeley, CA, 1948.* New York: Commonwealth Fund, 1950.

Goldfield N. "National health reform advocates retrench and prepare for Medicare." *Physician Exec* 1993 May–Jun; 19(3): 7–13.

————. "Truman and the medical profession: replay or lesson for the nineties." *Physician Exec* 1993 Mar-Apr; 19(2): 3–9.

Goldsmith B. *Johnson v. Johnson.* New York: Knopf, 1987.

Green M. "Comprehensive pediatrics and the changing role of the pediatrician." In: Solnit AJ, Provence SA, editors. *Modern perspectives in child development.* New York: International Universities Press, 1963.

Gregg A. Benefits of group practice. The Kingsley Roberts Memorial Lectures Series. New York: Medical Administrative Service, 1949.

Harvey AM, Abrams SL. *For the welfare of mankind: the Commonwealth Fund and American medicine.* Baltimore: Johns Hopkins University Press, 1986.

Hawn CV. *The Mary Imogene Bassett Hospital.* Cooperstown, NY: New York Historical Society, 1982.

Hay JD. "Self-demand feeding in the maternity unit." *Br Med J* 1952 Nov 29: 1180–2.

Hemmendinger M. "Rx: admit parents at all times." *Child Study* (NY) 1956-1957 Winter: 3–9.

Henderson RR. "Full-time practice in the community hospital." *JAMA* 1970 Jun 22; 212(12): 2106–7.

——. What is a community hospital? What is Hunterdon Medical Center? Presentation to a Hunterdon Medical Center Board of Trustees Meeting; 1965 Mar 26; Flemington (NJ).

——. Grant request for an epidemiologist. 1963.

——. Responsibility of the community hospital. Paper presented at the New England Hospital Assembly; 1961 Mar 21; Boston.

Herrick WW. "In the future: centralization, more group practice, more insurance and better teaching." *Hospitals* 1945; 19: 88–94.

Hunt AD. Parent participation in the hospitalization of children; a diagnostic and therapeutic aid. Paper presented at the 68th Annual Meeting of the American Pediatrics Society; 1958 May 8-9.

——. "An experiment in teamwork." *Child Study* (NY) 1957 Winter: 9–14.

Hunt AD, Parmet M. "Collaboration between pediatrician and child psychiatrist in a rural medical center." *Pediatrics* 1957; 19: 462–6.

Hunt AD, Trussell RE. "They let parents help in children's care." *Mod Hosp* 1955; 85: 89–91.

Hunterdon Medical Center, 1965. Publication on file.

Hunterdon Medical Center: the hospital, the staff and the community. A unique relationship. Publication on file.

Hutchins VL, editor. "Pediatricians' involvement in promoting Community Access To Child Health (CATCH)." *Pediatrics* 1999 Jun; 103(6 Pt 3): 1369–1432.

Illingworth RS. "Self-demand feeding in a maternity unit." *Lancet* 1952 Apr 5; i: 683–7.

Jackson EB. "A hospital rooming-in unit for four newborn infants and their mothers." *Pediatrics* 1948; 1: 28–43.

——. "The initiation of a rooming-in project at the Grace-New Haven Community Hospital." In: Senn MJE, editor. *Problems in infancy. Transactions of the 1st Josiah Macy Conference;* 1947.

Jackson K. "Problem of emotional trauma in hospital treatment of children." *J Am Med Assoc* 1952; 149: 1536–8.

Janson D. "Family medicine is made a specialty." *The New York Times* 1969 Feb 11.

Kaiser AD. "An experiment in improving medical care in rural areas on a regional basis." *Pediatrics* 1948; 1: 829–35.

Kasanof D. "Where country doctors learn and teach." *Patient Care* 1978 Jun 30: 118–46.

Katcher AL. "Caring for children." *Perspectives* (Hunterdon Medical Center in-house publication) 1986 Spring; 6(1): unpaginated.

Katcher AL, Grant EV. "Parents help care for their children." *Hospitals* 1961 Mar 1.

Katcher AL, Lanese MG. "Breast-feeding by employed mothers: a reasonable accommodation in the work place." *Pediatrics* 1985 Apr; 75(4): 644–7.

Katcher AL, Tileston B. Comprehensive evaluation of the handicapped child. Exhibit presented at Educator's Meeting; date unknown.

Keenan T. "A foundation perspective on Community Access to Child Health (CATCH) Program." *Pediatrics* 1999 Jun; 103(6 Pt 3): 1428–9.

Klatskin EH. "Choice of rooming-in or newborn nursery." *Pediatrics* 1950; 6: 878–89.

Kovi LV. *As ye sow: the story of an American rural community.* Flemington, NJ: Hunterdon County Board of Agriculture, 1961.

Lamm RD. "Marginal medicine." *JAMA* 1998 Sep 9; 280(10): 931–3.

Lee RI, Jones LW. *The fundamentals of good medical care.* Commission on the Costs of Medical Care; 1933 Report No. 22. Chicago: University of Chicago Press, 1933; reprinted by Archon Books, Hamden, CT, 1962.

Leman E. "Mothers make effective aides at Hunterdon Medical Center." *Hosp Top* 1966 Oct; 44(10): 95–8.

Leuck M. *A further study of dental clinics in the United States.* Chicago: University of Chicago Press, 1932.

——— . *A study of dental clinics in the United States: 1930.* Chicago: University of Chicago Press, 1932.

Lewinsky-Corwin EH. *The American hospital.* New York: Commonwealth Fund, 1946.

Linde SM. "When children need their parents most." *Today's Health* 1968 Jun: 26–9, 66–7.

Lischer BE. "Dental service in hospitals." *Hospitals* 1943; 17: 94–6.

Mannix JR. "Cleveland likes inclusive rates." In: Bachmeyer AC, Hartman G, editors. *The hospital in modern society.* New York: Commonwealth Fund, 1943.

Martell LK. "Response to change: maternity nursing after World War II." *MCN Am J Matern Child Nurs* 1995 May–Jun; 20(3): 131–4.

MacKenzie GM. "The social functions of the modern hospital." *Westchester Medical Bulletin* 1942 Dec: 7–11.

McBryde A. "Compulsory rooming-in in the ward and private newborn service of Duke Hospital." *J Am Med Assoc* 1951; 145: 625–8.

Means JH. *Doctors, people and government.* Boston: Little, Brown, 1953.

"Medical center emerges from a community survey." *Hospitals* 1955 Mar.

"Medical center for the rural practitioner." *Pfizer SPECTRUM* 1954 Feb.

"Medical center holds its own." *Med World News* 1975 Apr 7; 16: 987.

Menges R. "Country doctors get medical center facilities." *Med Econ* 1953 Mar.

"Metamorphosis of a satellite health center." *Group Pract* 1971; 20: 18–9.

Middleton J. "No salaried vs private practice wrangle here." *Hosp Physician* 1968 Nov: 74–80.

Miller LA. "The primary physician as manager of care and costs." *Patient Care* 1977 Dec 15: 9, 11.

"Miss Greenwood retires." *MiniMag* (Hunterdon Medical Center in-house publication) 1973 Jun; 4: 1–4.

Moloney JC. "The newborn, his family and the 'modern hospital." *Mod Hosp* 1946; 67: 43–6.

Moncrieff A., Walton AM. "Visiting children in hospital." *Br Med J* 1952 Jan 5: 43–4.

Montgomery TL. "Bedside care of the newborn by the parturient mother." *Med Clin North Am* 1948; 32: 1699–1709.

Morgan ML, Lloyd BJ. "Parents invited." *Nurs Outlook* 1955 May; 3: 256–9.

Muzzin LJ. "Understanding the process of medical referral. Putting the findings into perspective." *Can Fam Physician* 1992 Apr; 38: 817–21.

New York Academy of Medicine. Committee on Medicine and the Changing Order. *Medicine in the changing order.* New York: Commonwealth Fund, 1947.

Nyberg CE. "Survey of general practice in hospitals." *GP* 1951; 4: 95–8.

Örsten P, Mattson, Å. "Hospitalization symptoms in children." *Acta Paediatr* 1955; 44: 77–92.

Park EA. "The preservation of the ideal in a university children's clinic." *Can Med Assoc J* 1952; 66: 478–85.

——— . "The pediatrician and the public." *Pediatrics* 1948; 1: 828–9.

Parmet M. "The role of the full time psychiatrist in the general hospital." *J Med Soc NJ* 1960; 57: 562–5.

——— . "Flexible use of child guidance personnel in a medical center." *Ment Hyg* 1959; 43: 48–52.

——— . "The supervisory nurse's role in promoting mental health." *Am J Nurs* 1957; 57: 329.

——— . A child psychiatrist in a rural medical center. Paper presented at the 30th Anniversary Seminar Philadelphia Child Guidance Clinic; 1955 Oct 29; Philadelphia.

——— . "An added dimension for child guidance services." Oral presentation at unknown place; unknown date. HMCA.

Parmet M, Hunt AD, Rosen M. "Interdisciplinary organization around the pediatric patient," undated. HMCA.

Parmet M, Pellegrino ED. Treatment of the psychiatric patient in an open medical floor in a community general hospital. Paper presented at the Annual Meeting of the American Psychiatric Association; 1960 May; Atlantic City (NJ).

Parran T. "Voluntary hospital looks to the future." *Mod Hosp* 1946; 66: 73–5.

——— . "Voluntary hospital must expand activity to meet changing conditions." *Hospitals* 1945; 19: 41.

Pellegrino ED. "The identity crisis of an ideal." In: Ingelfinger FJ, editor. *Controversy in Internal Medicine* II. Philadelphia: Saunders, 1974.

——— . "The role of the local community in the development of health services – the Hunterdon experiment." *Industry & Tropical Health* 1961; IV.

——— . Quote. In: Trussell RE, Elison J. *Chronic illness in a rural area*, vol. III. Cambridge, MA: Harvard University Press, 1959: 302.

——— . "Role of the community hospital in continuing education – the Hunterdon experiment." *J Am Med Assoc* 1957; 164: 361–5.

Pellegrino ED, Parmet M, Henderson RR. "Emotional problems in the management of recent myocardial infarction." Paper presented at the Clinical Conference Hunterdon Medical Center; 1955; Flemington (NJ).

Perloff E. *Report of a Special Committee on the Provision of Health Services.* Chicago: American Hospital Association, 1970.

Pew Health Profession Commission Advisory Panel on Health Professions and Managed Care. *Health professions, education and managed care: challenges and necessary responses.* San Francisco: UCSF Center for Health Professions, 1995.

Powers GF. "Humanizing hospital experiences." *Am J Dis Child* 1948; 76: 365–79.

Rakove JN. *Original meaning: politics and ideas in the making of the Constitution.* New York: Knopf, 1997.

Rannels HW. "Combination in a single hospital service of gynecologic and obstetric patients." *JAMA* 1962; 180: 517–20.

——. "Obstetrics in a rural community." *Postgrad Med* 1959; 25: 180–4.

——. "Medical care and education in rural areas." *Bull Matern Welfare* 1958; Mar–Apr.

——. "Pheochromocytoma and pregnancy." *Obstet Gynecol* 1956; 7: 33–5.

——. "The role of the trained obstetrician in a rural community." *Obstet Gynecol* 1956; 8: 189.

Reinhardt UE. "The economist's model of physician behavior." *JAMA* 1999 Feb 3; 281(5): 462–5.

Richardson FH. "Rooming in: modern medicine goes old fashioned." *South Med J* 1952; 45: 131–7.

Richmond JB. *Currents in American medicine: a developmental view of medical care and education.* Cambridge, MA: Harvard University Press, 1969.

Ripley HS. "Psychiatric consultation service in a medical inpatient department. Its function in diagnosis, treatment and teaching." *Am J Med Sci* 1940; 199: 261–8.

Robinson GC. "The patient as a person." *Bull Johns Hopkins Hosp* 1940; 66: 390–7.

Roessel C, Greenbaum DS. "Upper gastrointestinal hemorrhage." *Med Clin North Am* 1964; 48: 1493–1502.

Rorem CR. "Hospital service plans and private insurance contrasted." *Hospitals* 1940 Jul; 14: 32–5.

Rorem CR. "Group hospitalization: Mecca or mirage?" *Mod Hosp* 1933 Jan.

——. "Sickness insurance in the United States." *Bull Am Hosp Assoc* 1932 Dec.

——. *Private group clinics.* Publication No. 8. Chicago: University of Chicago Press, 1931.

Rose JA. "The relation of the family to the hospital." *Med Clin North Am* 1952; 36: 1551–4.

Rosenberg C. "Trouble in a health planners' paradise." *Med Econ* 1978 Aug 7: 176–82.

Roth LG. "Natural childbirth in a general hospital." *Am J Obstet Gynecol* 1951; 61: 167–72.

Rothman DJ. *Beginnings count: the technological imperative in American health care.* New York: Oxford University Press, 1997.

Schenewerk GA. "Group hospital insurance." *Hospitals* 1940; 14: 38.

Schmidt HG. *Rural Hunterdon: an agricultural history.* New Brunswick, NJ: Rutgers University Press, 1946.

Senn MJE. "Role of psychiatry in a children's hospital service." *Am J Dis Child* 1946 Jul; 72: 95–110.

Shortell SM, Waters TM, Clarke KW, Burdetti PP. "Physicians as double agents: maintaining trust in an era of multiple accountabilities." *JAMA* 1998 Sep 23–30; 280(12): 1102–8.

Simmons H. Paper presented at the National Health Forum; 1978 Mar 7; San Francisco.

Somers AR. "Hunterdon – 'may it never be forgot!'" *N Engl J Med* 1979 Apr 26; 300(17): 977–9.

——— . "Toward a rational community health system: Hunterdon model." *Hosp Prog* 1973 Apr; 54(4): 46–54.

Sorum PC. "Two tiers of physicians in France: general pediatrics declines, general practice rises." *JAMA* 1998 Sep 23–30; 280(12): 1099–101.

Spence JC. *The purpose and practice of medicine.* London: Oxford University Press, 1960.

——— . "The care of children in hospital." *Br Med J* 1947; 1: 125.

Spitz RA. "Hospitalism: an inquiry into the genesis of psychiatric conditions in early childhood." *Psychoanal Study Child* 1945; 1: 53.

Stevens R. *American medicine and the public interest.* New Haven: Yale University Press, 1971.

Strauss H. "Health education in hospitals and outpatient departments." *Am Publ Health Nations Health* 1945; 35: 1175–8.

Sutton FC. *Hospitals* 1948; 22: 33–5.

Szasz T. "Diagnoses are not diseases." *Lancet* 1991 Dec 21–28; 338(8782–8783): 1574–6.

Tarnover SM. "Psychiatry in a general hospital of a small city." *N Engl J Med* 1948; 239: 466–8.

Thruelson R. In: Ladies Auxiliary. *378 recipes from Hunterdon's kitchens.* Quakertown, NJ: Quakertown Fire Co., 1953.

Terris M. "Joint housing of hospitals, health departments and laboratories." *Am J Publ Health Nations Health* 1951; 41: 319–25.

Thoms H, Wyatt RH. "One thousand consecutive deliveries under training for childbirth program." *Am J Obstet Gynecol* 1951; 61: 205–9.

Trussell RE. *The Hunterdon Medical Center: the story of one approach to rural medical care.* Cambridge, MA: Harvard University Press, 1956.

——— . "The hospital out-patient department in detection of non-manifest disease." *J Chronic Dis* 1955; 2: 391–9.

Trussell RE, Elinson J. *Chronic illness in a rural area. The Hunterdon study,* vol. III chronic illness in the United States series. Cambridge, MA: Harvard University Press, 1959.

Vali FM. *Access to primary care in New Jersey.* Princeton, NJ: Health Research & Educational Trust of New Jersey, 2001.

Van Ness E. "Lloyd Wescott and the power of giving." *Trenton Sunday Times* 1976 Jan 4.

Walker WF. "Opportunities in public health programs for community hospital participation." *Hospitals* 1940; 14: 28–31.

Ward R. "Is Hunterdon a model for NHI?" *Private Practice* 1978; 62: 69.

Watson BH. "Specialist–general practitioner cooperation in an obstetrical department." *Calif Med* 1951; 75: 261–4.

Wescott LB. "Hunterdon: the rise and fall of a medical Camelot." *N Engl J Med* 1979 Apr 26; 300(17): 952–6.

——— . "Reducing the need for inpatient care: a challenge for trustees [letter]." *Trustee* 1977 Aug; 30: 38.

——— . Annual report. Presentation at the Hunterdon Medical Center Board of Trustees meeting; 1976 Jan 23; Flemington (NJ).

——— . "Columbia – Hunterdon: similar but different." *N Engl J Med* 1976 Nov 25; 295(22): 1250–2.

——— . Address presented at New Jersey Hospital Association Achievement Awards; 1973.

——— . "The rural health care situation." Presentation; 1973 Feb 19.

——— . "Innovation in medical staff organization." *Hosp Med Staff* 1972 Mar; 1: 14–9.

——— . "Health care as viewed by the consumer." Paper presented at Rutgers Medical School; 1972 Sep 21; New Brunswick (NJ).

——— . "Family practice and the community hospital." Paper presented at the Association for Hospital Medical Education; 1972 Feb 4; Chicago.

——— . "The hospital governing board's responsibility in emergency department care." Presented at a meeting of the American Academy of Orthopedic Surgeons; 1971 Sep 12; Chicago.

——— . "The decision-making process in the hospital." Presented at the American Hospital Association meeting; 1971 Feb 5.

——— . "Hard facts about emergency service planning." *Trustee* 1971 Nov; 24: 1–6.

——— . "Community hospital–medical school associations." Presented to the Association for Hospital Medical Education; 1971 Sep 11; Atlanta.

——— . "A model medical center for comprehensive care in the community." In: *Contemporary medical problems in historical perspective.* Philadelphia: American Philosophical Library Publication #4; 1971: 220–35.

——— . Presentation at a meeting of the American College of Hospital Administrators; 1970 Nov 12; Greenbrier (WV).

——— . "The decade ahead – as a trustee sees it." *Trustee* 1970 Jun; 23: 10–7.

——— . "Discussion of the role of the community in developing improved health care." *Bull NY Acad Med* 1970 Dec; 46(12): 1042–7.

——— . "The community hospital in today's society." Presented to the Mid-Atlantic Hospital Association; 1968 May 16.

——— . Presentation at the 3rd national AMA–ANA Conference; 1967 Feb 23.

——— . "Planning a new hospital." Presentation; 1961 Jun 23.

——— . "Costs and returns to the hospital as a corporate entity." *JAMA* 1961; 176: 96–8.

——— . "A trustee looks at house officer training." *Trustee* 1961 May; 14: 1–6.

——— . "Capable trustees: product of sound organization." *Hospitals* 1960 July 1; 34: 51–3.

——— . "Should doctors be members of hospital boards of trustees?" Presentation, Public Relations Institute, American Hospital Association, August, 1958.

Wiles MB. "The nurse on the survey team." *Nurs Outlook* 1957 Aug; 5(2).

Williams TF. "Patient referral to a university clinic: patterns in a rural state." *Am J Publ Health* 1960; 50: 1493–507.

——— . "Cabot, Peabody and the care of the patient." *Bull Hist Med* 1950; 24: 462–81.

Wilson R. "Health center." *Mod Hosp* 1944; 63: 53–5.

Witke IM. "Teaching the public." *Mod Hosp* 1944: 57–8.

Wolf RE. "The hospital and the child." In: Solnit AJ, Provence SA, editors. *Modern perspectives in child development.* New York: International Universities Press, 1963.

Index

About the Author

AVRUM L. KATCHER was born and grew up in Philadelphia, Pennsylvania. He received his MD at Johns Hopkins, in 1948. His postgraduate training in pediatrics was at the Harriet Lane Home of Johns Hopkins and Mt. Sinai Hospital, New York City. Following service in the army in Korea, he practiced privately in Germantown, Pennsylvania. In 1959 he succeeded Andrew Hunt as Director of Pediatrics at Hunterdon Medical Center in Flemington, New Jersey. In private practice he has had special interest in child development and behavior. He is a faculty member of Robert Wood Johnson Medical School in New Brunswick, New Jersey, with the title of Professor of Clinical Pediatrics. Katcher is married, with four children and six grandchildren.

A Time to Remember is Katcher's first published book. He has published a number of articles in the professional literature, and edits and writes for the *Bulletin* of the Senior Section of the American Academy of Pediatrics. He has held a number of posts in that organization at state and national levels. Katcher has founded the county sheltered workshop, lactation consultation program, early intervention program and child evaluation center.

THIS BOOK HAS BEEN SET in Garamond. The font was originally designed by Claude Garamond (c. 1480–1561), who was taught his art by Aldus Manutius. Garamond's most praised designs were cut in Paris between 1530–1545, and are considered the highlight of sixteenth-century typography. The font was digitized for the computer by Adobe. It is this digiktized version that is used here.